THE MEDICINE FAMILY VISION

DEEP-HEART SHARING IN THE WISDOM & GUIDANCE OF THE EARTH

BY

JAI JONATHAN DAEMION

ajna media

EUGENE, OREGON

THE MEDICINE FAMILY VISION

DEEP-HEART SHARING IN THE WISDOM & GUIDANCE OF THE EARTH

by Jai Jonathan Daemion

PUBLISHED BY:

ajna media

PO Box 70133
Eugene, Oregon 97401-0107
Phone/Fax: (541) 937-1963 (11am-4pm PT)
Orders Dept: (toll-free) 1-888-255-AJNA
Email: ajna@sprintmail.com

Printed in the United States of America.
First printing 1997

Cataloging Data:
Library of Congress Catalog Number: 96-076583
Daemion, Jai Jonathan, 1944-
The medicine family vision: deep heart sharing in the wisdom and guidance of the earth / by Jai Jonathan Daemion
1. Parenting / 2. Spiritual / 3. New Age / 4. Self-help

PRINTED WITH SOY-BASED INKS ON ACID-FREE, RECYCLED PAPER

ISBN 0-9651534-3-6 : $16.95

WHAT OTHERS ARE SAYING ABOUT THE MEDICINE FAMILY VISION

"Jai's vision is unique in that it embraces...the capacity of children to grow into their highest sacred selves; parents and partners, however, are no less a focus. Daemion has poured considerable passion and experience into an epic elaboration of intimacy and life"

- Matthew Gilbert, in New Age Publisher's (NAPRA) Review

"At last a way to share my spiritual life with my children"

- Marika Denon, PhD (educational psychologist)

"Stories of the childhood we all would like to live."

- Stephen Anand (father)

"In the excitement of sensitive surrender, the constant primal wisdom of the earth and her creatures are discovered and trustingly shared by a family whose respect and love are extended to embrace oneness with all creation. A must read! This book challenges each of us to explore the possibilities of finding higher guidance in Nature."

- Joseph Sun Bear

"A process of profound simplicity and amazing depth. Highly recommended."

- Rebecca Rose Aarons (counselor)

"The Medicine Family Process brought me to a new softness of being in Nature."

- Tom Sharon (Medicine Circle participant)

"These children have a special combination of calmness and presence and joy that I have not met before."

- Robert Benson (teacher)

"Few teachers have ever touched me in this way."

- Stewart Walton (massage therapist)

TABLE OF CONTENTS

This book is dedicated to:
My Dear Pancha Mama friend,
Laney Stephens
And to the Mother Goddess
In all Her other manifestations
Through all the Circles of our Lives

ACKNOWLEDGEMENTS

This book and the Celebration of Family that fills it owes its first debt of gratitude to the mothers of my children - for full-filling them all with the Deep Mother-Love and nurturance which they return to me as great Trust and Openness… and the endless Love which fills our every Medicine Process… and all our sharing.

I also acknowledge the guiding reflection over many decades of my deep, wise-woman friend, Laney Stephens. And for their support and reflection during our beginnings in California and New York, and during our young-family 'rainforest years' in Australia: Norman and Robin Keegel, Jenette Williams, Kate Cameron, Daricha, Jennie Dell, Daan Spijer, Gary Kring, Sri Ramamurti Mishra, Ptashu Dauw, Jeanette Rogers and Jayne Sunbird. And thanks, too, to Leia for endless hours of re-reading and editing.

In California in the mid-70's - in the years just before I began my Fatherhood Vision Quest - I lived and traveled with a pioneering group of Tribal Shaman New Age Gypsy Minstrel Healers who lived simply with the Earth and gathered at an endless unfoldment of healing and spiritual festivals all along the West Coast (and beyond). Coordinating and facilitating these events was my full-time sadhana for many years. The Healing Circles that I offered at these gatherings grew from previous work at growth centers in London and California… and served as the heart-center foundation of all my future life-work of Shamanic Healing & Free-Ritual Circle processes. And wherever my medicine path leads, I will always hold the gifts of guidance and the many miracles of healing that took place in those early Free-Ritual Medicine Circles in special awe and wonder. So to all the free spirits of the **'ALL ONE FAMILY'**… I THANK YOU ALL! And with special heart: Kyle Story, Gabriel Olmstead, Joseph Sun Bear, Yashi Aga, Chela, Ouapiti and Jim and Jan Hall.

The teaching of medicine ways so often occurs through a kind of subliminal osmosis, through sources who are often wholly unaware of the great teaching that they have given. So in my work I honor all my Teachers of consciousness including: all the dawnings and all the darks of night; all the pains and celebrations of Heart and Spirit shared; and all the children and all the tribal peoples who have participated in my evolution. and the evolution of the new, *Free-Ritual Medicine Path* that is the subject and heart-song of this book… and all my present-future learning, teaching and life-celebration.

ABOUT THE COVER

The front cover design was conceived by Leia Daemion; snake art and photo-montage editing by Californian visionary artist, Phoenix & Arabeth. Cover type-setting & layout: Daan Spijer (Seventh House Communications, Australia).

In Australian Aboriginal lore, **The Great Rainbow Serpent** *was the bringer of all creation. This book is rich with many Snake-Medicine stories. So here we have 'Grandfather Snake' forming the Sacred Circle of the Native American Medicine Wheel, with the four directions cast in plumes of birds of the South Pacific Rainforests. And within his embrace are the children of this Medicine Family (and this book), with their sheer Joy of Life calling us to acknowledge their magic… and the Path they walked through their early years in a far-away, peaceful and ancient land.*

IMPORTANT WARNING! PLEASE READ THIS!

The methods of emotional and physical healing that are described in this book are based upon many years of intensive study by the author, of many modern and ancient healing path-ways, yogas, meditational disciplines, psychology and shamanism. And although every technique or approach described in this book is valid in itself, ***the subtle, intuitive skill that is required to use these techniques safely and effectively requires deep and intensive self-exploration and personal preparation, extensive training and, above all, clear Guidance.***

Because healing on this subtle level requires such highly focused energies and such finely tuned intuition/guidance, there is always a danger that an inexperienced individual may overestimate his/her abilities or insights.

AND THEREFORE: The author and publisher emphasize that in any situation of emotional, psychological or physical crisis, readers are advised to **PLEASE SEEK TREATMENT FROM A QUALIFIED THERAPIST OR MEDICAL PRACTITIONER IMMEDIATELY.**

- And may all your chosen practitioners be aware of (and so honor) the greater spiritual basis of all life and consciousness - and so understand the subtle energetics and spiritual components of all dis-ease and healing!

It is also hoped that this book can be an immediate help to untrained persons who seek to assume greater responsibility for their own health (and that of their children), by expanding readers' expectations and awareness of their right to more enlightened and more spiritually compassionate treatment by a new generation of more sensitive and wholistically aware practitioners.

This book has been published as an introduction to some new (and ancient) ways of approaching some of the many issues of healing and consciousness and relationship that every parent must face. This book is not intended to serve as a 'how-to' manual on any specific aspect of parenting or any process or technique of emotional or physical healing.

Therefore, the usual legal disclaimer: neither the author nor the publisher will be held responsible in any way for any outcome or events arising from the application (or misapplication) of any of the concepts or techniques of emotional clearing, healing or parenting described or alluded to in this book. Any reader who does not wish to comply with this warning may return this book for a full refund.

INTRODUCTION

HEY! JUST TRY IT!

Hello there! Yes, I know... 'no one reads the Introduction.' But let's try something new, together: let's begin the Medicine Journey of this book by starting at the same place and with something of the same head-set. Yes?

Have you ever noticed? No matter what we do as parents to progress our spiritual growth - be it yoga or meditation or pagan ritual or just trying for a more conscious relationship with the ecology of the Earth - there is one area where parents often talk about feelings of lack and failure in trying to find ways to share spirit-path with our children.

In their early years, of course, children cannot actually *comprehend* much of anything - though they can certainly *feel* the subtle energy changes in a well-meditated mom or dad. Then there is the time of middle childhood when they are often too energetic and impulsive to even be *able* to stop exploring-expressing long enough to 'feel a circle' or to deliberately focus their all-over-the-place energies on a medicine wheel offering... or even a simple before-dinner circle.

And then, in the pre-teen and teenage years, new self-identities become the all-important and all-consuming focus... so much that these young adult-children often simply *cannot* divert even the tiniest bit of their super-intense life-flow to accommodate the oldies' dreams of a unified and simply silent family circle.

So what can you do? Alas, so many parents respond to this grand enigma... by simply giving up! We make peace (somehow) with an ever-widening gap between our spiritual experience and our sharing with our beloved children. We 'try to accept' their need to be... well, 'otherwise' (i.e., contra to *whatever* we happen to be striving for that week). We reaffirm (mostly for parental benefit) that it is uncool to 'impose our beliefs' upon our children in any way. And so, so many families move through these magical years of Family with an unspoken loneliness and an unshared longing for *Deep Intimacy* that always seems somehow just beyond our reach, impossible to invite and already negated if we have to use 'parental control' or authoritarian power to achieve it.

This book is about finding ways into Sacred Space *together* with your partner and your family. This journey is about *de-mystifying* Earth-Spirit Shamanism: stripping away all that other-time, other-culture, much overdone acting-out of the empty rituals of other times and other cultures... until we discover anew, the deep essence of Guidance and Spirit and Circle and Initiation that is the true (and only) realm of Earth-centered Shamanic experience.

And when we open to trust *the absolute rightness of everything that happens*, on all levels of our feeling and experience, then we soon discover that 'shamanism' is an unduly weighty name for what can be the most natural and simple way of just being fresh with the world... of being so surrendered that we can actually begin to 'hear the littlest bird speak' and to feel deep message in the crashing torrent of a flooded river.

This way of opening anew to Nature again and again, this way of opening our freshness and receptivity over and over again (sometimes many times within a single breath!) is not new to our experience. In fact, it is very similar to the way all children feel-sense- imagine-wonder when they step into a beautiful forest or float down a magical river in a little inflatable boat. And because this process of Deep Surrender is so natural for every child, children immediately feel at home when they are *offered* adult companionship in this very special state of awareness. Knowing nothing.... Open to everything.... Reacting and relating to 'It All.' This *is* the natural shamanic process of childhood. And once we bigger children manage to shed our great mantles of expectation - and all of our 'neo-shamanic' or new-age-spiritual *programming* - then this simple and natural invitation awakens within our hearts and guides us into a new depth of communion with Nature.

This is a great gift of consciousness and Spirit (if you see a difference). For here we discover a new and ancient way of being that we have somehow always known was there. Through the simple surrender of the eternal child that is alive in each of us, synergized with all the empowered adult insight and awareness that we have gained for however many lifetimes we have danced and labored here... we can at last discover a way to be truly open to all the Magic that flows around us and through our experience... and newly receptive to whatever Meaning it brings. And so we have found a natural and simple *path-way* that leads us to re-union with our own innocence, joy, sensitivity... and a true re-awakening of pure Child-Wonder.

And just as soon as we find our way past all of our inner-held programming and are at last able to burst free into a beautiful, sunny meadow with all the spiritual freedom that is our common birth-right Gift of Spirit... when we look up from the flowers, we find our children are already there (or soon come running) to share this strange and wonderful way of simply *being in one-ness with Nature*... and with each other... and so open to the great wealth of endless Guidance that floods upwards through us from the Mother Earth and downwards in endless waves from the deepest realms of Space... and Father Sky.

Applying this simple process - which I have come to call, *'FREE-RITUAL SHAMANISM'* - as it emerges in this book, I know that you will find new hope and awaken the magic of *Deep Intimacy* within your family's experience. In fact this process - this way of non-doing and total surrender - works so powerfully within our usually pre-programmed and self-limited minds that often the problem is not 'how to get it to happen'... but *how to handle the sheer power and wonder of all that comes!*

Nature, in all Her workings, is our living path-way to the experience of Infinity: infinite understanding, infinite consciousness... and infinite Spirit. There is so much magic and guidance and power 'out there' in the natural shamanic world around us, that we have all had to *learn* to blind ourselves to this continual torrent of pure Revelation... just to be able to do the mundane things in our daily lives: as kids, to go to school; as adults, to do the breakfast dishes, manage our finances or attend a business meeting. And now, after all we have learned about 'spiritual path' and wholistic everything (or perhaps in spite of it) comes a gentle path-way sketched in dewdrops and sunlight and birdsong - an ever-changing kaleidoscope of *Sign* and *Meaning* and *Vision* that requires no textbook, no 'secret lore' and no 'certified training.' This is a path of such simplicity that often our biggest worry is how to process the great waves of amazement and wonder and empowerment that naturally come whenever we center our beliefs in no-mind Openness... center our willfulness in simple Trust... and set our only goal as Deep Surrender! This book offers every family a simple process for meeting and sharing these most powerful life-experiences... and ways to *celebrate* all that comes with Deep Surrender. And what comes is all-ways amazing!

Now... if we can only find a way to un-learn all the 'spiritualese' and psycho-babble and self-control and power-paradigms that we have conditioned ourselves to embrace... then we will be ready at last to really *meet* our children... in the temple of the Earth... and to walk through Her wonders hand in hand, learning together as we go.

And whenever you make this little step into Openness and Trust... I invite you to take a ritual moment to prepare: just close your eyes and try to *let go* of all your past expectations.... Open to feel the Earth.... Open to breathe in the Wind.... And then, when you are just as ready as you can be... open your eyes and look out very gently... *AND YOUR FAMILY WILL BE THERE WITH YOU...* wide open and wide-eyed - reflecting the Openness and the Surrender and the Readiness that you have achieved within yourself.

And *then* your *Medicine Journey Deep Healing Vision Quest Free-Ritual Shamanic Initiation* will have already begun!

><><

THIS BOOK IS A MEDITATION.

THIS BOOK IS WRITTEN AS A POEM.

PLEASE READ IT SLOWLY TO LET THE MAGIC IN....

><><

WORDS ON WORDS - A READER'S GUIDE

Some tips and points of perspective for your reading pleasure:

In this book you will encounter some unusual grammar and form. But not to worry! It is all for good reason.... It is a road sign that says:

'SLOW! CHILDREN!'

The utter simplicity of much of what follows may tend to lull readers into thinking that they can zip through it at their most mind-efficient reading speed. Bet you can't! These words are as 'poem' as anything. The meanings here are often interweave and wind around each other in circles and spirals. I promise you will enjoy the trip more if you proceed at a leisurely pace. And likewise...

BOOKS ARE LINEAR: They have a beginning and a straight procession through numbered pages to an ending... *but experience flows every which way*. I write to offer the awakening of Meaning in any reader. So... I wholly invite you to use this little volume as a gentle inspiration (and would be honored if it were, for you): pick it up and open it to any page... read what you feel to take in... slip and slide around within its soft envelopment... and *feel free* to drink it in however it feels best!

PACING MARKS: '...' or '-' are timing marks to invite a little pause - a separation of Meanings. A time to breathe and feel it through.

INSET LINES OF UPPERCASE TEXT: sometimes a little pearl - maybe a rallying point for a reader's memory to re-find a section - maybe something worthy of extra emphasis. Maybe a revelation. Who knows?

CAPITALIZED WORDS: Often I capitalize and/or italicize words that are ordinary in themselves, but are used here in 'medicine' context... as a hint to their special meaning: *'Breath'* is a living entity; *'Heart'* is Living Spirit; concepts such as *'Deep Intimacy'* are capitalized because they connote a higher order of being-ness or potential than the mere words themselves. The 'special words' and concepts of *non-authoritarian* shamanism are simple words of being, feeling and experience... and simple words of sharing. For example, the most powerful and primal dimensions of healing and personal sharing include the simple concepts of *breathing-feeling-touching-sharing- letting-go.* Very simple words for incredibly profound experience!

MOTHERS AND FATHERS: This book is a father's Vision, a father's teaching and a father's learning. You will notice that there is not much mention of (earthly) Mother-presence in the stories herein. And for the reason that my partner held herself gently apart from these adventures. A matter of choice. A matter of *path*. And, I admit... often an enigma and a wonder to me. Note that Leia has written a nice offering as *'A MESSAGE FROM THE MOTHER HEART'* - which appears as an 'AFTER ALL' on pages 393-394.

NAMES: Note that the children's names have been changed in these stories. With one exception, our family decided that I should use 'book names' for each of them... and we have picked these names together.

Happy Journeys!

Good Vision!

See you on the other side....

\- *Jai Daemion*

CHAPTER 1

THE MEDICINE FAMILY PROCESS

Ho! Great Spirit, I seek Vision!
I am Yours tonight!
Ho! Great Spirit, I seek Guidance!
Light my Way tonight!

A TIME OF GATHERING AT THE MOTHER RIVER

This is a time of great change. Our Medicine Family is in a wondrous, wide-eyed turmoil of change - change of place, of time, of feeling and of knowing. We have come to live in a new place: a wild, subtropical rainforest valley on the east coast of Australia, at the edge of the South Pacific Ocean.

This is a Deep Medicine Place and we have so much to learn about the elemental flows of Light and Darkness, Water and Air... so much to explore in the Earth and the Sky and the Mother Ocean, as we come to even deeper family intimacy and self-revelation in this river-anointed valley....

The weather here is different than anything that we have ever known before. The summer here is sticky-hot and intense. Now is the Time of the Wet. And now there is rain every day, week after week, pouring vast torrents of soft, pure Water-Spirit onto the steaming Earth.

The misted mountains which rim and cradle the Valley rise up and disappear in mystery into halos of cloud which enfold their peaks and swirl down the mountainsides on cold, clear nights. And from out of this shroud of soft, white cloud come long, thin waterfalls which crash into the valley floor below, then move quickly to join The Gathering of the Great Mother River merge together in great rushing surges of cleansing, flushing flood.

At this ritual time of gathering, the sensitively sculpted river world, with its ferned banks and limpid pools, swirling eddies, gurgling ripples and its quiet straight runs... changes totally within just a few hours. The lush ferns turn inward... the pools are swept clear of every flower petal... and the crystal clear river waters become turgid and dark from the effluent they carry as the Ancient Earth yields to the rains.

The River herself opens her arms to embrace these Earth-cleansing floods, allowing her belly and her bosom to expand as she receives and channels through her own life-flow, all the waters of all of the earth of all the mountains of all the valleys.

All of us who live by the river withdraw and wait. She closes our commerce and halts our busyness completely by flooding over the many bridges which cross and criss-cross her usually peaceful arcing course. And while she rages and celebrates her fullness, all living things must wait.

The turtles and eels and fish go deep and always swim into the current... to avoid being washed away to the sea. And all the land dwellers, human and non-human, seek and share shelter wherever they happen to be when the Great Rains come. For even the largest, strong-swimming rainforest reptiles - the huge pythons and lace monitors - will not enter the mighty River now.

For many days and all through the nights the rains will continue to bathe us all. The Mother Kali River rages and sings, crashes and soars, rushes and roars. Clouds come down and touch the Earth to help hold and focus the attentive silence of all living things... and the whole world seems poised on the soft-held Breath of Wonder.

><><

THE MEDICINE FAMILY VISION

THE MEDICINE FAMILY VISION is to walk among the magic, the beauty, the teaching and the wisdom of this living planet, enlightened by Shamanic Dances with every living being and opened by the pure wonder of the child-spirit that lives inside every one.

THE MEDICINE PATH offers every family a simple and natural way of feeling the Earth as our Living Mother Planet. This is a path-way which any family can use to find and share each individual's highest Vision... and to recover our natural sense of awe and wonder as we learn to live together in emotional openness and one-ness with the Mother Earth... as we learn to access the ancient knowledge of the medicine people and learn to reveal and nurture the deep, natural wisdom that which lives within every parent, every child and fulfills every Family Circle.

OUR MEDICINE PROCESS includes many things: the notion of spontaneous *Free-Ritual Initiations* and *Ritual Celebrations*... the conscious use of *Shamanic Sign* and *Vision Quests* and many kinds of active, kid-centered, meditational processes. We live in the endless magic of the *Circle* in all its expression: council circles, healing circles, celebration circles, dinner circles, guidance circles, clearing circles (and many more) - as the primary form and process that brings us into *Deep Intimacy* again and again... and guides all of our *Rituals of Sharing* . We also use many kinds of *Ritual Communications* and circle-based ways of clearing relationship conflict (and whatever else might inhibit our personal growth and family communion)... as we crawl and soar along our *Medicine Path*. Our goal is simple: just to *let go* and to open together to the magic of Nature and to the natural life-guidance and deep intuition which She all-ways awakens in us.

OUR CONCEPT OF 'MEDICINE' comes from the Native American peoples: Medicine speaks to all who would hear, of all that is healing and of everything that reflects and evokes the deepest meaning in life. Medicine awakens us to *Spiritual Vision* and invites us to journey through the realm of Spirit. Medicine helps us find our place in the living cosmos as the beloved children of Father Sky and Mother

Earth... and helps us find the Medicine Song and Medicine Dance to celebrate *'It All.'*

WALKING THE MEDICINE PATH TOGETHER

In this chapter we will introduce all of the basic elements of Medicine Process that we will be exploring throughout this book. As concepts, all of these principles are very simple. In practice... there is no end to their application or their variety... or the Shamanic Path that they illuminate. So deeper attention will be given to each of these essential elements in later chapters... with some nice stories to help illustrate how they work.*

The Medicine Path, however it may be called, is common to *all* tribal cultures. It is *The Way of The Shaman...* it is *The Way of Natural Earth-Magic...* and it is *The Way of the Medicine Wheel,* through which we learn to live in harmony with all things.

This is the *Free-Ritual Dance of all Life* which naturally evolves and illuminates our consciousness as we learn to *'Walk in a Sacred Manner'* on the body of the living Earth... opening to her guidance, her magic, her power... and learning to serve *her needs* as well.

And as we move through this endless *Dance of Free-Ritual Initiation*, we receive endless reassurance from all of Nature, of our own 'rightness of being'... and so we are freed from so much of our deeply ingrained cultural heritage of guilt and self-doubt and so become freer to grow into empowered and effective human beings.

By becoming aware of the Earth's state of crisis *without* dwelling on our despair at what has already been done; by searching for empowerment rather than reactivity; by opening to creative, pro-active solutions rather than wallowing in the horrors of our eco-unconsciousness of the past... the children of today *are* the promise of tomorrow. And those who can be *allowed* to grow into

---

* The processes and principles here are essential to learning this simple, non-authoritarian path. Since this material is necessarily conceptual (and didactic - i.e., of a teaching intent) some readers may find it less interesting than the medicine stories and the tales of our family's growing pains and wonders that it is preparing us for. But this is a gentle school... so if the going gets too ponderous... please feel free to jump around!

empowered adults with their natural sensitivity and consciousness fully intact... as beings of clarity and wholeness and peace who are all-ways open to the guidance of their own *Deep Intuition*, Vision and Spirit... are the only hope there is for the survival and maintenance of this planet... for all the Children of the Future....

In our naturally self-expanding state of awareness, every human being carries a birth-right heritage of wholeness, of union with *'The All'* of life... and consciousness: clear and unlimited in mind, full-filled in feeling, healthy and power-full in body, open and surrendered with in Spirit... and at peace with all being and consciousness... living in conscious one-ness with the Mother Earth and the Father Spirit as they move through their endless dance of being and becoming.

By any name, in any myth, in every culture and throughout all time... all natural peoples have known that this state of wholeness is the one and only goal of human life. This is the same and only goal of all the Indian *yogas*, of all meditation and of all shamanic ritual.

This is the Path of Re-Union with all Nature.
This is the Path-Way of Becoming Whole.

Here, we will call it 'Medicine' - the *Way of the Medicine Wheel*. And this naming and this Native American model is especially useful for *all* the tribes of the planet now (including yours), *because* it is a wholly open process which can include *'The All'* of every individual's unique experience.

Today we call it 'Medicine.' But you can call it whatever feels right to you. In the end there is only one experience or state of *one-ness*. And how you get there and what you call it is as variable as life itself! For those who notice it... every instant is a new *Free-Ritual Initiation*... in to *'The All and Everything'* that is yet to come.

What is available to us all - and *all* that is available to us in our mutual quest for healing, growth and ultimate wholeness - is the *Sign* and *Vision* and *Meaning* and *Guidance* that comes to every one who seeks to find a way to stop running through life without awareness... and that comes to everyone who will take the time to sit quietly upon the Earth and simply open in true surrender... to their own *Medicine Vision*... and to the teaching and the guidance and the wisdom that Vision will surely bring.

So, I invite you to walk with our Medicine Family for awhile as we explore the subtle realms of natural wonder and open to the direct teaching of shamanic Sign and Vision together... with the very young and the otherwise old... and perhaps your family will find new ways to awaken still more to the discovery of the Teachings of our Mother Earth... and to share the special wisdom of all her creatures and all her secret workings.

And as you move through this intimate journey with us... perhaps your family will also come to walk a little taller and find more feeling and intimacy to share... perhaps to open together into deeper surrender... and so to be full-filled with Wonder and Vision as you walk out in to the day-night sky together to meet the magic of the Living Earth which floats in our Living Cosmos... and so come to know firsthand the joy-full experience of *'finding place'* as children of the union of Mother-Father Spirit... and the inner peace and wholeness which this discovery seems always to awaken.

THE MAGIC OF LIVING RITUAL

Every day of walking the medicine path brings a new way to practice the special *way of seeing* that brings Sign and Meaning and Vision to us from the world-at-large. Every new event, every daily chore, every interaction with other people brings a new opportunity to relate this new process - this new way of being - to *everything* in our lives. And the formless form that weaves all of this magic together... arises from the *Living Rituals* that we share.

Every ritual that our family shares springs up spontaneously from whatever situation we encounter. What we know as 'ritual' is not somber, heavy or 'occult.' It is never pre-structured or directed as it unfolds. Whatever springs up afresh and brings new Meaning to us... and so we know it as 'Sign.' And every sign is an indicator, an alarm, a flag, a guide... that points the way to new and subtle *Meaning*. And as human consciousness dances through life... *anything* that we experience in this way can be our *Medicine Sign*.

How we relate to these signs and how we interact with them is the *content* and the *process* of our journey. What we actually *do* to discover, feel-through and express this relationship is our *Spirit-Dance* (in eastern yoga terms, our *lila*). Thus each special moment has ritual significance *only* because of what it awakens in us and the closeness that comes from acknowledging and honoring and sharing together... the most meaning-full experiences of our lives.

When any small moment of improvised ritual dance helps anyone's meaning to be revealed (and shared), then we can all feel how our own 'ritual dances,' our own, little, one-act plays and our moments of shared wonder and communion bring us into ever deeper, feeling relationship - with ourselves, with each other, with all of humanity, with all other sentient beings, with the Earth and (if we are very fortunate) far beyond, into the presence of the *unified mass-consciousness* of the *Living Universe.*

SNAKE-SWIM DREAMING

Even at its best, Process as concept is merely *Medicine Word.* It is in the dancing-through of these concepts and dimensions... that the awakening of *medicine* actually occurs:

It is an early, long-summer evening. The valley of the river is just beginning to slide into the shades of dusk. But it is still too hot to want to do anything else than laze and play and swim.

Slowly, the mothers gather their trailing lines of ducklet kiddies behind them to wend their way up the winding grassy path to the dusty cars and vans which will carry them to wherever they feel at home. This is a favorite place on the river for many families....

It is also our family's favorite 'magic place' where the river turns slowly and ripples around a shallow sloping pebble beach... and then plunges deep into peaceful, green darkness near the opposite shore, where overhanging reeds and ferns shade its deepest secrets. And from these rushes emanate the most amazing things: amazing birds, huge goannas, mystical snakes of all kinds... and even, at times, a soft-furred platypus or two.

Now sometimes we are all aware of being a family of spirit... and sometimes we are not. During hot-sun afternoons of splashing around with dozens of naked children and mothers (and a few dads thrown in for the mix) our 'great medicine rituals' often take the form of 'good old fun' and we just play and play and play. Just like today!

But even in the highest moments of our most excited river-play-splashing, we know that Medicine is still around somewhere. And we know (and we trust) that magic will come to us in its own time.

And as long as we can remain in this state of *Deep Trust* we can be free: if you know you will not 'miss out' on anything you need to experience... then you can give yourself totally to whatever is happening here and now.

In its own right time, play-time softens into peace-time... loud voices of celebration let go into listening... and well-tired bodies sink into *Dreamtime Vision* almost without even noticing the change. As the play-time of excited self-expression slowly changes into the stillness of evening, the medicine path begins to glow and summon us to walk in ancient ways of mystery. And this evening, just at dusk, such Sign came....

Perhaps in our excited play, we missed some of the early signs... but it does not matter at all, for I know that: *we will always see the signs that we need to see... and all the Sign that we can.* And no matter what subtle signs we might overlook... we will usually *feel* the primal changes of the Sun and the Moon, the elemental Wind and Rain. And on this special evening, the moment of our inward turning (the feeling that always awakens us to the inner worlds of subtle Earth-magic) came just as the sun dropped to kiss the mountain-rim lip of the valley's ever-open mouth....

The air cooled slightly, the side-light of the sun turned everything warm and orange-toned and for many of the happy and play-filled people at the river this meant it was time to go. But for us it meant that a magical time of stillness was about to descend upon the river, healing it of the scrapes and gentling it from the turmoils of the long day of water-play. And then, all at once, a strange (and familiar) feeling of heightened meaning filled the air around us... and was immediately felt by every one.

The new feeling meant that something was about to happen. Sign was here. Of course! And we all knew it at once. I felt the little ones looking up with excited eyes and hearts. We were all beginning to prickle with anticipation... but we could not yet know what was going to happen, because we could not yet *read* the sign.

The families-at-play scenario continued to fade with the dimming daylight. We were being left alone. We settled into a silent vigil, each of us watching-feeling-hearing our very separate views of the evening dance of birds, fish, frogs, wind, light... and the reddening clouds. And still, in this difference of experience, we were as one being: like lovers entwined in each other's arms but thinking far-away thoughts of other times and places, making duality from oneness... and back again to oneness in their timeless re-union.

The electric chill of unfocused adrenalin surge still hovered around us and within us as we waited. It is always difficult to describe shifts in the prime *dimensions of experience*. But at that moment, the living spirit-being 'Time' began to stretch out, to give way to non-linear flows of non-time experience in pure and open space... and from this I knew that we were *very* close to a special meeting. And then it happened:

A thin black line emerged from the gloom of reeds across the river, waving gently in the still air, looking, looking... everywhere.

"SNAKE! There! Shhhh!" I said, barely speaking above a snake-breath-sound. Heads bobbed and necks craned to quickly scan the un-scannable complexity of the dark-river world. Children see *so much*... that they often cannot see anything specific at all!

Time was still fluid. We had time enough... and we made space within that liquid time for every one to have a chance to see the snake head in the reeds, looking... looking... looking....

Now I knew that Snake cannot hear. Snake has no ears. So we could *'talk snake'* aloud without scaring it away. But Snake can *feel* so much! My first "Shhh!" was to still any chance of snake-frightening movement. We were still. At last we were all tuned in: we could all see Snake and its subtle dance. And so it was time for The Meeting.

I waited until Snake entered the water. Ami was the only sure and certain, long-run swimmer at that time... so I softly invited her to follow me. We entered the now black-skinned River silently, slithering in like snakes ourselves, until we were eye to eye with this beautiful being.*

Snake stopped its gentle arcing tail-stroke. We stopped. *Everything* stopped: birdsong, kid-talk, windsong... even Time itself seemed to slow and then shudder to a halt.

We hovered in this no-time floating world for...ever. Snake absorbed our warmth, our size, our breath, our air-taste from its place

---

* Australia has some sixteen or more species of venomous snakes - or maybe even more (they're still trying to count them all)! This particular snake was a very common Red-Bellied Black Snake. And because it is so common, bites (which are rarely fatal) also occur. But *any* venomous snakebite will affect your health and self-integration... forever! This species grows to about eight feet in length, but it is a peaceful ally and not vicious or aggressive... as long as it does not become afraid.

of totally motionless holding, perhaps thirty feet away.

Motionless: treading water with its tail and body moving gently against the wind and current, but holding its neck and head absolutely still and fixated upon us... absorbing us in its own inner way, revealing nothing at all. And we were absorbing Snake: every pore of our bodies eager and frightened, loving that beautiful being... and trying to find trust to go with our eager love. And then we did.

When Snake decided we were all-right beings to share its evening swim, it began to move slowly toward and away from us, swimming downstream in a slow diagonal from its side of the river, to ours. It did not hurry. It did not worry. It just flowed broadly across the surface of the evening waters, pulsing perfect, arcing waves of energy in a wake behind its head as it swam.

And we swam with it. We swam slowly up behind it until we were within six feet or so of its tail, staying careful to remain beside it as well, so it could see us clearly and know by our position - or our speed... or our smiles... or our gentle breathing... or our infra-red or bio-electrical pulsing... or our open hearts... or whatever - that we posed no threat (and, indeed, wanted none in return).

Sometimes 'it all' comes together. Sometimes everything works! This *Ritual Meeting* was like that: we swam beside this great Black Snake for a few minutes which stretched into forever and we were completely at peace. [In fact we were somehow safer within that snake's energy field than if we had thought ourselves to be alone in the water... because we knew that no *other* snake would harm us as we swam with such an ally].

That evening, Ami got to meet and feel the great and powerful beauty of Snake for the very first time. I was thrilled all through my permanently nine-year-old, snake-enthralled consciousness to have been allowed so close to such a magical being.

It is sometimes hard for humans to feel the great Medicine Power of *Snake*: Snake is a deep and beautiful, primordial being. Snake has been succeeding at living on the earth for millions of years. And Snake carries such a painful weight of guilt-induced biblical (and pre-biblical) human fantasy. Heavy, archetypal symbolism assails Snake from every culture and every land: death, fear, deceit, treachery....

In old Australia, the Rainbow Serpent was a bringer of Creation for the Aboriginal *Koori* people. And in our early western civilization, there was thought to be a great serpent that encircled the

Earth, while the earth was balanced on the back of a great turtle! So, for all our fear, we humans also share some deeply implanted genetic programing that feels the beauty and the magic of Snake.

Beyond all of our ingrained fears, Snake is one of the most amazing of all living things. Snake is a *fully integrated* life-form. Fully evolved. Fully capable. There are no 'loose ends' in its design... or in its consciousness. Nothing contradictory or unknowable in its body, its perfectly precise movement... or its Spirit: *Snake is always absolutely true to its nature.*

And so the great Black Snake is pure magic to behold... as it swims so cleanly across the sky-lit waters in the magic-time of evening light... and darkness.

From being so close, and feeling so assured that we *could* stay this close, we were able to relax and find some long minutes to share a truly bonded relationship with that beautiful snake.

Now, snakes can swim *very* quickly. But this evening we were *invited* to a meeting: Snake did not swim away from us (or attack us) in fear. Snake swam *with* us. And so Ami and I still carry with us the *medicine power* of that swim together - and some of the medicine power of that archetypal being.

As we finally reached the river's edge (Snake and Ami and I) the long black body finally slid unceremoniously between two rocks and moved out of sight in the dense reeds of the riverbank.

We might have imagined that it paused, turned its sleek head ever so slightly and somehow acknowledged what we had shared - perhaps with a meaningful backward glance, or something like that - but Snake needed no Sign of parting.

Thus Snake ended the audience and our *Medicine Dance* on its own terms - with a flick of its tail as it disappeared without a sound, without stirring so much as a single twig or leaf or reed. It was with us - so close we could hear the small wind-waves licking at its skin as it glided through the waters - and then it was not there! Simply and inexorably... gone. And there was no external Sign of our experience... except what we each carried inside.

Wonder, slight confusion, excitement, perhaps even some uneasiness at not knowing where the big snake was now, as darkness moved in still closer around us... and all at oncc!

We swam back in silence - well, nearly silent, little exclamations bubbling up, recounting the joys and the thrill of our encounter like ancient tribal warriors returning from a great hunt.

There on the riverbank was our family... sharing in the rush and glory of the Great Medicine Hunt! Shrill excitement cascaded outward from all the bouncing heads of bobbing curls, with arms flapping in endless excitement. Such power-full medicine. Such a simple joy! There was no containing it.

It did not take long - perhaps only a few seconds - until the Medicine Power of our ongoing experience had moved from River-Snake to the children and the family (once again). The mini-shamans at the river's edge had been so excited and so scared as they watched our ritual meeting with Snake... now their great rush of energy met our return with such bubbly and silly and all-at-once chatter that we all laughed about it all the way home.

And Snake... well... Snake was out there somewhere, perhaps fondling the wonder of it all, too, in Snake's own way. And Snake-Mind? Well... who knows what Snake could make of such a tender meeting there... while he thought he was just swishing through black-river waters in the evening-cooling air...?

LETTING GO - AND FALLING IN TO WONDER!

For many years, now, our family has been (more or less) consciously exploring new kinds of awareness together. As our basic tools, we use naturally occurring phenomena of Nature and consciousness in order to feel-through whatever we might encounter as we move through life.

On one evening's *'Medicine Walk,'* [see Chapter 5] we might deliberately 'let go' of *looking* around in the dark of night so that we may open to *seeing* whatever might come out of the darkness and into our minds' inner image-in-ation.

Then we will form a Ritual Circle on the Earth and take the time to share how it felt for each of us... and so find out if any aspect of the experience was felt in a similar way by every one. And whenever this happens, we know that we have found powerful medicine!

On another day of great wind, we are invited to allow our senses, our breath and our feeling (intuition) to soar on the Grandfather Wind to new heights and to expand our awareness as we fly across the Earth on the mighty winds... like spiders... like fairies... and Spirit!

Perhaps another sunny afternoon finds us playing in the Mother Ocean, perhaps reaching out to feel what dolphins might experience as they move from elemental Air to Water and from the Light in to the Darkness... and back again, endlessly linking these dimensions of being and experience.

To feel like a dolphin we found that we just need to breathe and move like a dolphin. And once we are flowing through the waters, then all we need to do is open our awareness to discover *'Dolphin Consciousness'*... and then it just comes through! And once we 'catch on' - then the dolphins come zooming in close to join us in newly intimate sharing.

Where do our hearts and spirits go when they are given such *Free-Ritual Invitation?* Whenever we make time to share our separate journeys in such welcome intimacy... we find ourselves bathed in yet another revelation of our inner feelings, selves, purpose and process.

Aha! *Revelation!* Now here is another essential building block of the Medicine Process. The concept of 'revelation' is an ancient notion that is fraught with patriarchal, biblical associations. Let us see how revelation might be active in our lives in a new (and maybe fresher) way:

Many people who aspire to use some kind of 'shamanic process' to nurture and direct their own self-evolution tend to pounce upon any revelation, whenever it occurs and try to hold it as some kind of fixed Meaning - as if by freezing an inspirational image and holding on to it very tightly, they will gain some permanent in-sight as to their 'ultimate destiny.'

For us, *Deep Revelation* is simply the natural guide-dance that is here and available for every one... who will but open to it and let it flow through. This ongoing experience of Revelation, then, is fluid and all-ways changing. It is the basic stream of Guidance that is there for all of us - to help us *'find place'* in every present-time moment on this very present Earth. It is also the flow of constant invitation, reflection and association that combines to show us *the Way of the Medicine Path* and the *Process* that we need to make it all work for us. This path - and the process through which it evolves - can be an amazing gift to anyone who wants their life (and their family) to be truly intimate, meaningful... and effective.

THE MEDICINE OF ALL LANDS

The word *yoga* means 'union.' In the East, this refers to the union of *body, mind* and *spirit*. In the West (and including Indigenous American cultures), this 'union' is often felt to be a whole-being integration of *four* elements: body, mind, *emotion* and spirit. But however it is conceived or symbolized, the notion of achieving this same-and-only Union - the *one-ness* that we all seek - is common to *all* spiritual paths.

As our medicine path-way unfolds in all of its infinite variety... we have come to recognize that this process is a yoga in itself. The specific *form* of yoga that anyone might use to move toward their re-union with Spirit and Infinity is not important. In fact, it simply does not matter at all. It is the *new awareness* that matters. And when we experience spiritual breakthroughs... it happens at levels far beyond even our most sophisticated intellectual analysis.

So, whatever path we choose to follow is not as important as *how we walk* that path. For in the 'how' lies the ongoing revelation (revealment) of the Process. And it is how we move within our process that either holds us rigidly fixed (and un-growing) or expands and liberates us with endless discovery and new awareness.

We have found that within this simple medicine process, we have everything we need for whole-family growth: all the resource... all the tools... all the gifting... all the ritual... all the revelation... and all the guidance that we could ever ask for... to help us to share the most profound intimacies and to learn whatever we need to keep growing together.

This is a path-way that has parallels in many cultures and through all times. The medicine path that we follow includes and integrates many elements from the East and from the West. Just for now, within our little tribe, I am the only one of us who knows of these things. But that is not a lack. For beyond the few terms and notions that we are presenting here... *it is simply not necessary to share 'concept' with children in order to share Deep Medicine experience.* And *this* is why this Free-Ritual Medicine Process is so wonderfully suited to deep family sharing.

Even though my family is still too young to formally meet and acknowledge any formal sources, our path-way of discovery often includes many of the elements of traditional Eastern path including: *Taoism* (the dance of polarity, the energies of *yin* and *yang*); *tantric yoga* (the yoga of polarities and sexuality); *yoga pranayama* (breath-yoga); the meditational movements of *Tai Chi* and *Aikido*; and energy channeling, fire rituals, water purifications, Ayurvedic

(Indian) and Chinese medicine (acupuncture) and Buddhist meditation... to name some major influences.

These Eastern processes and path-ways naturally synergize with many specifically Western therapeutic and wholistic healing modalities including elements of: Neo-Reichian energetics (and specifically the Bio-dynamic Therapy of Gerda Boyesen) - various polarity and magnetic healing systems - color healing (chromotherapy) - radionics - iridology - nutritional healing - naturopathy - anthroposophical healing principles - homeopathy - allopathic (conventional Western) medicine - Gestalt therapy, encounter and other experiential and group communications processes.

I also include as influences, my own experience of several decades of 'intentional community' formation and my work as a consciousness celebration ritual-maker (while always learning from the ritual traditions of many other lands and times) as building blocks for the ongoing evolution of my personal approach to *New-World Shamanism.* I also honor the Native American traditions of the Medicine Wheel (and the concept of 'medicine' itself, of course), the *inipi* (sweat lodge) purification ritual, the *Vision Quest* and, above all else, the foundation awareness of all humanity as the beloved Children of the Divine Union of the Living Mother Earth and the Father Sun. Father Sky, Father Spirit... by any name, the currently less recognized, equal-but-opposite father-force which dances endlessly with the Earth and Waters... awakening life and consciousness in us all.*

Other lore from the indigenous people of other lands also finds its way in to our Circle and our Free-Ritual adventures: 'Dreaming' wisdom from the *Koori* people of Australia; the Hindu-animist death and rebirth rituals of Indonesia; the spiritual warrior consciousness of the Maoris of New Zealand, the Kahuna of Hawaii and all the other Pacific Islands peoples; the shamanic lore of Thailand, the ancient

* The lists (above) are not meant to imply any particular level of personal mastery of any or all of these dimensions, but rather to identify and 'credit' important *sources* and *resources* which have affected and nourished my own (often bewildered and staggering) journey through the realms of yoga, meditation, healing, shamanism and Spirit.

wisdom of Tibet, (etc.).

In fact, of course, everything that I have personally experienced inevitably affects everything that I have to offer my family.

It feels very important to emphasize (once again) that with the exception of these specific and basic principles: *Medicine, Sign, Vision, Materiality, Spirit, Breath and Feeling*, my experiences from all my travels of the past and all through the complex names, systems and philosophies which I have personally studied are rarely (if ever) even mentioned as my family explores and evolves our Medicine Family Vision together.

Understanding the 'why' of this feels very important to the success of this present work... and the possibility of other families coming to use the Medicine Family Process that we are sharing here:

I do not avoid these 'metaphysical' concepts because they are in any way irrelevant to our Process. In fact they are absolutely vital and intrinsically *connected* to all of our family's explorations, even now. It is simply that they are never mentioned to avoid lumbering our simple magic with the many complex concepts that come with this esoteric lore. But there is another important reason for this careful omission: *it is all simply unnecessary!*

The many elements that combine to bring us Medicine, including: *guidance - lesson - revelation - healing - ritual - initiation - power -* and *Spirit* (and more), arise very naturally within every individual's experience of life... without the need for *any* special incantation or sophisticated, pre-learned rituals.

And every individual's blocks to living in the realm of pure Medicine Wonder - like every individual's blocks to whole-being enlightenment - *all* arise from within our past programing and inherited (biological and cultural) predispositions.

Without a single book, without quoting any gurus, teachers or 'ascended masters,' we (and you) can go as deeply as any of us dare to venture... into the magical realms of collective consciousness... into Medicine... into Spirit... into learning the *Dance of Medicine* and learning how to *'walk in a sacred manner'*... together! Nothing more is needed than the simple openness and surrender of the innocent child that lives within us all... and a little shaman guidance from time to time for each individual to evolve a self-guiding Process to dis-cover the Guidance which will light the Way Home.

So... Yes! I try to spare my children from as much of the dogmatic, 'new age,' spiritual consumerism which so distracts and delimits our slowly evolving cultural consciousness... as much as I possibly can.

All that *we* seem to need to share together on our deepest levels of intimacy and self-unfoldment and to continue to grow as a Family-of-Spirit derives directly from our Ritual Dance with the Mother Earth and the Father Sky... from whatever we dis-cover in our feelings... from our faltering steps across a fallen log at night... from falling together into the stars and open space of night... from a ripple on a gentle stream... from the raging thunder and the deep peace of the Mother Ocean... from the effect on each other of a father-word or a child-laugh or the song of a magical spirit-bird.

We follow a path of experience which needs no name, no history, no esoterica and no vocabulary except the primal expression of our feelings-thoughts-wishes-communion... and a very few notions of process. You know: *sign, meaning, vision...* etc.

As my children grow in mind and understanding, they will (perhaps) be eager to use more of my experience of other lands and times and peoples (and, still later, to find their own)... so that they might knit together for themselves a world-view which includes the wealth of all humanity, all traditions and all cultures.

And/or they will have heard so much from me over the years - in passing, as it were - of other ways and other tribes that they will take all of that as 'given'... and then head off into realms that I have never imagined... perhaps (I always hope) to dis-cover even vaster realms of medicine, Spirit and consciousness than anything that I have ever experienced... or imagined.

And if, someday, they return to me with a new perspective to teach, some new feeling to share, some new songs to sing, some new way of walking-moving-soaring - some new appreciation of Spirit - and come to share it with me (the by-then aged medicine man of their very first memories), it will be a great returning and a great ritual re-union for me!

And when they come to visit me... perhaps the undemanding, non-conceptual freedom of our present, *Free-Ritual Shamanic Process* will also then pay off for me... and I will so appreciate not having to learn the dogmas of all the beliefs and all the theories of all the cultures they have seen... in order to share my children's New Medicine Teaching... and all that they will have become!

MEDICINE TOOLS FOR CONSCIOUS CHANGE

Medicine is everywhere... Revelation is all-ways a surprise... and *Medicine Process is the Living Path*:

Sometimes we find ourselves waiting for a magical moon to peek out from a pillow of clouds. How we wait... how and if we can stay focused... what we do while we wait (tend our process)... and above all, what we *feel* while we are waiting is the stuff of every Moon Walk.

But if we ever *try* to wait... it usually happens that long before Grandmother Moon ever emerges from the cloud that rides the winds to hide (and reveal) her... we find ours'elves off and running in an entirely new direction! For we, like the Moon herself, are subject to the winds of change... and we know these *Medicine Winds* may blow us any way at all.

So the Grandmother Moon, the impish Cloud Brothers - and in fact, all the phenomena of weather and place and relationship that swirl around and through us - never become, for us, *fixed* elements in any pre-ordered dance.

No... they are merely the momentary *tools* of our medicine process... the catalysts of our family's growth... the 'strange attractors' that evoke changes in our consciousness from within and from without.

And in fact, every sign, every process, every altered state and every incoming phenomenon in *'The All'* of our experience might be regarded as a *Medicine Tool*. Medicine tools are everywhere and all around us: we need only know how to put them to use!

So sometimes we wait for the Grandmother Moon. Sometimes we drift in silence on the Mother-River at platypus-time. Sometimes we follow a leaf as it is blown across still waters by an unseen wind. And sometimes we look deep into the ways we react to each other. But whatever we do... and whatever it is... it is all Process. And within that process... *everything that we can consciously use to affect our medicine experience is a Medicine Tool.*

At other times we use the light trance states which occur naturally whenever we gaze at a bubbling stream or de-focus eye-vision as we let cloud-shapes float through our awareness, bringing whatever images they will bring to play through our very different, individual perceptions. Process. Phenomena. Tools. Medicine.... *Magic!*

What might be different here from the workings of any other family of day-dreamers? Perhaps only this: that we consciously work to become more sensitive to - and find out how to *use* - these tools. We are endlessly exploring: how can we use the natural state of 'trancing' and what brings it on? How can we use the bubbles of the diving platypus, the rhythm of the great python's glide - and everything else in Nature - to deliberately *move beyond* ordinary ways of seeing... to move together beyond the ordinary dimensions of real-time vision... to move together beyond whatever we knew before... in to whatever we have to learn.... to become whatever we are coming to be?

Sometimes late at night, even medicine-children have scary dreams! And then, whoever awakens with the Dreamer gets to explore with them the spontaneous working-through (the *Gestalting*, we might say) of dream-time fears and images. More medicine process... and still more *Medicine Tools of Change*.

Here, the new tool may be an invitation for the child to re-live the frightening experience there and then, within the arms of mother-father-family. Perhaps we will invite the child to *be* each element of the dream... to *go through* the whole, scary mess... until the whole drama is 'worked out' and all feeling is gently and wholly cleared... and deep and peace-full sleep can be found once again.

Through all our dances and dramas, it is important to note that we never try to talk anyone *out* of feeling. Why does anyone ever say, "Everything's all right!" to a dream-frightened child? How can anyone else possibly know what ancient (or future) experience might have been awakened in anyone's frightening dream? No... it is not 'all right' until it is *all* right. And that takes time... and caring... and processing... and *Process*.

But we also know that dreams are tools which we can use for furthering self-revelation. And we have found that if we take the time - respecting the content and the medicine power of the dream and allowing *it all* to be processed-through - there is all-ways new understanding and rich new learning to come from every moment of supportive invitation and the care-full dis-charging of every night-dream scare. New learning for the dream-scared child, to be sure... but also new learning and new meaning for all who have shared in *The Ritual Medicine of Healing Dream-Fear.*

TOOLS COME WHEN TOOLS ARE NEEDED

Sometimes we concentrate on special ways of hearing, smelling, feeling or dancing. Whatever we might do as a dedicated meditational action, the tool seems to spring into being directly from the needs and potentials of the situation.

You need never fear the rightness of whatever tools come to you. Whenever medicine tools appear to us - whenever any sign, feeling, ritual or vision occurs - we have learned that it is *always* safe to pick up these tools and *use* them.

Shamanic medicine tools do not appear from nowhere and they do not appear at random. Nor do they ever seem to appear when they have no use or meaning.

Sometimes you will be able to see exactly how they work and what they may facilitate... and other times their ultimate function (their use-fullness) might remain hidden in some inner need-of-the-soul which has not yet surfaced in your experience. And then they may seem arcane, displaced and bizarre. But even this feeling of strangeness and 'inappropriateness' can be a Sign... and a Guide.

For if you follow the medicine path with great care and integrity, you will come to *know* without a doubt that: *whatever comes... comes for a reason* - though it may be 'reason' which only makes sense to you long after the whole event has unfolded.

And though the words are simple, it is sometimes hard to Trust that:

There is an ultimate 'rightness'
In all things of Medicine...
And in all experiences of Spirit.

Thus it is all-ways inherently safe to explore *whatever* comes to us in our medicine quest for meaning.

And through this process... and in good time... the *invitation* that lies within every experience, the *essence* of everything that flows through awareness and the *meaning* of every sign... can-may-will be revealed.

The rightness and wholeness, the completeness and the infinite (experiential) resource of the natural world is all-ways amazing! I have come to realize that medicine tools are all-ways evoked by our needs. Sometimes the tools come first and the arrival of this resource sometimes awakens the need... which soon arises in our experience.

It often happens like this: one day you happen to find a ten dollar bill on the path... and then later discover that you left your wallet at home and need the ten dollars to complete some important connection. Or, perhaps one day you notice an empty burlap bag waving from a branch in a tree as you walk underneath. And a little further on... you find a friendly snake who would come with you to see the medicine children *if* only you had a way to carry it home....

I know you get the point: the tool often heralds the need. Find an interesting tool... and sometimes you can puzzle for a long, long time: "I wonder what need-lesson-initiation will be coming along that will make use of this...?"

To be able to recognize and utilize a medicine tool it is not necessary that you be able to analyze it or categorize it, either by its *process* or by its *effect*.

In trying to describe the medicine process, we might sometimes use sophisticated concepts of de-focusing, trancing, channeling, meditating or talk of being able to *'read sign.'* But it is *never* necessary to name or rationalize (in psychological or spiritual terms) these different experiences - or these processes of consciously using breath, sense, mind - to be fully able to utilize whatever tools or techniques you may discover (or be given).

In the realm of medicine, whatever works... works. Whatever you experience... whatever you can feel... whatever you imagine... is *real*. And sharing medicine is to share this deep respect for the real-ness and the rightness of each other's feeling-being-experience.

Medicine tools unlock the doors of our ignorance and help us stay on the medicine path. A key may be of any color or any material. A key may be called by many different names by different cultures. But if it suits the lock... it will let you through the door. What matter how you name its form or substance... if you understand its *essence* and can put it to good use? And the same may be said of all science, all medicine lore, all wisdom... and all Spirit.

It is basic to the path-way of Free-Ritual Shamanism that we are sharing here, that whatever we experience as sign inevitably focuses our awareness and evokes a response (and so we know it as 'sign').

From our reaction (from whatever we feel), meaning comes. And to aid this process, ritual action-tools appear or are suggested (awakened) intuitively. And so we may use the *action-tools* of breathing-feeling-sounding-moving-stillness (or whatever) and/or we might use *elemental tools* such as a special rock, a tree or a stream to help awaken our awareness of the meaning of any sign.

And somewhere in and from that meaning... may come the *Vision...* which guides and teaches and enriches our experience even further. So *what* we might do in response to any particular sign or situation is all-ways, for us, a direct response to our inner feelings of meaning. And whatever we can access as a medicine tool... can be *anything* that helps reveal this meaning within our awareness.

But it is also important to remember that: *this whole process is completely circular:* what we pick up as a medicine tool may be sign in itself. Perhaps the ritual tool that we use to reveal the meaning is itself the meaning (and the revelation) that we need to find. To extend this even further, perhaps it was *all* sign and the 'real' meaning - the deepest and most profound meaning of all - will only be revealed many years from now.

Anything is possible... and we can never know for sure! But there is a great security in this complex simplicity as well: for if you cannot (ever) know for sure what 'means' what... then all you have to do is *stay open... to everything...!*

And it is all-ways a Circle: if everything is sign... then everything is a 'tool.' And if everything has meaning... then every experience can be pure *Visionary Revelation.*

Wherever you begin, it is all a perfect circle... moving outward and inward in two directions... to Infinity. And there is no way - and no need - to fit this process into the cold, linear logic of cause-and-effect thinking. Because it is all real and it is all happening at once and it is all... *experiential magic!*

Living and growing and walking together as a medicine family... it is always *experience* which brings us our intimacy, our feeling and our guidance. And as long as we remain focused on experience as the *content...* and experience as the *teacher...* then it is not too important if (only) one or two of us are aware that falling into a light trance as we watch raindrops patter on the river is actually a profoundly energizing state of meditative opening and an (open) state of light hypnosis and a way of naturally inviting-releasing breath to flow away on an infinite out-breath, bringing waves of relaxing, orgone energy streaming through the whole body-mind... or whatever...!

No, to find your own sign and meaning requires none of this sophistication. And it is this genuine simplicity and natural openness which brings such beauty... and such purity... and such amazing power to this process, to this way of being... and to our family as we simply walk down a country road together at sunset... being and feeling and sharing *'It All.'*

AND EVERYTHING IS PATH...

No matter what occurs when we face Nature with an open heart; no matter what we share in exclamation as we fall off a balance-log into a happy, bubbling brook on a hot summer's day; no matter what we think about between times of wondering if we will ever find a real Vision to re-solve any of life's mysteries or to help in a time of special need... no matter what it may be...

It is all Path... It is all Lesson
It is all Yoga... It is all Medicine
It is all Experience... It is all Consciousness
It is all Spirit!

No matter what you or your family are sharing at any particular time... no matter where you are... no matter what you may think you are doing: whatever is happening in your experience moment by moment is a *New Invitation* to find the reality and the power and the magic of life.

But we are all so busy... no one (myself included) can claim to be 'in process' at every moment of every day. But there is space - there *must be* space - in this whole-being process for whatever we really need to do. Too busy for regular spiritual practice? Too busy to listen for every new invitation and sign? Plagued with killer 'patterns' and 'trips' that always distract?

Hey! No worries! You can miss one (or a thousand) of life's invitations. There will always be more to come. But also: once you realize that this endless stream of invitation and revelation is running through your every moment of experience... then why waste this special Gift of Grace... that we so lightly call 'life'... and 'consciousness?' Why waste even a single instant of the natural revelation that can fulfill us with every breath we take?

We all tend to look far and wide for experts and answers that come from somewhere *outside* our own experience. But in the end, experience is the only thing that you can count on for sure. For experience never ends. Experience runs in seamless infinity, wall-to-wall. And the only walls that exist in our experience are those which we have allowed to be programmed into our mind-sets. *Every* new experience is a new invitation to feel and grow and learn and share... together. And so we have this very simple free-ritual recipe which is at once our path and our process, our learning and our goal:

'Trust It... Be It... Feel It... Share It... Know It...
And let It All change You.
And then Open to Celebrate all the Change that is You!'

LIVING THE PROCESS

To walk this spiritual path so filled with sign and meaning and vision there is only one requirement, only one dogma, and it is this:

'Let everything be important.'

Try it! Treat everything which feels meaning-full on any level whatsoever as an essential element in a totally new and wholly unique Free-Ritual Dance which is unfolding within and through your consciousness... now... and now... and still... and all-ways... forever!

Honor all Feeling
And you will be One
With your own Inner Ritual...
And then you will be 'Living the Process.'

If you can honor your consciousness by welcoming *everything* which comes through your experience, you will be as clear as you can possibly be with/in your own experience.

And no matter what spiritual practice you might undertake, no matter what new technique or teacher you discover, nothing more will ever be asked of you - nothing less will ever be enough - than whole-hearted commitment to this simple reality, this simple choice of whole-being total integrity: *to be as open as you can be at any moment*. Nothing more... and nothing less.

If you can actually *live the process* in this way you will already be headed directly toward that whole-being transformation (real-ization) that the ancients called 'enlightenment.'

Wherever your consciousness is right now... whatever dimensions of awareness you are inhabiting right now... if you are on your path and making any headway at all... then your ultimate 'enlightenment' - i.e., your wholeness, total self-integration and natural one-ness with all life, consciousness and Spirit - will naturally follow.

And so you need only to retain your focus and your integrity and work through all of the experience which time and Spirit will bring to and through you. And ahhh...! Doesn't this sound neat and simple...?

Think back on all your previous attempts to find guidance and growth through one system or teacher... or another (and one after another). Remember all that experience of endless striving and never quite being fully met... and you will probably realize that you have already discovered that most spiritual paths contain built-in dogmas that inevitably restrict your experience (and so sharply limit their worth).

Sooner or later, at one level or another, every 'system' - and the dogma and control that comes with it - will oppress your *freedom to feel* and your *freedom to be*... whole.

But here is something different! This medicine path is different: within this non-discipline of free-ritual medicine there is time and space for *whatever* you are, whatever you may need and whatever you may feel... about anything and everything.

You can fall down, be lazy, forget your lines in the Divine Comedy and spill your drink on the host. It matters not at all. For we all come to see that there is *lesson* in everything... and every lesson is an essential element in what we are becoming to be. And as we move through these endless lessons, we are all just as worthy and just as blessed as any being that ever was.

If you are on your path and even barely able to move at all... crawling pitifully along toward some unseen goal which (you must hope) will lie just over the next hill... or the next one... or the one after that...

If you are on your Path
And if you are moving at all
Then you can take heart!

Celebrate your great fortune and the consciousness which is unfolding (however painfully, however slowly) within you! For you are already *one* with your path: you are already *living the process* of unfoldment and you are already becoming whole... as time and experience unfolds and reveals... your living consciousness.

Alas, as we all know... all of these things are easier said than done. Total openness, whole-being integrity, whatever: it all sounds just fine. But it can be a very difficult road to walk... and sometimes a path that is almost impossible to find.

But in this harsh light of the reality of our all-too-human consciousness, there is one saving grace: it is *The Power of Us* - the deep nurturance and profound guidance that comes when we are (usually very suddenly) awakened with a start.... by the revelation that explodes in our inner awareness and says: "Hey! We don't need to be alone! We can walk this path *together!"*

And then we know that we *can* reach out and hug each other tightly. Suddenly we are newly accessible and available to share in everyone's dramas and everyone's breakthroughs. Now we can support each other as we have never been supported before. And as we sink even further into this amazing state of *Deep Acceptance*... we begin to learn to trust that our way is all-ways, somehow, guided by a force that we may only know as the nurturance of the cool Mother Earth and the warming of the Father Sun. Known or unknown by any other name or face... this is the Great Spirit of the *Medicine Wheel*... of which we are *all* an essential part... and which is the whole of the living cosmos... of *us*.

FEAR & GUIDANCE: ENTERING THE SACRED POOL

Whenever you first begin to experience things which are 'magical' in their appearance - when you first begin to discover sign and meaning which seems to spring forth spontaneously from every charged situation... when you first find yourself 'making-ritual' with no intention whatsoever... and when these free-ritual expressions first begin to awaken true medicine vision within you - it is often frightening to suddenly find that you are thrown back (again and again) on your own experience as your ultimate resource and your *only* reality.

Beginning this process can be very hard. There is so much room for self-doubt and negation of even the most amazing revelations! But if you persevere, accepting whatever you can (and whatever you dare) of all the 'medicine' that is swirling all around and through you - allowing whatever you can of all these new ways of being, seeing, feeling, knowing, growing and becoming... and tasting and dipping into all these new dimensions of *sign, meaning, vision, ritual* and *guidance* at your own pace and in your own time - you will eventually begin to evolve a new reality for yourself. And with that will come... your own Shamanic-Spiritual Guidance.

In time, whoever opens to the medicine way inevitably discovers that there is guidance... and that guidance is everywhere! Everywhere and all the time: in every sound, every birdsong, every cloud and every feeling.

SO EASY TO SAY... ALWAYS HARDER TO BE

So... this is the Process that guides our Heart Family through all the crises and celebrations that arise from our explorations in the Realm of Medicine... and through all the other dramas of big-family life. It is such a simple and open model... and yet our little tribe still struggles with even the simplest experiences as we try to apply this Process to everything we meet... to everything we feel... to everything that we share... and to everything that we are. And even though we (sort of) always believe in our one living medicine principle that: 'our experience and our feelings will guide us'... there is still so much room for doubt and confusion... there is all-ways so much more to learn....

For now, the little ones (of course) tend to look up to me as some sort of ultimate reality-fix and process-keeper... and I, in turn, look into infinity and turn to Spirit with the same naive trust that they shine on me.

Sometimes our trust is rewarded... and sometimes it is 'rewarded' in disappointing ways which feel a lot like simple abandonment. Like when we leave the hazy path in innocence and have not yet noticed how far we have strayed... until we fall into an abyss. Medicine or no... there is still pain and suffering and doubt and confusion for every one. So please believe me when I say that as I share this simple medicine path here, with what may sometimes seem a too-simple optimism and a simply naive sense of surety... that I do *know* that it is easier to *tell it*... than it is to *live it!* Not just for the 'beginners' on the path, but for all of us. For on the medicine path - yea... on *every* spiritual path, it is important to remember:

Every teacher is also a learner... of slightly different lessons!

Whoever you are, and for however long you have been consciously following your own medicine path... you are just like me and we are like every one: we are *all* still meeting our every next Initiation, day by day and breath by breath. And time and time again, we all find that we have only our own very fallible fantasies of what is what to guide us... until some clearer guidance comes... until we learn to read the sign that will evoke the meaning that will open us to the vision and revelation of the Deep Change that we so long for....

But as you struggle... and as you join all those who are waiting-looking-hoping at any single instant for some sign of guidance, your own *integrity* will be your key and your best resource-center as you plunge into every new dimension and confront every new obstacle that you encounter on the path.

Such as we can... we move through our medicine journeys always trying to maintain the highest sense of response-ability. And yet our own standards of performance must be very self-accepting and very forgiving, as must always be with mini-shamans so young and eager and clumsy... and with daddy-elders who meet their different lessons with all the same uncertainty....

As our medicine family wends its way up a quiet river in the moonlight, we open to all the deep magic of this earthen world. It is simple. It is sublime. It feels so 'perfect.' And yet, even in the midst of all this 'rightness of being' we are still and all-ways struggling somewhere with the endless interface between our egoic human selves... and the simpler splendor and wholeness that (we somehow know) is all around us.

And even in the littlest ones, medicine power and integrity grow and deepen with every dip of their paddles and with every sun-ray that pierces the clouds of ignorance which hide the shaman that lives within us all.

STEPPING STONES ON AN INFINITE PATH-WAY

As our medicine family moves through its playtime - dreamtime -

needy - time - loving-time rituals, we notice that all the medicine-sign-vision-ritual that we share seems to move through four distinct phases:

First there is *THE TIME OF GATHERING:* the time of *letting in* new experience (through de-focusing, breathing, listening or whatever).

Then comes *THE TIME OF SHARING PROCESS:* looking at *how* we are approaching this experience, how our individual choices of actions/words might be affecting our overall experience, each other, etc.... and sharing all our reactions to each other's process.

Next we find *THE TIME OF SHARING MEANING:* sharing whatever each of us felt, imagined, saw, wondered (etc.) - through words, song, dance, mime (or whatever) - and *allowing* our individual meanings to emerge. Once we know what we each feel... then we begin to look for any larger, deeper *Collective Meaning* that we all may be able to feel... together.

Once Meaning has arisen... once meaning has been explored and shared together... then there comes *THE TIME OF CHANGE:* when we let the new meaning flow through us, inviting the growth and change and new understanding that it always brings. And the more wholly we can share these separate and inseparable elements of every medicine dance... the more we grow and the more we learn to trust this process... and so come to trust even more deeply, the endless revelation of our medicine vision.

And there you have it: four concise stepping stones on the medicine path! But, like most linear hierarchies, this one falls into a shambles and self-destructs in its own alienated abstraction as life unfolds its ultimate and all-ways amazing reality. Within the circular process of the medicine wheel, things never seem to proceed in a strictly linear way.

Often we find ourselves absorbed in *'talking process'* even before we are able to move toward a river in explorational openness... or we find ourselves busy with pecking order business before we can even get around to sharing our experiences of some sign which is clearly shining on us all.

And though it takes time and great caring... in this way, we strive to align and clarify our energics, share and stabilize our intentions and allow our mind-flows to merge as wholly as possible *before* we 'talk to a fairy' or disturb a shaft of magical light shining through a spider's web with our sometimes very eager and innocently invasive curiosity.

'Talking Process' includes sharing our primal experience of anything that feels meaningful as well. Who gets to tell next what they saw, who is willing (or unwilling) to wait for the little one(s), how we can maintain our own experience and keep it alive while waiting for others to share theirs: this is all *Process*.

And whenever we 'come apart,' whenever we lose our focus, our one-ness, our sense of a moment's meaning... or sometimes (well often, actually), even our basic social animal sense of sibling courtesy... then there is nothing else to do but freeze the frame right there... and get right into it!

In this way, Talking Process often *becomes* the sharing... becomes the sign... becomes the meaning... and finally evokes all the change that is to come that day!

Sometimes the external phenomena - like the brave shaft of rainbow light splattering through the trees and smack into our noisy tribe-of-all-ages - becomes the trigger of more primal stuff: who stepped on the magic mushroom-sign in trying to see the rainbow light? And who pushed whom while elbowing in for a better view? And who had to squeal and laugh and scare the precious medicine bird away before everyone else could see it?

IT IS ALL PROCESS! It is all Life. And there is nothing else to do... but follow it through.

For us, this is the basis of our hope of lasting family-tribal intimacy: if anyone really *feels* something - be it beatific enlightenment or egoic confusion or primal night-fear or sibling rivalry and anger, we will *always* find Ritual Place and make Ritual Time to meet it. There will always be an elder available to serve as guide-helper-facilitator. There will always be a Circle (usually the family, but often a larger circle at festivals, gatherings and in our circle-making in many different communities) to enfold and full-fill the need. And there is always this *Medicine Process* through which all needs and all experiences can be met and felt-through and shared... and released... to leave us all and each as open as we can possibly be... to feel the very next moment's revelation... of new sign... and new meaning... and new vision... to share.

And who will get to tell their story first this time...?

BRAVE EXPECTATIONS

As we squirm and writhe and grow through our family years, what we expect from ourselves (and each other) is simply this: to fully live-out and process-through our responses to *everything* which is meaning-full, with just as much sensitivity and clarity and openness and as we can manage at that particular instant. No more. And no less.

Thus we are committed to being as fully surrendered and receptive as we can be. And we are committed to putting in whatever time and attention is required to clear through our obvious and accessible blocks - our defenses against simple surrender and openness - whenever they arise.

But we also feel that it is important to respect the 'rightness' of everyone's experience... so we try to allow everyone to be exactly *what* and *who* and *how* they are in their feelings and their experience at any moment.

Too tired to wait in stillness while Daddy inches toward mutual acceptance with a giant monitor lizard...? It's all ok! Perhaps the lizard needed to hear the little whimper of complaint to set it free from the trance we shared so that it could go somewhere else it needed to be right then. As Australians often say - in quick, ritual dismissal of even the barest chance of meaningful conflict: "No worries, Mate!"

Just as surrendered and as relaxed and as trusting and as focused as we can be at any time. No more and no less. Let ourselves space out into ego-talk of other times and places while we are pledged to float down the Mother River just at dusk in stillness and openness, waiting for a sign of Platypus Medicine? Why not? We're free to feel, aren't we?

Sure... but then our 'medicine' that day may be about reminding each other that we may be wasting that particular here-and-now moment of charged possibility - a moment which will never come to us again in this same way. And instead of blending in with Nature so that we can find sign and meaning there... perhaps we will actually hold Platypus away that day as we play around in mind-less-ness, splashing and laughing our way through the material plane of all-too-everyday Life.

But there are times for Platypus Magic and there are times to remember yesterday's delights - and splash around all over the place while we share them all.... And who's to say which time is which?

To the Old One who can appreciate the rare chance to share medicine with magical animals on the silent river waters, it makes better sense to talk about yesterday over dinner... and to honor the short time of our medicine sharing with precious silence.

Sure... it makes sense enough. And in fact, most animals demand it! But such adult logic may not make the lineup of tonight's show, if any kid-mind spontaneously soars off on a different tangent. And who's really to say which is the right course at any moment? Just now, I usually go with the kids....

TIME AND TIME AND TIME AGAIN

Sometimes our family process moves very slowly and feels painfully ponderous to everyone. Sometimes so much so that it feels to us that we are somehow disadvantaged in comparison to other families who seem to just chug along their way, swinging through the material world like busy, care-free, playful monkeys with an endless source of vines to swing on... while we to spend so much time and energy working out our feelings, our fears, our love and our attitudinal dramas, that we seem to have less time for organized activities than other families. Less time, energy, money (and/or willingness) to speed around every day getting our kids to-from typical outside activities - piano lessons, dance classes, riding lessons, sports, etc.

And it is true: even during school times we still average a few hours *per day* just spent *'in process'* - processing-through our experience of the many elements of life, work, learning, medicine, path, healing, sharing, relating, communications, intimacy, earth-lore, external relationships... and school.

We usually meet in the morning for a great cuddle - a family heap - on our largest of family beds. The bed in my bus-studio is about eight by nine feet in size and piled with bouncy, cuddly pillows and magical medicine blankets from a long past of travel in wondrous lands.

Then we meet again at eveningtime, as the littlest ones get tired ("but I'm only tired in my eyes") and squirm and wriggle into mommy-daddy arms and legs and caresses.

And as each one falls into dream-time, they know that they will be awakened sometime later and dispersed to their own beds. As the family grows, our late-night logistics become more and more ponderous: biggies had to learn to make the 'long walk' on their own feet... and now are even reaching out to help carry the little ones.

So, yes, we sometimes feel that there is not time for all that others seem to (want to) do. But whenever we look at *how* we are spending our family-time together... all of us (so far) reaffirm our direction and we all feel deeply privileged to be a part of such a loving and caring tribe.

And so we celebrate a heart-circle-based tribal family lifestyle in which *there is time* to feel-through and work-through whatever comes up... in which we are committed to making space and place to include and honor everyone's experience... and yet we somehow always still find time to go exploring in *'The Great Unknown'* of the world-at-large... on medicine walks and river raftings... and school trips and going to the store as well.

In a way, it is just like the old platitude that says: "There is always time enough for the things that really matter - and we are *all* free to choose what matters!"

What choice of meaning will our medicine family make today, I wonder, when we are all together again at evening time...?

><><

And what choice will YOU make...
For your precious family today?

If your choice be for feeling 'IT ALL'
Then yours is also a 'Medicine Family'

And Guidance and Revelation will surely come
With every Breath and every Song you share!

And as you Surrender in to Sacred Parenting
We Honor You and Thank You for your Father-Motherhood:

We thank you for the Medicine Gift
That you give to your children every day

And we honor you as this gift spreads outward
To be shared with all the Children of the World.

Thank you for this Gift of Child Healing
That grows your children deep and true.

And for the Great Healing that it will surely bring
To all the Children of the Future.

And for the Healing of our Mother Earth!

><><

CHAPTER 2

FREE RITUAL WONDER

RITUAL IS A NATURAL WAY OF BEING

Anything can be a ritual. Any breath, any movement, any act of perception, any communication, any sharing or any inner focus. Anything at all. For *Deep Ritual* lies not in whatever we might *do* but in how we *feel* and how we *are* as we do... whatever we feel to do.

To enrich any moment of our lives with *Ritual Meaning* we only need to focus on two acts of will:

Firstly...
We assign ritual significance
To everything we do, to everything we feel,
To everything we sense and to everything we are.

And then...
We try to trust whatever Sign and Meaning may come
And we try to Surrender
To Accept whatever Impulse or Feeling may arise
As the Guide-Dance Revelation
That shows us the Way
Through every Living Ritual...
Through every Dance of Life.

From within this surrender in-to trust, *everything* is Medicine Ritual. And whatever happens, we take it as 'a dancing lesson from Spirit.' And we can know that whatever comes to us will be exactly appropriate to our needs and appropriate in its timing.

From within the deep openness of true *Ritual Surrender,* everything that flows through our awareness is all the medicine that we have to see, to feel, to learn from, to share... and to celebrate.

But beware! This Process sounds so simple that it is all too easy to overlook the many obstacles and points of great struggle that arise so suddenly and overtake us wholly by surprise!

It is 'easy' to do whatever we feel to do... but it is sometimes hard to discover its deeper meaning.

It is 'easy' to take risks and to make playful ritual when we are in a light and jovial mood among close friends... but very much harder to take risks when our most honest inner impulse is to do or share something that is embarrassing, wildly outrageous or even, perhaps, aggressively provocative.

Likewise, it is easy enough to 'hold focus' for a few moments and to 'play with' this notion that *everything is ritual.* But to hold focus through those endless dead spaces that drag on and on, while we wait for meaning which does not seem to want to come, is very, very difficult, indeed!

And then there is the most painful irony of all: whenever we are close to any amazing breakthrough - exploring new meaning, new dimensions of awareness or whatever - is precisely when we are *most* likely to feel distracted (to distract our selves) and when we are most likely to feel so egoically uncomfortable that we will leap to follow any distraction that arises... from inside or from without.

Given all of this, it is never a simple task to make the commitment that will begin a vision quest... or to make ready to become living channels for the subtle guidance that we may believe will always come to reveal the meaning of every surrendered free-ritual experience.

It is hard enough for adults to assign such complete surrender and maintain the near-perfect focus that is often required for the real meditation, magic or vision to happen. In fact it is one of the hardest things that we ever have to do.

But when we try to share medicine ritual with children... well then, *watch out!* For now, every distraction known to humankind - and many more that no parent has ever before imagined - suddenly become the very 'stuff' of life itself. Whatever may happen is 'all part of the ritual,' of course... but lookout! Once we add some free-child energy to any ritual mix, our form-less freedom can reach critical mass in an instant from anytime... and break into wild explosion all over the place!

It is an honor and a privilege to share medicine with our children... but it takes a special kind of facilitation if the Medicine Eagle is ever to fly... *toward* any Family Circle!

Many parents report that they have always dreamed that 'there must be some way to include the children in our most precious moments' - but feel that they have never quite found any way that really works.

After three decades of sharing medicine family vision processes as they are evolving in families in many lands, I have come to understand that through the care-full use of very flexible, gentle, open and non-authoritarian *Free-Ritual Processes*, we can indeed find the way to include our children... and to learn with them... and to learn from them... and so to full-fill our highest visions and dreams of what deep family sharing can be.

CHILDHOOD GAMES, RULES AND RITUALS

All children love rituals. In fact almost every children's game is a ritual in itself. Games like 'musical chairs,' 'pass the parcel,' 'telephone' (Chinese whispers), 'Simon says,' 'Captain may I?' etc., are all exciting *because* they are *Living Rituals*.

If we look more closely, we soon see that virtually all children's games involve the use of *Fixed Rituals*. Now, whether it be a child's game or a somber religious ceremony, Fixed Ritual can always be known by its three cardinal elements: all fixed ritual requires 1) adherence to specific, *pre-existing rules* and 2) demands that participants follow a *pre-set form*. And if the rules or the form are violated... then the ritual is believed to have been ineffective (at best) or even dangerously blasphemous (at worst).

The other common element of fixed ritual is 3) the presence of a patriarchal figurehead or ritual leader - which can be male *or* female in gender - who oversees the ritual and judges everyone's performance and to what extent they have fulfilled the rules and re-created the pre-set form. School teachers, bosses, the police, priests, etc., all fulfill these functions within our culture-at-large.

When they play alone, young children's games are usually very simple: just enough control to provide an outline of form (structure) and to regulate the process of playing the game. The pre-set rules thus provide an infrastructure, a foundation from which wide ranging experience and even wilder flights of fantasy can be launched. And how free the children feel will determine how far their free-range fantasies fly. (And, too, how able they are to soar into new experience within the minimal form and rules will reflect how peace-full or rebellious they are inside).

Chinese whispers (or 'telephone') is a good example of a simple ritual game. Passing a whispered message around a circle in one direction only requires very few and very simple rules: the message is to be passed on as accurately as possible; it is passed in one direction only; and players must whisper to each other so that others cannot hear.

But as basic as they are, these three simple rules do many things: 1) they effectively control the flow of energy and attention; 2) they ensure that everyone is included and that everyone gets a chance to participate; and 3) they allow for the message to be innocently distorted (which is the fun of the game) in a linear mode, without the complexity of cross-circle interactions, whole-circle synergy etc.

In this game, it is the unpredictability of how each child might distort the message that makes the game spontaneous. And this ritual of 'ordered spontaneity' is every child's introduction to the world of free-ritual interactive experience.

Because the rules of these games are simple... the fixed rituals which result from 'following the rules' are usually very simple rituals. But it is this very simplicity of *fixed-ritual behavior* which allows for such great variation in *free-ritual experience*.

If the rules become many and complex and difficult to follow, then there is so much attention and effort needed to act within the given structure... that there is little space-time-energy left for the spontaneous magic of true free-ritual experience.

FREE RITUAL BEGINS WHERE FIXED RITUAL ENDS

The concept of self-unfolding 'free-ritual' is one of the sweetest flowers of my ongoing work with shamanism and medicine ritual. So I would like to share it in more depth with you here.

Whenever we find ways to keep to the barest minimum the 'rules' that inevitably limit our personal and spiritual freedom... and when we can learn to use rules just to create a somewhat stable framework from which we can all leap into *'The Great Unknown'* together... then free-ritual takes off where the fixed ritual ends... and our experience takes off too... becoming wildly unpredictable... very intimate... and a lot of fun!

When our family shares any medicine ritual, or when we try to feel the magical experience that can come from swinging on a rope or floating down a warm summer river, we try to keep any operating rules as simple and easy to remember as we possibly can.

First, we use some fixed ritual: we agree to walk close together; we decide beforehand who will hold the light; we decide who will first step out on a tree that has fallen over a stream, etc.

We know these agreements as part of our process. This is the formal beginning of what will soon become self-evolving, Free-Ritual Process. And this is the initial phase, the *Ritual of Agreement*. After the basic agreements are established, the process continues to unfold as we are faced with dealing with... whatever comes next.

In fact these *material* agreements that often begin our medicine process are not based upon 'rules'... but evolve from very simple *preferences*:

We *prefer* not to talk when we are approaching something magical - a green-glowing earth-sign, a strange reflection in a moonlit pool... or whatever. We prefer not to climb over/on a fallen log until we try to *feel* whatever sign and meaning it might hold for any of us as we come to meet it in silence and openness.

And as we evolve and expand our operational choices (material preferences) together, through direct experience, whatever we agree upon today as 'good process' (all too) easily becomes the *Fixed Ritual Beginning* of our very next medicine experience.

For example, once we discover that it is better to wait a moment so that we can cross streams or fences together or to avoid using a flashlight unless we have to, then these choices tend to become loosely fixed in our process. But 'fixed' only so long as they seem to work for us... fixed only until we choose to try something new... and fixed only until they are formally changed by a new agreement.

In this way all of our fixed rituals are constantly (i.e., pragmatically) changing and growing. Whatever fixed rituals we use have been discovered by us as we move together *'in-process,'* as we would say. And whatever rituals we may adopt as beginning points or basic structure for our next free-ritual experience... we are clear that:

All of our Rituals only exist to serve our Process.
We have no need to serve them!

Like our rituals, our current understanding of process is always evolving and changing. And wherever it stabilizes - even for a fleeting moment in the swirl of our ongoing explorations and our very different individual mind-spins - then we know that we have discovered a fixed ritual that *works*... for now. When this occurs, we find that we are truly sharing on an equal and mutual basis, and this helps us to feel *centered* and *unified*. And so we find a starting point and a foundation for our next leap together into *'The Great Unknown.'*

Thus our *Moving-Circle Rituals* (we call them *'Medicine Walks'*) usually include some form: some in-formation of how we will order our beginnings, how we will proceed, how we will conduct ourselves (if we can only remember what it is that we agreed upon...), etc.

But because the form is ultimately always change-able and because each of the simple agreements which serve as any moment's fixed rituals represent ways of being which we have learned will directly enhance our overall experience... our process seems rarely to get bogged down in pointless ritual observances or meaning-less rules. We only use our first, formal agreements to provide low-keyed and minimal structure - as an ideal jumping off place for magical free-ritual explorations and initiation rituals of all kinds.

You can go out for a walk with your children with no real intent and they will discover something new and amazing *every* time. And/or you can add a few elements of fixed ritual: like suggesting that everyone stay (sort of) silent until something wonderful happens, or agreeing not to use flashlights in any way that scares away the birds and animals that everyone wants to hear and feel. Little things. Simple agreements.

And as these elements of agreement are added, by consensus, one by one, you will be evolving a precious wealth of *living process*.

This collection of agreements-held-in-common need never define your *goals* - for they can remain as wide-eyed and open as the children themselves.

But even in this openness, your evolving process can help you agree upon the *'how'* of whatever you do: how you walk together, how and when you talk about your experience, what principles of safety are needed before you cross the edge of a ravine... or whatever. And in this way, minimal rules become medicine tools to maximize everyone's freedom and aid in the flow of all shared experience. If we all agree to be quiet... then *everyone* gets to see the wallaby before it thumps its feet on the earth in warning sign... and jumps away to disappear through the jungle wall!

Proceeding in whatever adventures you may undertake, with this kind of simple, formal agreement and whole-family consensus will all-ways help your family to bond together more securely... creating deeper levels of *trust, inclusion, commitment* and *surrender.* Whenever these elements are free to synergize and dance together... *Deep Intimacy* is the inevitable and amazing result!

Holding and treasuring your *Ritual Agreements* (your process) as special rituals-of-sharing will also give your family the confidence of knowing that they can work-through any problems which might arise as you look for medicine signs together... and throughout the flow of your daily life.

And when the medicine works (even in the face of sometimes amazing and bizarre encounters) making-ritual of *honoring your process* as you walk the medicine path together will provide new ways of meeting whatever might come along and help you to move gracefully and intimately through the endless cycling of *sign-feeling-meaning-vision-revelation*.

So... we might say that your own family's particular fixed rituals are whatever elements of process you *agree* upon all together... and the free-ritual is what you actually *experience* and how you feel to share it within that sacred space of simple openness and wonder... sharing in that special way of *deep surrender* which turns any simple evening stroll into a profoundly moving Medicine Walk Family Vision Quest.

EVERYCHILD'S WORLD OF FREE RITUAL ADVENTURE

To further illustrate this important difference between fixed ritual and free ritual, we might notice that however any ritual action may be construed or represented, every fixed ritual is a *formal observation* (of custom, rules, expectations, etc.), while free ritual, by contrast, is a *spontaneous celebration* - of whatever comes when creativity, intuition and whole-being self-revelation are allowed to run free.

All children love *Rituals of Freedom.* Acting-out *anything* can be fun... when we are allowed to let meaning run free. And so it is with adults, too: the less we restrict ourselves with self-limiting *form*... the freer we can be to feel and appreciate the *content* (the essence) of every new experience.

The less we structure any important moment... the more room we leave for the pure magic of *spontaneous revelation*. The less we pretend that we can ever know what is to come... the more open we will be to whatever actually happens.

In this way the wide-open potential of our conscious experience can be freed to crawl out of its usually pre-defined limits and to *let go* of its pre-conceived content... to celebrate the free-ritual of meeting-feeling-sharing-knowing what I call, *'The All and Everything'* (i.e., all life, all being, all consciousness and all Spirit).

And with this New Freedom also comes the realization that *Experience is truly infinite* - in form, in feeling, in dimension, in extent, in subtlety, in power, in beauty, in vastness.

And once *this* little reality explodes into our awareness, then we can open together to the revelation and celebration that:

Medicine is everywhere and all the time.
And Medicine flows through Everything...
Through everything we Do and Feel and Breathe
Full-filling everything that We Are
And Guiding us to 'The All' that we are to Become.

Children respond naturally to life-affirming rituals of all kinds. But adults rarely speak to children in terms of *Free-Ritual Process*. Too often we only talk in terms of specific fixed-ritual obligations, like: "It's time to put on your shoes because we are going out." Or, "It's time to get ready for school or you will be late." Or... "We need to go to church every Sunday if we want God to love us."

And meanwhile, beyond and underneath what we are actively sharing with our children, and even while we are preaching those fixed-ritual dogmas that seem to be essential if the everyday scene is to be even remotely workable... the mini-shamans are busy finding *Free-Ritual Meaning*... everywhere!

A shoelace becomes a snake, going in and out of holes in the shoes and then dancing with another snake into a pretty bow (or not). A belt follows belt-loops around the race-track of the kid-pants until it meets itself in the very middle and is the grand winner. A book slides off the table and, for a mere instant, time slows and then stops completely and the child opens to new, *Free-Ritual Vision...* and in that moment perhaps discovers through Deep Intuition, the very essence of the great power of gravity.

As getting dressed merges with breakfast and the far-away considerations of school, child-mind is *always* absorbed in trying to bring everything all together at once. And the child laughs and sorrows inside when s/he cannot remember to put on *both* shoes or cannot manage to hold everything in both hands at once.

And so every child learns of the eternal frustrations of living in a finite body-mind... and how we always have to reach a little further to accomplish what we want... and the need to accept what we cannot. But through all of this essential learning... the process of *Deep Surrender* and the wonder of spontaneous discovery is alive and throbbing and active in every child, through every instant of their endless experience.

And all the while we harried adults may be too captivated by the material plane - the clock and the stove and the lost shoes and all - to even realize that this pure and endless magic of consciousness-in-evolution is unfolding non-stop and in all directions within our children's experience, feeling and Spirit... right beneath our very feet!

Then the ancient ritual cry-of-the-parent goes out: "It's getting late! You have to get ready for school!" And the very urgency that the child feels in the parent's call (and the child always feels it all)... fans the fires of *Free-Time Free-Ritual Magic* even further... and all is readied for another run through the infinite variety of pure child-mind wonder:

"Hey! Cool! My shoelace never looked like *this* before...! I wonder what would happen if I...."

"Wow! I can balance one shoe on the very edge of the window sill while I tie the other one... if only I can keep my other elbow from...."

Caught up in our ritual parent-panic-push it is so easy to overlook the simple fact that medicine process and the family circle magic *never ends*: that the sign and the meaning and the endless vision which *is* the natural magic of consciousness goes on and on and on...

whatever else is happening.

If ever we forget this bottom line truth... then we might just miss the Morning Medicine Show:

"Get ready right NOW!" We're getting louder and more strident now... and things are getting very power-full now. And our very intensity brings new vision to the ever opening child-consciousness: new images come... new ideas come... faster and faster and faster....

"What is *'now?'*"

"What is *'ready?'*"

"Am *I* 'ready?'"

And then, without warning, a few alien space-travelers might sneak out of the side-mind gaps in the retro-rocket backwash of kid-concepts and hazy real-time understanding, make themselves 'ready' (whatever that is) and blast off into ever-new adventures... while child watches engrossed and in pure and open wonder... and the time-school-parent drama intensifies (everything) even more.

Shoelace snakes continue to writhe and squirm, decide they hate each other and, even having tied the knot, refuse to be tied down to any long-term relationship.

A glance at the clock-god shows that time is not a simple linear progression - that it almost stops completely when Dad is angry and then jumps ahead of its own free will all over the place when a guy is only trying to tie his shoes.

With any luck, and just in time (or maybe only a little late), all of the time-less, free-ritual magic is brought into process-driven alignment with the fixed-ritual real-time world... and we are off to school... again and at last! And so it is. And perhaps inextricably so. And so the week (and childhood itself) goes by....

But after school... at night before bed... on sunny Saturday mornings... there are other ways that we can come to be with our children. For these moments there are ways of learning to 'walk together in a sacred manner' in the way of the Ancient Ones - ways that admit, accept and affirm the child's whole-being experience (and our own)... of endless magic, deep intimacy and the great medicine of free-ritual experience.

Whenever the real-world, time-fixed rituals subside, even for a few moments, we can share a medicine walk together. We can share a dreamtime fantasy-meditation together. We can share a moment of pure wonder together. And *these* are the moments of free-ritual sharing that no child (or parent) will ever forget.

However and whenever it happens in this infinitely complex dance-of-family-life, just as soon as we let go of fixed ritual structure and surrender into *Free-Time Revelation...* then we are right *in* the flow of the Medicine Wheel. Then we have immediately entered the realm of magic. And then we are already 'walking the medicine path.'

And the only thing that will be certain after that... is that *there will be* sign... and *there will be* meaning. And if we can but hold our hearts open against the weight of all our conditioned disbelief and resist our endless material plane self-distractions... vision... and Spirit will surely come!

YES!
If we are but Open and Patient and Trusting enough...
Every Medicine Dream will come True.

DEEP UNION IS ALL IN THE SHARING

However it may happen: watching the toothpaste swirl down the drain, losing mind-self in the dance of a shoelace, or whatever - *Sign* and *Meaning* and *Vision* can be a very private (and sometimes even lonely) experience.

But when it can be shared within a family circle... then every sign is felt to have come to the whole circle. And whatever meaning is found by anyone... will feel meaning-full to all. And through this *Ritual Sharing of Meaning...* we are bonding with each other and aligning our energies to ride together into a free-ritual future... which *no one* can imagine or predict.

The fixed ritual left-brain establishment may issue the decree: "We are going to school." But if we can learn to hold such rigid *in-form-ation* very loosely and tenderly and allow it to blow free with the winds of adventure... who knows where our free-ritual experience of 'going to school' might take us...? Hmmm?

Certainly not you.... And certainly not me!

This is the Way of the Medicine Family. This is the way of following - with all the awareness we can muster - the *Living Path of Free-Ritual Revelation.*

And this is the path-way to discovering the ways of medicine: how to walk lightly on the Mother Earth... how to feel her teaching... how to begin to heal the wounds she has suffered from the passing of so many care-less feet... and how to really feel love for each other at the deepest levels of our spiritual beings... even through all of our confusions, reactions, unclarities, blocks and always-blind strivings.

As we walk this path together there is a *Deep Knowing* that often floods through us: we come to *know* - that our being here together as a family is not merely some 'accident-of-birth'... that we are together here-and-now as a medicine family for reasons of Spirit which we cannot (and need not) fully comprehend.

And we come to realize that we are *all* the teachers and the students of each other... and that our medicine way is all-ways self-revealing and self-evolving and self-full-filling in ways that no fixed-ritual dogma-of-expectation has ever been... or could ever be.

As long as we walk in the dignity of knowing that we are being just as open as we can be - no more and no less - then we can feel deep trust that we are all and every one, the beloved children of the Mother Earth and the Father Sky.

When we are deeply secure in this spiritual union, then our every step - be it clumsy and unsure or brave and strong - feels so sacred... so blessed and so wholly affirmed.

THE ONLY DOGMA OF FREE-RITUAL OPENNESS

Still, we of this medicine family - and 'we' all of humanity - are all so, well... h-u-m-a-n. Sometimes there are so many distractions and so few invitations to remember that we can ever rise above the material plane of busyness. And so, sometimes we all lose our way for awhile. We simply forget. Maybe we do not even notice our loss right away. But sooner or later, we come partially awake with a great rush of confusion. And as soon as we do... then the realization begins to form inside our awareness... that we have to do something (anything!) to break out of this rut. We realize that *we have to do something* to find our path and to inspire our vision once again.

But on the medicine path... the 'how' of this recovery can be less confusing than it is when we travel other roads. For once we have internalized the 'always and everything' gift of free-ritual process... we know (if we can but remember) that we can simply walk away from confusion and contradiction, close the door behind us and head out into the evening light and try (just as much as we can, no more/no less, etc.) to open once again to whatever sign and guidance may come to us now... and now... and now....

And just as soon as we get back to that simple place that I have come to call, *'Deep Surrender'*... we naturally find that we are freshly empowered once again to ask those basic questions that form the very Heart of this medicine process. And whenever we ask, from this space of deep openness, the answers seem to come easily and clearly... and just as fast as we can let them in:

> "What is Medicine Process?"
>
> > *"It is the Revelation of our Open Love and Trust... learning how to move together in close-heart consensus and mutual support."*
>
> "What is Medicine Sign?"
>
> > *"It is the appearance in your Awareness of something special, whatever you feel as Power-full and Meaning-full to you."*
>
> "And where can we find this Sign?"
>
> > *"Anywhere, in all things and in all experience. Sign lives in every expression and every working of Nature... in your every experience of the Mother Earth, the Father Sky and the Living Cosmos beyond."*
>
> "And what Meaning comes from Medicine Sign?"
>
> > *"The Meaning of all things and all Feeling and all Experience."*
>
> "And what Vision will come from this Meaning...?"

And then, perhaps, we become suddenly distracted (or suddenly enlightened) by the gloss of a reddened leaf, the down of a milkweed's puff or the slow cascade of a great waterfall. And all at once, as we startle and turn away from question-and-answer learning, we can see once again our Medicine Vision of One Family... One Tribe... and then all of humankind as *'ALL ONE FAMILY'*... living and working and loving in peace and trust - living so gently and caringly upon the Earth.

This is our Way.
This is our Learning and our Teaching.

This is the only Dogma
Of the Free-Ritual Medicine Path

And this IS the Living Process
Of every Medicine Family
Of all Tribes and of all Times.

THE RITUAL POWER OF THE LIVING CANDLE

There are many kinds of ritual tools that can help to bring *focus* to any ritual moment: a drawing of the Medicine Wheel in the sand... perhaps placing a flat stone in the center to receive offerings... finding a conch shell to call us to-gather... or just holding a crystal or a vessel of water. Or perhaps it might be the lighting of a living candle flame:

When the candle is first lit, it feels like a free-energy system that 'gives' light. But if we watch a little longer, we begin to see the energetics much more clearly: the light is just the magnificence of a very complex being.

Beneath the glow there is an endless dynamic of heat and melting wax... the capillary action of the wick as it draws molten wax up from the wax pool to be vaporized near the flame... the re-shaping of the candle body from wax that runs down from the overheated pool... and, of course, the magic flame that dances around its darker hot-gas center, evoking, expressing and celebrating the elemental Fire.

While everyone explores the enlightenment of the candle and studies its Process - the physical *energetics* of the living candle - the multi-dimensional candle works a far subtler magic on everyone who watches its light-dance.

It is the flame of a candle that naturally attracts all eyes and so as soon as the candle is alight, the circle naturally comes to perfect, one-point focus, all together and all at once - without need for 'rules' or special leadership. *Fire brings immediate attention*: everyone is here. And everyone is ready... for whatever is to come.

Whatever is shared by everyone in any ritual circle awakens and strengthens our feeling of *the power of US*. And we have found that a candle will *'hold focus'* in any circle (almost) better than anything else. And so it is that in our little tribe, we have come to use *the power of the Living Candle* to consolidate and energize many kinds of ritual sharing.

When a candle is brought in to any circle, there are a few important moments. If we recognize these ritual *Moments of Power* we can use them creatively as conscious turning points and gentle guidance in whatever ritual is to come.

It seems that whenever we place an unlit candle in the center of a circle, a wave of *expectation* flows immediately through everyone. This is a *Time of Arousing* that can be used to settle and focus the circle.

As the mini-shamans settle into their expectant waiting - "What is this candle for? And I wonder who will get to light it?" - there is a natural *letting go* that occurs in every one. We begin to let go into our out-breath and so begin to relax and sink downward, into our belly-centers, into our inner selves... into the Earth... into the Circle... and into each other.

And so, without a word, *The Placing of the Candle* has begun the process of surrender... and so begins to open us to the experience of deeper communion.

The next *Moment of Ritual Power* is when the candle is to be lit. Since everyone is already highly aware of the candle as it stands tall and strangely unlit in the circle-center, holding the potential energy of everyone's expectation... then it is certain that whoever moves to light it will immediately become the center of the circle's attention and focus.

And so they do! Without any need for direction or agreement or fixed ritual 'rules,' as soon as anyone reaches for the matches (or a burning stick), all breath-energy-hope-wonder is immediately raised and poised: "What will happen next...?"

We know that lighting the candle is an act of both giving and receiving *The Power of the Ritual Tool*. It brings everyone still to hear what we have to say... and it also awakens the fire-spirit-flame.

Thus we have found that this is the prime moment to *consecrate the circle*... a prime moment to offer wishes or blessings to one or all who are there... a prime moment to invite the circle to *project* its energy-caring-healing (etc.), to serve the needs of any who are present and those who are far away, those who are alive (embodied) or those who are somewhere else, 'in Spirit'... a prime moment to *Make Offering* to Spirit or to the Living Mother Earth... a prime moment for any act that leads us together, into a truly sacred space.

The fixed ritual that we use, each time we bring the flame to awaken the living candle medicine tool, begins with: "As I light this Candle...." And the free-ritual that soars from that fixed beginning may urge us to say or do anything at all: "...I bring all my love to all the people who are close to this family who are not here."

Or: "As I light this Candle... I hope that we will have the most wonderful Christmas that we have ever had."

Or: "As I light this Candle I invite this circle to help Joah with his angry feelings and to help Joah and Beny find their brother-love again."

Or: "As I light this Candle I honor Sian's new name and wish her life to be beautiful and powerful forever."

Really... this formless form works for anything. Once *'The Lighting of the Candle'* has begun... it can be lit and re-lit again and again. And if this is to be done, then whoever lit the candle may also blow it out after it has burned for a few moments and when their offering is complete.

In medicine ritual terms, both the lighting and the blowing out of the candle create a kind of *Ritual Seal*: lighting it 'seals' the wish or consecration and blowing it out gives yet another chance to make a special wish or offering:

"As I blow out this Candle I send my wish out to the Air and the Sky with the smoke so that it will all come true."

Or: "As I blow out this Candle I send its warmth to everyone and I send my wish to everyone so that they will hold it in their hearts."

And then the candle (or the matches) can be passed around the circle - or just placed once again in the center of the circle so that anyone who wants to can make a wish or offering as they light it yet again.

If the circle is small and (especially) if it has a particular focus - like a special *Naming-Circle Ritual*, for example, then we often pass the candle around the entire circle after every lighting. Then, as each person holds the candle, they can add their own, special energy to whatever offering or wish was just made, giving each projection that much more power.

But also... as each person holds the candle, they can draw some of the candle's 'spiritual warmth' into themselves (like Eastern *yogis* do) as still another way of sharing in the *Ritual Energy Exchange*.

As any Candle Circle unfolds, it is sometimes hard to tell where the fixed ritual leaves off and where free-ritual begins! The sameness of the opening statements ("As I light this Candle...") is a fixed ritual tool. The passing of the candle may also be a fixed ritual form. But as any individual lights or holds or passes the candle... then there is open space for *Free-Ritual Offering* of any kind: a prayer, a poem, a wish, a song... maybe even an elaborate dance.

Ultimately, you see, it is *all* Offering. It is all Medicine. It is all Ritual. And the living candle serves our free-ritual process in the same way that a drinking glass (or the ocean) may carry water to our ritual circle:

Water is *Water* and fire is *Fire*. Beyond that, what we do with it - that which becomes the *content* of the ritual expression - is all-ways a free-ritual response to whatever anyone might feel at that moment.

Nothing more need be fixed. And usually, no additional guidance or direction is needed: the ritual will be, like every free-ritual experience, whatever it will be. Nothing more... and nothing less.

And we know that whatever will come will be medicine enough!

><><

JAI'S MEDICINE WHEEL CONSECRATION

I begin every Medicine Walk or Ritual Circle with this 'two-part' Medicine Prayer. It works as a complete *Consecration* (Ritual of Making-Sacred) for any Time of Medicine - and opens us to whatever Meaning, Revelation or Vision is to come. This is a *'Tantric'* prayer because it naturally honors (and evokes) the primal forces of *yang* (the masculine) and *yin* (the feminine)... Shiva and Shakti... spiritual high and spiritual depth... *Father Sky and Mother Earth*. This prayer celebrates our *Gift of Knowing* - that in our open Surrender we are all beloved children of this Universal Dance, this ultimate Spiritual Union. And so we are all worthy of all the nurturance and Spiritual Guidance that we shall ever need. This is *Free-Ritual Offering* - so the form of this prayer is never fixed. Change it for every offering! But however it comes out, *Ritual Consecration* goes something like this:

"Father Spirit be with our Circle...
Bring us your Clarity, your Sensitivity, your Empowerment -
Your Guidance, your Light, your Gentleness...
And the Blessing and all the Power
Of all the Fathers and all the Grandfathers and all Spirit...
To Heal us... to Guide us... to make us Whole...
That we may Heal each other, Heal our Mother Earth,
And all the Children of the Earth... for all time to come...
In Openness and Surrender to the ONE-ness that WE ARE...
May we walk in a Sacred Manner, gently on our Mother Earth.

Holy Mother Earth receive us, your Beloved Children...
Full-fill us with your Infinite Nourishment and Love.
Help us to feel your Teaching, your Deep Wisdom
And the Eternal Blessing of The Universal Mother.
Help us to be true to our Feeling and our Needs.
Help us to find the Strength and Endurance
To give birth to New Ways, new Depth and new Openness...
For every One... for all Living Beings...
For our Living Earth... and for all Her Children."

And then we make a 'seal' that roots this Sacred Word in the Earth and sends its Light upwards to the Sky... perhaps one (or all) of these:

"This is my Offering... This is my Prayer... I have Spoken."

CHAPTER 3

FREE-RITUAL IN THE MOTHER-SEA

BENY SKY MEETS THE MOTHER SEA

It was a slow, sunny, sultry day when Beny Sky met the Mother Ocean for the very first time. We were driving northward along the Pacific Coast Highway when we passed over a rise and the sparkling blue-green water and white-foam light of the South Pacific Ocean filled our eyes and our hearts... and, as always, with virginal wonder. And no sooner had this Vision exploded in our awareness... than yet another Medicine Pilgrimage had begun.

On that day, Beny Sky was exactly one year and one month and one day old. It was also the day of his paternal grandfather's seventy-second birthday. And on that trip we were traveling with Beny's godfather. So it was a special time to be moving through wonderland together. And today, Beny was going to meet the Sea.

We left the van high on a bluff and made our way in silence down a narrow winding path through sand dunes and rocks to the broad, white and empty sands of the secluded crescent-shaped beach. Small rocks moved out into the water from a point of land, and there the limestone cliffs overhung the beach giving us the feeling of being in a secret grotto, far removed from any artifacts of culture or time... except those which we carried in to this magic-place ourselves.

We walked in silence, mostly (or, you know, that kind of 'intended' silence at least). Anyway, even during the deep reverential silence of such a ritual walk, there is still space for some good laughs when little shamans roll down a long sloping sand dune... and even more when Daddy follows, head over tail.

Finally we came together for a moment of real silence at the waterline - poised at the earth-sea interface for a moment to touch hands and invite *'the Spirit of the Mother-Sea'* into our Medicine Circle - to invite Her healing and inspiration and guidance.

This is something we always do. It is part of our medicine tradition. It is our ocean-*sadhana*. It is spiritual path. It is our way: whenever we meet Ocean for the first time in any day, we always hold hands for a moment before anyone enters the water.

We do this in a line or a crescent, facing the open water, rather than in a circle. This way no one has to turn their back to the sea, like they would in a round-round circle. And also, we do this because the sea *is* a circle: by standing at the edge of the water hand in hand, we are making a circle *with* the only-one ocean which encircles our entire planet.

When we had made these little offerings to the Mother Sea (and of course felt blessed in turn by her as well)... we moved to a place where rocks poked out of the sand and formed small tide pools and rivulets of water as the surf breathed in and out. There we gently walked Beny into a few inches of very shallow, very warm and very shiny water. He sat down/fell down and just looked all around at this liquid jewel which flowed all around his hands and his legs... shimmering and dancing and bouncing Sun-light up into his wide-open eyes.

Pat-pat splashes, submergence of a finger, a whole hand... a laugh... and Beny said he was 'one' with the great ocean. I looked for a stone, a shell... a *Ritual Object*... a Sign. The others did as well. All that each of us knew for sure as we searched, is that the right object would reveal itself to us. And we knew that this ritual object would be a material-plane vessel in which many memories and all of the energies of this moment would reside. This would be strong medicine for Beny Sky to take with him on his way....

I found a rock. Ami found a shell. Kira-Sparkle ('Sparkle' was a recent self-chosen add-on which proved to have a very short life-span) found a crab claw that was no longer in use. I offered Beny my father-blessing for his life with the Mother Ocean, inviting his surrender to the living sea and hoping we could invoke some overt nurturance-sign from the ocean herself.

One by one, everyone offered Beny their affirmations and prayers. We passed the ritual objects so that as each person spoke (or simply held each medicine object in silence), their energy and their spirit would full-fill this token... and make it powerful as lasting ritual medicine for Beny Sky to keep in his medicine pouch for a long time.

When the stone had made a full circle around his family, the last to bless it passed it to the Beny. He splashed it in the sea once... and then promptly popped it in his mouth... and then he laughed. And so the softly poignant solemnity of the ritual changed in a flash: Beny was doing his already established magic of bringing fresh lightness and mirth to our family. And now, too, the *guidance* of the ritual had changed: moving from my/our direction to Beny assuming his rightful place as shaman of his own first-ocean baptism!

We all followed along, laughing and celebrating his power with him as we each took turns washing the stone in the sea and then sucking pure ocean-magic out of it.

Many stones and shells and sea plants and crab claws were passed and blessed and patted and tasted that day. But eventually it came time to move on, time for the daddy-droid to organize the infinite walk back up the bluff to the sun-sweltering van and get the all-and-everything of us rolling northward - toward the equator, toward the even hotter Sun - once again.

In our Circle, and even as we were tasting it, we had all agreed that the first-stone of Beny's ritual was to be the one we would keep for his medicine bag. And as we began to wash off loose sand and get ready to leave, we stopped our busyness for a moment to pick up the stone... and it was nowhere to be found. It was simply nowhere: not in the pool where we sat, nor under the sand nearby. It had simply gone back to the ocean of its own volition! Perhaps it would lie in wait for another three billion years for another cherub shaman who to find the magic stone when s/he came to meet the Ocean for the very first time....

We were all happy that day. We had taken Beny Sky to the Mother Water and the ocean had baptized him, over and over again, as it unfolded surprise wave-splashes for him, one after the another, in endless variety.

True, we had 'lost' the ritual object which we had imagined we would save for Beny. But of course there was really nothing lost... except our materialistic expectation. Beny had met the sea and Beny was still laughing... all the way up the trail.... And he was still laughing as we drove away, heading on up the coast to the 'Rainbow Region' in the tropical North.

As we rode along in silence for awhile, we were each thinking of the ritual we had shared. Well, most of us, anyway. Beny was probably not thinking about it at all. I was full of feeling: what a great privilege it is to shepherd these children into such meaningful moments... and then to watch them take over the shaman's role and guide themselves (and all of us, in fact) through the most intricate and spontaneous free-ritual magic... and out into the light of our ordinary realities again and again and again.

Moments like these really affirm the profound openness of this approach to sharing medicine and ritual and initiation... with anyone.

And whatever he *thinks* he is thinking right now, as we drive along the road and myriad new stimuli wash through his senses... somewhere deep inside, his first ritual meeting with the Mother Ocean has been imprinted upon his spirit.

And whenever and however he meets the sea through the years and decades to come, somewhere on a deep, inner, cellular level, he will be reiterating and re-experiencing his excitement, his surrender, his first ocean-prayer and his *MotherSea Initiation*, through every cell of his being. For now Beny Sky will know the Ocean Spirit forever more -

And the Mother Ocean will know him!

SWIMMING RITUALS AT THE EDGE OF FEAR

Fear is the only stopper. Fear is always the block. Fear is the end of every opening and the end of every moment of pure Wonder. Fear underlies every dis-ease. Clearing fear is the prerequisite of all healing. And exploring and dis-charging fear is the ultimate path-way to health and wholeness, by any name or in any discipline.

Fear can be met anywhere, can be processed whenever it comes... and can be released whenever it can be met and *felt-through*... forever.

It is now two years since Beny Sky first met the Ocean. Beny is now three and we have returned to Byron Bay to live with all who have come here from around the planet to share the simple splendor of this peace-full, Aussie place of blue-ocean-dreaming.

Today, Beny Sky meets the dancing light of the little shore-waves with excitement and joy. And today Beny Sky still meets the deepening cold waters and the wildly swirling foam of the surf with his natural human fear.

As I swim him through Light and Dark, I try to feel the very *edge* of his fear. We move back a bit and play in the safe place until we have a good strong bond of trust with each other and with the Mother Sea. Then we take a few more steps out. We go a little deeper. The waves are a little higher, a little stronger now... and somewhere Trust inevitably gives way to Fear.

I hold him tighter, I bend to his level to share his view and the coldness of the growing waves with him, to better empathize with his experience. I speak of *primal trust* as a warrior and as a father - re-minding him of my soft care and my deep love and my daddy-strength... and I promise him protection from every danger... from every danger - every danger *except* his own, inner fear.

And even as I do this I am moving backwards very slowly, one step at a time towards the safety of the shore. And so we retreat from the fear-full place. Yet still he cries and complains and tries to get me to turn back so that I am actually facing the beach. Aha! We are in safe space... but Fear has followed us even into these gentle, shallow waters!

Once (and however) it is has been triggered, our subjective experience of fear bears no relation whatsoever to objective reality. Once Beny is afraid, it does not matter whether we are in the darkness of the ocean deep or on the safe, dry land. *Fear must follow-through its own inexorable progression...* from blinding tension... to simple openness and clarity.

To process it through, we look around together. We see the water is only four inches deep and we laugh at ourselves for being so silly and afraid... and so we try to put Fear to rest. But it is not so easy as that, because -

Fear can sometimes be put to rest...
But Fear cannot be put to sleep!

Once he has become saturated with the all-over cringe of fear, *all* water feels too cold; *every* wave seems too high and too strong; and no embrace of mine seems able to bring security. Sure... we can laugh at our fear and feel real grown-up-manly from the safety of the shore. But when any sliver of a pesky water imp suddenly licks at us from behind, or a loud wave crashes far off shore... Fear leaps to attention again and fills every cell of the body-mind with its sickening chemical messages of doom and dread. Yuck!

So it is that we cannot ever really banish Fear just by going into shallower waters. It is a good lesson to learn: the pervasiveness of Fear is as real as fear-its-self. You cannot deny it. You cannot pretend it away. You cannot decoy it and distract it's attention. In fact, in very actual fact, and even though it seems the furthest thing from all desire and all common sense:

Whenever Fear arises, there is nothing else to do
But to meet it, clear it... and let it pass through.

And then... when Fear finally becomes transparent to your Vision and your Touch and is no longer felt by your belly when you slide right through its domain... only *then* are you truly free of Fear... and only then can you be really clear... and so be open to feel... something else... anything else.

To really *meet* and *clear-through* our ocean-fear today we have to move in and out of the surf many times. We do it laughing, we do it hugging, we do it crying. We try everything. Still the Fear. Live the Fear. Feel the Fear. Drink it in. Taste it. Breathe it in and out... whatever it needs... until you can finally begin to hear the *New-Life Invitation:*

"LET GO, My Son! Run *toward* it! Dive right *into* it! FEEL IT ALL! Feel all the Fear that you feel. Feel all the Fear that you are. Drink in all the Fear that ever was and all the Fear that ever will be. And then, when you are ready... whenever you can... make that leap of trust and *LET IT ALL GO!"*

If it becomes too much to bear, we can always go back to shore and strengthen our Trust. We can play with the sand for awhile, tell Mommy tales of our bravery - perhaps even *'talk-courage'* before we find true Courage for our selves and so prepare ourselves... to go back to into the *Sea of Fear* yet again. Back into the coldness... back into the roar of the open waves... back into the very frontier of that *Ritual Place of Fear*.

Now we are there. Now we are in the primordial Deep. Waves are swirling and crashing all around us. This is the home-center of Fear. But wait... where is it now...? Where is that Fear now...? I don't feel it! I don't feel afraid anymore, Daddy! I am Brave! I am Sure! I am Strong! I am... suddenly...

"Daddy! No! Go back beessh!"

"It is just another wave, Beny. We will be ok. Yes, it will be cold. But it will be friendly. And we will be ok!"

A splash, a swirl, a clutch, a cry: it is *not* ok! No, it is not 'ok' yet.... And so we move back to shallows safety to comfort a salt-stung eye and to smell the beautiful warmth of a tousled sun-warmed head of curls as it nestles into Daddy's huge and still-somehow-reliable arms... and we wait for the confidence to try yet another wave... to try to dis-cover true warrior 'braveness' once more... and yet again....

THE PRESENT CLEARED HEALS FUTURE FEARED

Whatever the issue, whatever the particular arena of our confrontation, we are in the process of meeting and dis-solving *Primal Fear*. And this fear-clearing process always takes time... and always deserves all the time that it needs. And Guidance says: *"HEY! GIVE IT TIME!"*

There is always time enough in this universe for care-full growing. It cannot be done to clock-time or given just a few minutes of ritual attention. No... not if we are to really plunge into the bottomless abyss to meet and clear-through *all* the fear....

To be really healing and deeply effective, the process of meeting-discharging-clearing-healing fear must be entered as though it will last forever, without impatience and without any pretense that we can ever know what is to come: TOTAL SURRENDER is the only thing that works.

But ours is a very human-tolerant path. And for us, 'total surrender' (like total openness) means 'just as much as we can... no more and no less.' In and out, cry and shout, laugh and cringe, gingerly test and somehow celebrate: *Guidance all-ways comes as we move through the Free-Ritual Dance*. And the guide-dance may suddenly feel complete at any time....

My children and I have been through many such *Dances of Fear* together... and we deeply respect that there will inevitably be many more to come. Today I dance with Beny Sky and I know that we will both know precisely when Fear is fully freed and when this water-dance has accomplished its transformative, healing magic.

And so it is that both felt it when the all-clear finally came: "Hey! All of a sudden... *everything* is ok!" And at last... we have succeeded.

And then at the very apex of our self-satisfaction came the inevitable zen-daddy message: "Ok then, Beny Sky... now let's try going further out!"

Today Beny and I dance with Joy at the ocean's edge... and today we dance with Fear. Both are such natural states of being. I prefer joy, if given a choice... and I want to give my son that choice. But fear is everywhere - all-ways lurking at the far edge of all that is familiar and all that we have already mastered. Joy needs much help to stay strong in the very face of fear. And I do hope that I am helping in its nourishment....

I want to show my children how to dance *through* their fears. And here at the edge of the known world we can explore this new way of dancing together: moving in and out of the growing waves, bobbing up and down in the deepening waters, feeling the coldness of the sea and letting it be all right to feel cold. Minute by minute, wave by wave, hug by hug, and a laugh at a time... we learn to *Dance the Fears away.*

After meeting the Mother Sea and clearing through his ocean-fear in this way - however many days of ritual swims with Dad it may take - Beny Sky will come to know his power. And he will come to know his real limits (not his fear-limits) and he will be able to explore the sea for himself... be able to explore the sea and everything else as well! He will be better able to feel his own limits-of-sureness... and most of all, I hope, he will have a *working process* which he can use to move through every fear, letting them go one by one, until he can find real freedom... and real peace. The deep sea today... the dark of night tomorrow... and perhaps deep space in decades to come. Who knows where Joy (and fear) will lead him?

It is *so* important to respect our fears and to allow Fear its rightful place in our children's lives, without dismissive denials or ridicule. For little ones (or big ones) on the medicine path, perhaps this little pearl - this little mantra - can be both guide and invitation:

'WHEREVER IS FEAR, MEANING IS NEAR!'

Hey! Find the Meaning! Take the time! There is a lifetime ahead for this three year old boy to swim in the waves... but *only this one moment* to choose the path of ritually *respecting* and *honoring* Beny's fear... or to default to our reactive impulse to try to deny it, to push it away as though it was somehow 'unreal,' unworthy... or simply unimportant!

Beny's fear of the waves today is the fruit of all of his past fears... and this fruit contains the seeds that will flower each time Beny comes face to face with Fear... through all time to come.

If we meet it now, here, today, in this arena of gentle green-blue crystal surf cascading onto a warm, sun-streamed winter beach... then my Medicine Son will have his fair chance to grow up whole and strong and soft and deep, respecting and honoring Fear as a shamanic sign of all-ways deeper shamanic meaning... and knowing the medicine way to *move through* Fear into the clarity of peace and trust... and openness.

It is to this Song of Openness and to the heart-beat of our shared love that I dedicate my Medicine Dance with my little son in the surf today.

> *"Dance long, my Little-Big-One, Beny-Sky. Dance strong on your growing feet. Sing loudly of your fears and grow strong in your courage! May you shout and chant and dance through your Fears-of-the-Day... and laugh and sing through your Fears-of-the-Night!*
>
> *"Dance through your Fear of the Darkness and so find your Fear of the Light. Dance and sing your littleness and so celebrate your Medicine Power. Dance and sing of your* becoming*: Whole and Free and Strong and Big and Clear. Dance and sing your Chant of Warrior Courage evermore... and know that I am all-ways here...."*

And to help it along for now... at least for now... for this beautiful child-spirit, I will be all-ways here....

FREE-RITUAL WITHIN THE BIRTHING WAVES

Now we must weave our story-web through another moment in the Circle of Time: it is another clear day on this soft ocean bay. I am swimming around in the gently breaking surf with mask, fins and snorkel while the *shamanus minimus* play in the shallows. It is a day of powerful archetypes - very hot sun and very cold ocean... and underwater visibility which seems to stretch forever in all directions.

The bare white-sand bottom lit by the million-prismed diffractions of the evenly breaking wave above dances in my eyes and the constant swirl and heave of the swell and the break rocks my body in its perfect, womb-time rhythm.

If you watch the waves from underneath on such a day, the cosmic pulse of the *Tao* (the dance of *yin* and *yang*) is revealed in every dimension of this inner-outer universe of to and fro, give and take, push and pull, in and out - totally revealed in this infinite power... and celebrated in this infinite simplicity. And in this universal *lila* (holy dance) of these primal male and female forces, there is always something new to see... and always something new to learn.

The shore break this day was rolling perfectly straight toward the beach. When the crest could bear its own weight no longer, it rippled over into white-faceted jewel lights of froth and bubbles which danced in the sunlight in an unbroken line across my eyes and poised above the emerald-green water for an endless breath before falling into clamorous confusion as it raced into the shallows to wet the squeals and cries of all my babies who were playing there.

As I ducked underneath the break to let the mother-wave wash gently over my head I could see the whole side of the ocean fall away into a sheet of sliding, silver water... which I suddenly realized was moving in two directions at once!

The main wave was falling away toward the beach, as waves usually do. But there was another movement on top of this wave... a more etheric motion which perhaps involved only a few molecules of solid water in its dance. This was a sort of 'reverse wave' which appeared to slide upwards across the top of the falling sheet of beach-bound water like a visual membrane of etheric Light and Water... a placental energy-membrane through which each wave was released at its moment of birth.

For many eons of several minutes I stayed in this privileged place of total aloneness within the very birth-temple of new waves, bobbing up and down slowly with the unconscious surfacing-clearing-breathing-sinking rhythm of snorkel-breathing... just watching and feeling this endless cycle of the ocean-womb birthing new waves and drawing back a membrane of elemental Light and Water to let the new waves breathe in bubbles of fresh, new Air... until I *knew* it well and surely, inside and out: it, them, me, *us*.

SHARK-FEAR CLEARING-RITUAL

When the surf returned once again in my vision to its more usual persona of one-way waves breaking on a beach, I moved on, sliding through the azure sea and swimming outward toward some always interesting rocks that I knew well... and the embarrassed wreck of a coastal freighter which had been wallowing around too close to the earth a hundred and thirty years ago - when a great storm sank sixteen ships in these waters in a single night.

I have been to this wreck countless times over the past eighteen years and I have watched it change profoundly in its one-way slump toward total dis-integration. With each visit, it shows me more of its bones and its viscera. And wherever it opens a space, life floods in and claims every bit of surface in its wild profusion of color and movement... and consciousness of all kinds.

A few days ago, our shores were suddenly ravaged by the incredible forces of a tropical cyclone far to the north. Everything was moved. Everything was different. Amazingly, half of the great old ship had been raised right off the sand and rotated a few degrees, breaking the spine of the great beast. What a force it must have taken to do that!

And today, the old derelict lay in total surrender, huge ribs of rusting steel and boilers and pipes and rails strewn all over the ocean floor.... And on this day I knew that it was finally and certainly dead!

Walking on the Earth, we so often move in a two-dimensional world: most of Earth's landed inhabitants run around on the ground or climb trees of very finite height. True, a few species take to the air and so extend our awareness of three dimensional space. But as we move around on our earth-plane, we quite naturally judge all animals against our own physical size: 'little' is whatever we have to stoop to look at. And 'big' is anything which is longer or taller than our own bodies.

But to swim in the Mother Ocean is to move through a *three-*dimensional world which is alive on *every* level of being and consciousness. And 'big' and 'little' scale in every direction - almost to infinity.

As we move through this new realm, floating in this world of Inner Space, our experiential universe is a very small sphere - the size of which is sharply described by the relative underwater visibility of any particular day. And at the very center of this sensory sphere lives a small, frightened and helpless... person. We are the foreigners in this alien land - breathing (if at all) through bizarre mechanical apparatus, peering through artificial lenses and often carrying buoyancy gear - all of which greatly limits our movement and, of course, our Vision as well.

The human sense of hearing is better suited to air-borne soundwaves. Here it is cluttered and confused underwater by bubbles and regulator noise. And in this realm, our sense of taste and smell is confined to rubber, plastic, saltwater and dry tank-air. Our sense of touch is often clouded by textured gloves, boots, fins and a thick layer of neoprene wetsuit which leaves us able to only grossly sense the water temperature... and the most in-pressive underwater currents... and often little else.

Still, swimming *at all* at these depths is a grand miracle. Being able to be so close to the lifeforms in this magical realm is an incredible gift... on any terms.

And so we flounder around, wholly immersed in a long-alien element. We swim around, up, down. We float, we hang suspended in space with vistas stretching to the limits of sight in all directions. We look at whatever our eyes can reach. We touch what we dare without gloves, other things with care and some things not at all. We dance with gravity and the flow of the swell and the deeper currents... and we move through life's most amazing light-show of dazzling sparkle, shimmering silver sheets, penetrating shafts and lapping waves of rainbow diffracted sunlight.

But even as we move around in this swirl of endless Wonder, it is always with some risk. For there is one thing we simply cannot accomplish in this three-dimensional underwater environment: *we just cannot be aware of what is happening all around us at all times*!

Front-rear-left-right-up-down: it's just too much to manage on a continual basis. And wherever our awareness goes, trying to force eye-sight ever deeper into the ultimately impenetrable gloom... we are necessarily *not* looking everywhere else. And sometimes this can be the scariest thing of all!

As we penetrate the blue nothingness (or total darkness) which always defines the far edge of our little sphere of awareness, we meet myriad other living beings that dance and flit all around us as they appear from the gloom (and disappear into it) from any direction - around, above or below. And so we get to swim and dance and play with whatever is friendly in the ocean that day: whales, dolphins, groupers, schools of silvery darting fish of all kinds, turtles, rays, moray eels, sea snakes, squids, jellyfish, octopi, cuttlefish, blowfish, reef fish... and, of course, somewhere out there... somewhere there is always *SHARK!*

I happen to be one of those people who is always aware of Shark whenever I am free in the sea. Shark is a great and power-full archetype. And Shark is a living *fact* of the open ocean.

Shark is very good at what it does: clearing the sea world of damaged and derelict units of all kinds. And yet... even at our very best moments of oneness and grace with the Mother Ocean... we humans are hopelessly derelict and really 'un-cool' as we lumber about in this world of incredibly sleek and fast beings-of-the-waters.

Have you ever seen penguins on land? And have you ever seen film of the amazing speed and grace of penguins swimming underwater? Well, that's us: we are like penguins on land whenever we go into the sea. And there is no hiding our great helplessness. Shark *knows* this. In fact, believe it: *everything* in the ocean knows this!

By some contract with Grace we humans are not often eaten by sharks. This is more than a little surprising when you consider that our bodies (muscles) are constantly broadcasting a great fusillade of pulsing and swirling bio-electrical energies into the water as we grope about for air and flounder around, trying for some pitiful progress against the surf or underwater currents. And these impulses all say:

"Non-oceanic meat-based presence! Barely navigable hulk of flesh here! Seriously dysfunctional lifeform here!"

Far beyond our pathetic, little, sensory sphere-of-awareness, these subtle messages are flashed across *vast* stretches of underwater space-time. And Shark is always there... and Shark is always ready.

Shark is amazingly sensitive - precisely fine-tuned for just this sort of input coming from great distances away. And still, somehow, we can (usually) swim in the ocean - and actually more safely than we can walk across any city street. And the only way to do it (on the street or in the ocean, for that matter) is to surrender in to *Deep Trust.*

I have met real-time big-shark when scuba diving, but never when snorkeling. Scuba gear gives you an advantage... but not enough to get you up to 'even' with all those who actually belong there. With a scuba tank you can turn around, sink down, wait, etc. But when you are free-diving, you have to keep surfacing for a re-birthing breath of that good ol' elemental Air every minute or two. And so you are very vulnerable indeed!

Surfers spend long hours sitting on their boards, just waiting for the 'right' wave... and usually without being able to see much of what is happening just beneath them. And as they wait, their hands and feet hang into the water, sending out a 'small-meat' electro-image. Surfers are very brave. They are playing the odds... and they know it. They accept this and just focus on their art. And any trouble is always only there for the 'other guy' to deal with.

But very occasionally, they don't catch exactly the wave that they are expecting! Sometimes Shark catches them. Usually not with malice. Never with anything personal 'in mind.' Just a huge explosion of power and the surfer is knocked right up into the sky by the force of the strike... or torn apart in an instant by a mouth that works with absolute precision and dedication to its work. While the shark behind the mouth just closes its eyes (the nictating membrane) and allows its ancient genius to perform.

Sometimes Shark is savage, but often it is not at all intent on doing any harm... more likely lost in mindless meditation - or 'dreaming' of some distant day and a nice cold and peaceful ocean to swim in... when this present clean-up job is done.

As we come to explore the experience of Shark with less and less prejudice, we are beginning to realize that perhaps *most* shark attacks do not result from a shark trying to eat a human - but are the result of sharks merely 'tasting' a bit of human body to *see* if it is really something good to eat. Once 'tasted,' the human is often passed by. But even the smallest nibble from a Great White can so easily ruin your whole day!

Today I swim with Shark. Known-to-be-near Shark. And lately (let's face it), really bitchy Shark! There have been two very serious attacks on surfers in these waters in the last few days, both within ten miles of where I am swimming now. Neither fatal. Neither pleasant.

These separate attacks were not from the same shark: one was a ten foot bronze whaler and the other a larger tiger shark. Both occurred to the south of my home bay... and so it is to the south that I found myself directing most of my shark-watch energy. I always watch out. I am always careful. But I usually do not feel *afraid* as such. But today was different... and Fear was very near.

Anyway, on this day I wanted to see how the wreck had been

changed by the big seas that had come from that tropical cyclone up north, in the Coral Sea. I wanted to see what new-old lifeforms might be hanging around. I wanted to be part of the adventure that the Ocean had already experienced when the king tides and massive waves stirred and changed... everything. So I moved into the deeper water very purposefully and with my open-water wonder fully open.

As I swam out from the shore I was cautious as usual, but not too scared - or at least, not fully aware of the load of fear that I was carrying with me. But as I got farther out, I suddenly noticed that no matter how I dived or turned or spiraled... *all* of my sensors remained sharply focused in a southerly direction. And when I noticed that so much of my sense and consciousness was absorbed in compulsively probing the southerly gloom... well, then I saw that I *must be* deeper into fear than I had realized. Sometimes fear is like that - you have to feel it head on to even know that it is there. And *inner* fear - well that's almost always a total mystery.

Fear in the water just compounds any other signal or personal image problems you might be having with the shark-works. We all know how it works. It is just like being afraid of a very mean dog: you can tell yourself not to let it 'smell' your fear... but Dog will probably have sensed your fear before you even felt it... and even now is probably 'smelling' you *thinking* about how to mask your fear... and already knows your whole story inside and out, including what you have been eating for the past week.

Any animal sense which goes beyond our own gives that animal an unknowable and eerie advantage. Often, when we are out in the 'real world' of Nature... in the night, in fog, in storm (or in the ocean), we are as beings robbed of all senses. While every other animal around us seems highly sensitive and fully functional, we humanoids often cannot find avenues of understanding through any of our usual sensory channels. And being underwater can so easily awaken this chilling experience of unequal (and unfair) helplessness....

But now I knew that I was carrying Fear - a foreboding sort of distracting worry. Overall, it was still ok. I put it away with the self-reassurance that I would be careful... and a little medicine ritual to invoke stronger Guidance. And so fear calmed inside me... but only for awhile.

And then, just as I finally reached the first hulk of the wreck, a deep shudder stuttered through me. A cold water chill? A nameless premonition? Whatever: *Fear was back!* And even though I could bear it... still, it was not being cleared... it was only being *managed.* Moment by moment I needed to use Fear's cue to re-search my situation and continually assess this environment.

Caught within Fear's inspiration, I was suddenly flashed back to something that had happened long ago at that very same place. It was on a still summer day when the waters were cloudy with jellyfish and jellyfish sperm - and yes, it *is* amazing, this one-day ritual of jellyfish sex! Anyway, the visibility on that day was very poor. As I dived down to peek in the side of the holed hull that day, I saw something that was very large and very dark move quickly away from me in the murky gloom... staying just beyond the reaches of my pitiful, human eye-sense vision.

Whatever it was, I may never know. But the mystery - and my fear - both came to a head later that day when I was swimming back to shore and met a friend returning from a scuba dive, with his charter boat full of tourists.

He called out to me with some excitement and said, "Hey...! Were you just at the wreck? Did you see anything down there? When we passed by it a few minutes ago, I thought I saw something really *big* moving around down there.... But it went out of sight before we saw what it was!"

We shared some talk and some jokes as we went through the various (knowable) possibilities, with me bobbing about in the swell: unusually big ray... baby whale... dolphin... perhaps a misplaced dugong... or maybe a *shark.* And even as we spoke, I was unconsciously imprinting a *'LOOK OUT! DANGER!'* Message onto all of my present-future experience of being at that wreck.

And now, some ten years later... this unconscious programing was still alive and well, always ready to re-play whenever I swam near that gaping hole in long, dark shape of the hull in the water... and perhaps especially at times like this, when there were such disquieting rumors from the south!

I have learned a lot about Fear. Fear as a presence... Fear as an entity... Fear as a guide... and at least the tip of the iceberg of the personal-cultural load of experiential and mythical fear that I carry inside every cell. I know that whenever apparently irrelevant fear arises, there is often a good reason for it - and clear and logical reason at that. But until Fear manifests in a particular *context of experience...* its logic is almost impossible to understand.

Today, my old-fear memory could merely be a re-play... and/or it could be providing a *vehicle* (a channel and a rationale) for some newly *intuited* fear to ride on... as it rushed through my body-mind. Bottom line: *FEAR WAS NEAR!* And all I knew for sure... is that I didn't really know its 'why.'

But the day was sunny and bright and my children were playing on the sand not too far away and waiting for me to wave to them from the protruding communications tower of the ship, as it broke through the surface and reached for the sky at low-tide. So I moved on... surrounding myself with all the Trust that I could muster.

THE GIFT OF TURTLE DREAMING

And then, just as I reached the mast, I looked over the drop-off formed by the side of the ship and there saw a small sea turtle swimming lazily around, just below my feet. I waved to the mini-shamans as agreed, but could not see if they waved back. And when I returned to the greater intimacy of the underwater view... there was Little Turtle, still, swimming about as friendly as could be!

It is amazing how fast sea turtles can move when they want to. Even one of this size - a female, it felt to be, with a shell of perhaps twelve to sixteen inches long - could easily outswim a diver... if it wanted to. But this turtle did not want to go away from me. So I swam a little ahead of it and reached down and gently-firmly grabbed its shell, gently folding one of its back legs under my hand.

From this position, the turtle could quite easily have thrust out its back leg and pushed my hand away.... But this day, it did not. Instead, it *allowed me* to move it upward with my arm outstretched, until it was directly in front of my mask. And then we began to swim around the wreck... together.

Like all turtles, sea turtles breathe air. So of course I held the turtle near the surface as we went on to 'explore' the area together. Sometimes I would lead us in a new direction and Turtle would just coast, letting her flipper-feet hang loosely while I did all the work. Sometimes she would lead me... pulling me to change direction and even helping me by doing some of the propulsion work. What a team!

It was a good game. But it was also more than a game: for very soon I noticed that things were becoming highly charged. Everything began to feel *different*: powerful... sacred... *magical*!

As we swam together, Turtle and I, our energies blended so well that we became as one being, moving in slow-dance synchronicity through the water. Fish that would usually dart away as soon as any human approached now made no attempt to flee. Schools of fish which usually suddenly change direction many times as I approach them now let us swim right through their clouds of soft color and shimmering sparkles of light... without any sign of caution or fright.

All this was different. And experiencing this new state of non-intrusive acceptability would have been medicine enough for that day. But then I noticed something more: while I was swimming with Turtle, I just *knew* that I did not need to fear Shark! And as soon as this realization hit me, I felt a real jolt as I completely let go of all the tension and energy that had been maintaining my half-conscious shark-vigil to the south.

At first I thought that this was because I was so involved in my innocent turtle fun that I had merely forgotten to be afraid. So I deliberately washed the child-like state of play-bliss from my consciousness... *looked for my Fear* of Shark all through my body-mind... *breathed into* my species' primordial dread of the deadly Great Shark... and found... nothing there at all. Nothing to catch my breath or cloud my experience of Trust and Openness. And although I make ritual of looking searching every nook and cranny for that ancient shark-dread that lurks inside us all... I knew that there was simply none inside me.

Somehow... Turtle and I were Free in the waters - just as free as Turtle already knew how to be, I realized, long before we ever met.

And so, in the ways of ancient times, I was *taking medicine* (the teaching) from my meeting with this little turtle. As I swam and played in that soft blue sea that day I was being purged of fear that had been borne and passed on through countless thousands of generations of my people.

Turtle was protecting me right then, true enough. But beyond our fear-less play, Turtle was also passing on to me some secret that turtles already know - or, more accurately, some way that Turtle unknowingly *is* - about how to live with Shark and how to play in Shark's domain without attracting Fear.

I could feel my accumulation of ancient shark-fear releasing, flowing out of every cell of my body-mind as we swam that day, round and round, up and down, inside the shell of the wreck and back to the surface again. And as my fear washed from me, I felt so grateful for this Medicine Gifting. I sank into such a profound state of child-like, grateful love with Turtle... that I soon wanted to share her with my children on the beach.

I 'asked' and she seemed to agree - perhaps with some reservation, I don't know. But a giant, eager child with a magic turtle to share can be pretty convincing. So together we swam toward the shore break... and the beach that lay just beyond.

Now I recognize that this is asking a lot from an animal whose whole security-sense depends upon being free-swimming in a sea of some reasonable depth. Shore-breaking waves are hostile things to most sea creatures - and to many of us land-based lifeforms as well! And to a turtle, the beach is a dangerous place: if the drying sun doesn't get you, the dogs will. Let alone what the eager humans might do to any turtle who carelessly clambers out of its protecting waters.

But turtles don't think about all of this when they are being invited-coerced-carried-pushed (or forced) to swim toward the shore. In fact, one of the real beauties of turtle-consciousness is that they don't *have to* actually 'think' about anything at all! Their wisdom of the dangers of the waves and the beach is pre-programed - lying dormant in their *no-mind* state but fully ready activate long before there is any immediate danger to Turtle.

Turtle reacts to being invited/pushed toward shore by wanting to go back. No value judgment: no personal rejection intended. The inner ROM (read-only memory) program says: *"In-shore motion = threat --> action: dive and swim back to deeper water. Exceptions: egg laying."* Nothing more and nothing less. I know because I have read this far into the Turtle-ROM chip. (Once you discover how totally pre-programmed most animal species are... a whole new world opens up... and another closes down... forever).

But on this day, Turtle *let me* be childlike and Turtle *let me* swim us both toward the break and the shore... so that I could show her to my tribe - like any bright-faced kid bringing treasure home to Mother.

So Turtle let me carry her homeward. And I was at once both trusted and trust-worthy with her very Life. Occasionally as we swam, she would make a little, token "No, go back to Sea!" gesture with her flippers and back feet... but then she seemed to be somehow reassured and easily surrendered yet again to my gentle invitation and my eagerness... and we would go on.

Children are sometimes very silly. And in my childlike moment, I was as silly as the silliest of all. I was so eager to reach the shore with

Turtle in my embrace... that I did not notice that I had passed the outer break between two fair-sized waves. Suddenly, just as I was holding Turtle up above my head so the kids might see her from the shore... I was rudely hit from behind by a large, clean-breaking wave. A ton of purposeful water washed the turtle from my grasp and, no doubt, sent her spinning end over end along the bottom... with me rolling along not far behind.

I knew that even before she stopped turning, she would have been swimming strongly back into the surf, hugging the sand and moving out to sea with all of her strength and all of her pure and ancient, pre-programed and reflexive wisdom.

And then after I surfaced and while I was rubbing my eyes and spluttering, I knew she would be clearing the break and settling down to long-swim speed for several minutes until she was back out among the finger-shaped rocks - where something about the light and shade and myriad fishes would flash signal the "All stop!" signal. And her adventure with the big and silly human kid would be over - perhaps with some tiny piece of the drama filed away in short-term turtle-RAM memory (somewhere well out of awareness) to be recalled if I ever appeared again (very soon).

Even though I sort of knew that she would be long gone, I swam back out through the surf myself, just to try to swim *with her* a little longer... just to honor our connection. In case she happened to be waiting for me out there... I did not want to disappoint her. But alas, she was not. And so I turned back slowly to shore... coasting over the swirling white-sand bottoms while little stingrays rippled and scooted below me on the sand as my shadow passed over them.

When I was properly beached and back in my dry land element once again, I talked to happy children about the Sea and the Turtle and the wreck. Later, as we watched the star-light blasting out of a moonless, clear black sky on this most easterly point of this most ancient of all the earth's continents... we talked about shark-fear past... and shark-fear passing... and my *Ritual of Initiation*... by a gentle little friend, by

'The Little Turtle who was not Afraid.'

><><

CHAPTER 4

SIGN AND MEANING AND INTER-SPECIES DREAMING

MEDICINE SIGN IS THE PROPHET OF VISION

Medicine Sign is everywhere... all around us... just awaiting our experience of *Vision* which will bring to life the *Revelation* of its special *Meaning*. Once again, these are the four basic elements of this very simple process of shamanic guidance.

But while these basic elements themselves are simple enough to understand, they are also inseparable. And the ways in which they interact and combine and synergize... well that can sometimes be very difficult to understand. In fact, these prime elements are so wholly interactive within our experience that it is virtually impossible to experience just one 'element' of this wholistic process without plunging right into *'The All'* of the shamanic realms... and so right into the 'The Great Unknown!'

To make things even more confusing to those who would like life to manifest in clearly linear chains of 'cause-and-effect' relationship... this process is also *circular*. So none of these basic elements of the process can live or function in isolation from the others. One becomes another becomes the last one becomes the invitation to yet another dimensional leap... and so on... forever. So as we move along this path, our awareness dances freely around the endless, Free-Ritual Circle of the Medicine Wheel, touching and moving through these four, basic, elemental experiences in endless variation... and eventually awakening deep guidance (and consciousness), from within and from without.

Thus we can say that 'sign evokes meaning, meaning evokes vision and vision brings revelation'... or we can spin the wheel in reverse and say that vision brings meaning to the revelation of sign... etc. And it is all the same: it is all part of this non-linear and formless medicine process.

Even though the experience of this process is *wholistic* - here that might mean 'all at once' and 'all interrelated' - there is also a practical sort of chronology that often occurs as we voyage in these lands. As things usually occur, it is the discovery of sign that awakens us to begin the process. Each new sign is the invitational impulse that urges us toward meaning-full experience yet to come. So... sign is the *initiator* and also the *catalyst* that evokes meaningful experience from the ordered chaos of all that is around us. And in this sense... sign can be both the *materialization* and the *herald* of our every next experience of medicine vision.

This *Medicine Word* is sweet. This Word says it all. But beyond Word... there is all our direct experience. And the experience is far simpler and far more complex than any words can tell. The real-time experience of the *Ritual of Meeting Sign* often flows something like this:

At any moment, as you go about your life, you might encounter an unusual object - or a very ordinary object which you suddenly notice in a new way. Perhaps it is in an unusual position... perhaps it is illuminated in an eye-catching way... or perhaps it is something which seems immediately to have some timely, symbolic sense.

This new experience which just popped into your awareness could be anything at all: an energy phenomenon, a special look from another person, an unseen pebble that made a sound as it bounced away from under your foot as you walked... or a new way of seeing your own front door.

Sign can be anything at all. But whatever it may be, one thing is always true: just as soon as you notice it - the very instant that it leaps out of the white-sound background and into your foreground awareness - it has already become *your* sign for that moment. And just then... this sign may be the *only* real guidance that is opening to you!

And so, again and again, you set out on a new quest. For once you notice sign... then you have begun the process. And now you will urge to discover: *"What does this new-sign have to say? What does this sign mean... to me?"*

You may feel a strange sensation inside-outside which comes with a whisper of the Spirit Wind as you walk through an otherwise still night. Sign? If you feel it... it is your-sign now!

Yes! It is all-ways like this: first comes the Sign... and then comes the Wonder: *"What does it Mean?"*

You might hear a sound where there seems to be no sound-source. Or you may hear a great etheric chorus in the song of a single marshland frog... and feel a new vibration in his love-call which pulsates through wholly new dimensions of feeling within you. If it *affects* you... if you *feel* it with an unusual intensity... then *it is sign*, plain and simple.

And it simply does not matter what the material-plane source of this new stimulation might be. In fact, it matters not at all. For in this realm there can still be objectivity... but it rarely matters at all! What matters is only your *experience*. What really matters is only this: that you are *feeling* something in a completely new way.

Let the feeling flow in to your whole-being experience. *Let it grow* within this safe place of your trusting acceptance. And hardest of all to do: just *LET IT BE*.... just let it come... to be... *you*.

Drink It in
Breathe It in
Let It become you.
You can dis-cover Meaning
Just by 'breathing-in the Sign.'

MEANING CHANGES MEANING CHANGES YOU

Just as soon as the meaning of any sign reveals itself to us... just as soon as meaning comes clear... we all naturally want to hold on to it. Fix it. Seal it. Make it 'mine.' Wrap it up and take it home to share at dinner time....

But meaning is not an object. Meaning is not 'fixable' and meaning is *never* stable. Meaning is a wave that passes through your experience... and then keeps flowing on. Left to run its own course... meaning will all-ways change. So the best you can do is to just let it change within you. And the guiding questions - coming from within you and/or from somewhere far beyond, will all-ways be the same:

"What is the Meaning for you?
And how are you feeling it... now...?
"... And now...? And now...? And now...?"

Let the meaning change as it will: meaning is never fixed. Meaning is never absolute. No! All meaning is relative to your experience.* In fact... *meaning only exists within this state of dynamic relativity*. Experience all-ways changes. And experience all-ways changes us: instantly, constantly, in all ways and forever. So just let the meaning - *your* meaning - change with you. Whatever it may be:

You Are your Meaning... and Your Meaning is You!

Meaning will come and go as your experience flows through time. If you want to stay in touch with meaning... you will have to allow it to change... and you will have to *follow* it. And through this emotional-spiritual 'Quest for Meaning'... *you will be changed.*

To go with it, to feel it, you will have to surrender to *whatever* is meaning-full to you. Become Meaning's lover. Become Meaning's disciple. To live your highest vision: become the *living expression* of all the meaning that you feel. For meaning is *'The All'* of experience.... And everything which has meaning to you... synergizes to become your Sign, your Vision, your Guidance... and your Medicine.

Perhaps, just now, it is the hug and smell of your own child, filling you yet again with all the joy and love and magic of parent-bliss. Perhaps it is a sun-rise which seems to last forever and beckons your awareness to meet and inhabit some new dimension of experience that has been awakened inside you. Perhaps it will be a carpet of leaves and flowers aswirl on the surface of a river after a great Grandfather Wind sweeps the forests and gathers forest's offerings for the Mother River.

* A note for shaman-philosophers: Realizing that *experience* is the ultimate reality for all beings of consciousness leads naturally to awareness of four primary dimensions or elements being: mind-body-emotion-spirit. Understanding the circular interaction of these elements through experience leads naturally to an original philosophical paradigm which the author has called, *'Wholistic Phenomenology.'*

Or, less romantically, perhaps it may be a fleeting image that leaps out at you from a video screen... a door banging in the wind, far away, like a shaman's drum... or the shape of a stain on a piece of dirty laundry.

No matter what has entered your awareness: *IT IS ALL SIGN!* That is... it is all sign *if* you can *'read sign'* and find way to reveal its special meaning - meaning that is always yours alone to know.

Beyond our ordinary, physical world of sensation and material objects lies the more subtle *'Realm of the Shaman'* where *everything* is real... where *everything* has meaning... where *everything* is alive... and where consciousness flows everywhere, throughout *'The All and Everything'* of the living universe. And in that expanded state of being...

All Meaning is Sign
All Meaning is Medicine
All Meaning is Magic
And all Meaning is Sacred.

SIGNS UNSEEN, MEANING UNFELT

Sign is a chimera. Sometimes right out there and waving at you... and sometimes hidden behind many layers of the veils of our own unwillingness to see. Sign comes and sign goes: will we be there to acknowledge it or will it slip by unnoticed in the swirl of all our perceptual overload... and inner confusion? The answer, of course, is 'all of the above.' For Sign is like that: sometimes you see 'em... and sometimes you don't. And sometimes the experience is so exquisitely private to your feeling... that no one else will *ever* see the light of Meaning that blazes all through your inner awareness. But these unshareable moments are very special - they feed the heart and strengthen Self like no other experience in our lives! And in the end, whether others share your sign-sense or not doesn't matter at all. For Sign manifests in infinite flow... and there is always more to come.

So there is nothing to lose in this game. There is Sign and Meaning and Vision enough for everyone! If you happen not to notice something - an unusual object, a strange phenomenon of nature, a ray of magic light or a fountain of symbolism that flows from a magical flower - there is no failure in that. And there is no blame.

You can know that sign was there... is everywhere... as surely as you can know anything at all. But if you did not notice it just then, then just at that moment, well... it just wasn't sign for you! And in that absence of awareness, *Meaning* was just not there - just then, for you. 'No worries!'

In this free-ritual medicine work, there is no 'ought to be otherwise'... there need never be any blame for what was not seen. We all see exactly what we need (and all that we can bear). And no-one can see any more....

So we need not worry about sign unseen or meaning un-felt. There is no loss: you cannot 'lose' meaning which you have not felt. And sign is everywhere and all-ways... so there will always be more!

As experience flows through your life and your life flows through the magic of Time, some sign will be known and some will not. All that you can do is to *encourage* your own openness: to be as open as you possibly can be at any particular moment, to the whole-being awareness of any and all meaning-full experience that may come to you.

All you can do is to prepare your self-Self as an empty vessel to receive the input which will inevitably channel through whatever openness you can realize: emotional feeling, sense-feeling, mind-think... and Sign... and Meaning... and Vision... and Guidance.

Some of these will come. In fact, all of these will come, in their own time and in their own way. If we can just open to receive... *anything* may come through. We cannot predict its form or content... and we cannot pretend it away.

We cannot tell how we will feel it. But if we meet it in trust... we need not fear it... or push it away. Just by making the conscious choice to be 'as open as we can' to receive whatever sign and meaning and vision we can, we are already *worthy* of whatever comes through. And 'come through' it certainly will!

VISION-DANCING WITH THE SIGN

Here are some vital keys that can help your quest for sign become a continual *Vision-Dance* through an endless procession of sign:

Wherever you feel the presence of meaning (maybe even before you know what it is), you can be sure that there was a sign that pointed to that meaning. Did you notice? And wherever you dis-cover any vision-sign of meaning-full revelation... you can be certain that there will be others nearby - in time... in space... inside.

If you are patient as you breathe in sign and give it its full moment of surrender, focus and wonder... that sign will point the way to another sign... and that to another... and that to another.... and the process-ion will go on... forever.

Of course, sign may manifest through different perceptual channels or be felt through different experiential dimensions at different times... and it does not matter at all:

I can point my flesh and blood finger at a sunset which I may see as a pure flame of Spirit-Light... or as a phenomenon of photons, light-waves and atmospheric dirt... as I overlay my particular meaning on the real-time event.

Is it flesh that I point with or is it the energy of the awareness that lives within? Is it 'me' pointing to the physical sun... or is it the Father Sun beaming into my finger. Of course... it is 'all of the above.' It is whatever we can feel, whatever we can imagine... and so much more that goes far beyond our finite mortal awareness...!

I can try to be aware of all possibilities... honoring every meaning which passes through my awareness as real. And perhaps, even as I am processing all of this input and this multi-dimensional flow of interactive meaning... perhaps something in the sight of me just standing there in awe of the living cosmos will, in turn, be sign for someone else... and I will never even know.

Perhaps a particular slant of my arm, a sun-ray splintered by a single strand of my hair, the way my bare feet fondle the Earth as I stand there, will change the lives of some other being forever.... Who can know? *Sign is everywhere!*

Today, perhaps, the meaning of the sign you feel is to re-mind you of a love which you shared long ago and have long-felt as finished. But even as you remember it you bring it to life once again in your experience... and in the other person as well? Who can know? Experience love and the archetype of Love comes alive within living experience.

Perhaps the meaning of your sign today is that this love can never die away... and will live forever in the realm of mutual inner feelings. As an exercise, you might try to follow the 'how-it-works' pathway and see how such a casual and unconscious gesture from deep within another person's very different experience can take you on such a great journey of meaning.

Try and try with effort and you will never quite see the Way.... But *Trust the Meaning* you have found... and you are already there!

To look for a straight-line (linear) path-way for any feeling is to focus on the material world of cause-and-effect. But which is more important here, the path-way of the associations... or the true revelation of the love-feeling within/between you and that distant friend?

It is an easy choice to make: the path-way of the physical sensations which led you to this moment of experience is all-ways meaning-less in itself. But the *Revelation of Meaning* always brings feeling and wonder and new awakening. So which has more medicine power? And which is more real?

Like an electronic circuit, sign is meaning-less until the *emotional energy* of Meaning flows through it and awakens its magical functions. But for every electrical circuit board, its function is built in to its design. This means that just by looking at it (if we can read such things), we can already *know* what it will do when energy passes through it. And this is where the metaphor ends: for when you open to *sign* and *meaning* and *vision*... and once the energy begins to flow... you can *never* know what will come!

And whatever comes - at any instant in your real-time experience - there is only one (more) thing which you can know with certainty about the process of your own self-revelation. And it is this: whatever you are experiencing right *now*... will soon change, continually, completely and inexorably. For throughout all life and all awareness: *Change is the only constant.*

Since sign and meaning and time and awareness are ever-changing - and since nothing in the living universe has a fixed meaning - you cannot stop at any point in time-space-awareness-life and feel that you have understood 'everything.' In fact... you cannot 'stop' at all!

The evolution of consciousness is *'The Path of Eternal Becoming.'* It has no beginning... and it has no end. It is all *process*: flux, flow, progression, evolution. And so it can never be a stepping-stone, follow-the-leader, pre-established, straight-line course to any predictable end.

No indeed! Process is multi-dimensional and omni-versal (in all, through all, of *'the all'*). Process is everywhere, all of the time... and forever.

Wherever your vision takes you, wherever new awareness

ventures... sign will be there, meaning will be there. And the process *is* the adventure. And the process... well, it just flows... and flows... and flows.

Living in this eternal flow, living within a *Dance of Endless Change*, hearing 'different drummers'... and learning how to *'read sign'* as it passes through you... this is the process that the ancients described in such simple words, as: 'walking the medicine path.'

THE PROTECTION OF PURE INNOCENCE

We are all accustomed to shifting quite autonomically (spontaneously and without effort of will) through myriad *dimensions of experience* with everything we do - with every new feeling - with every breath - with every thought. This constant dimensional shifting is natural to our multi-dimensional consciousness. The mix of all of these interactive dimensions as they play through our consciousness - their constant re-blending and re-prioritizing - is experientially infinite... and is actually the experience of infinity. That is:

Our Living Experience is our Door-Way to Infinity.

And so it is, too, in the medicine realms of sign and vision. As you dance with Change through *experiential infinity*, you can open to every sign and open to the revelation of its meaning in openness and in trust, without any prejudice or fixed expectation....

You can walk tall, secure in knowing that each sign will point you to another... and that to another (etc.)... through the whole of your meditation... through the whole of your vision quest experience... and, in time, through the whole of your life... as you walk the medicine path.

To walk the medicine path, you do not need to know where you are going - indeed no one can know - or even where you have been. Your only certainty is to devote yourself to *'walking in a sacred manner'* and to attending the process that is your only guide as you move from sign to sign.

Wherever you are led... through every new dimension of experience, through every new meeting with every conscious being or entity... through the ever-changing flow of infinite feeling... through one lifetime... or through a thousand lifetimes... through all the change which will come your way... this one assurance can accompany you:

Wherever you will travel on your Medicine Journey...
If you go in Good Faith and with an Open Heart
You will always carry with you
The perfect Protection of your own pure Innocence.
For every experience is New... and...

'WE ARE ALL VIRGINS TO OUR EVERY NEXT EXPERIENCE'

FEAR IS THE SIGN OF MEANING

The endless Circle of the Medicine Wheel goes on and on and on: sign comes to you *for* your own enlightenment. Vision enlightens sign with meaning. In fact, no matter what it is, any phenomenon only becomes sign when it is empowered by personal meaning.

Beyond this... all sign that comes to you is a Gift of Spirit... a Gift of Grace. It is your guidance that gives you sign as you walk your medicine path. You bring it into your heart of awareness because you intuitively feel its medicine power. And within your Open Heart Center... its meaning can be revealed.

Empowerment is the attraction, even before the meaning is clear: the empowerment of Spirit. The empowerment of Guidance. The empowerment of Love. But too much power can be terrifying! And this is a very natural response: the greater the power, the greater will be your fear... until you learn to *surrender* fear and to *transmute* fear... in to the protection of *Pure Innocence.*

Wherever meaning flows deepest... to be sure, fear will be all around you. But fear, too, has some very worthy functions: fear sharpens your reflexes, heightens attentiveness and effectively washes away all the petty distractions which usually impinge upon your awareness from inside-outside your self.

Endless sign flows past for you to read the 'medicine story' of all that is meaning-full to you. The story of your life, your awareness... and your becoming. And the more important be the sign, the more powerful be its meaning... and so the stronger be your natural fear.

So as you approach your deepest experiences of meaning... do not let *primal fear* scare you away. For fear, too, is sign! Fear-Sign heralds the presence of great power... and so, awakens us to great Meaning.

The Herald of Fear sings out loud and clear:
'Where there is Fear... Meaning is near!'

Fear is all-ways sign... of great meaning. Breathe in your fear. Let your vision dis-cover its meaning. Feel it through... deeper... deeper... on every level of your being. Let it move your body, thrill your mind, sharpen your senses and enlighten your spirit. Let the natural wisdom of your body-mind flow inward-outward all around this *Sign of Fear*.

Dance through all the subtle path-ways that fear-full meaning may describe: breathe in your fear. Feel your fear. Meet your fear. Breathe *through* your fear. Dance with your fear. Clear your fear.

It will take lifetimes of diligent work to clear through it all. But that does not matter at all... for now, just here, just *be*-ing you, here-and-now...

'There is simply nothing else to do
But to Open to Fear and Feel it Through!

And as you move through fear and its surrender... and its release... and its transmutation... and its *celebration*... remember, also, this:

You need never fear *any* sign which comes to you! Others' signs cannot be seen by you... will not be felt by you... and so will not confuse or distract you in any way. Every sign that you experience is all-ways your-sign to feel and to know. Every sign that comes to you carries only *your* meaning... and has come as messenger to you alone, to escort your awareness to the meeting of your own self-revelation (your own self-revealment).

And fear will surely arise. Bide its meaning and learn to walk through its flaming gates. You can often find your way through fear if you can come to know (*from experience*) that every sign that you will meet is, somehow, *exactly appropriate* to your needs and your capacities at that moment.

That is to say (as so many have said before): *"Every lesson suits the learner?"* And it is all ways up to us to find out how....

Sometimes it is hard to see this when you feel overwhelmed and out of your depth. But remember... Sign is sign *because* it is meaning-full *to you.*

Your sign is your meaning. As such it is your destiny to move-dance-swim-crawl-surrender-explode through whatever and all revelations of meaning you encounter. It is an endless flow that may begin with the sign of a single leaf cast by a magical wind to a very strange place of landing. It may begin with the sound of a faraway voice changed by the elemental Air and the Wind. It may begin with the special drift of a feather floating downward to settle in your open hand... or a spark of Fire that dances your awareness in to a new dreamtime dimension... or the smile of a stranger who was always known... or the glint of an only crystal in a pile of stones... or the inspiration of a lightning bolt crashing *up* from the Earth at your feet... or the smell of a crushed blade of grass... (deep inside, you already know so well this medicine poem of infinite possibility).

Whatever it will be... you cannot escape that which is meaning-full to you. You can *resist* seeing or feeling sign. You can *resist* the revelation of any meaning. But you cannot escape your own, inevitable opening in to New Awareness.

For this path-way is the process of *'The Becoming.'* And this is the evolutionary destiny of every conscious being. However you come to know them, meaning and that which we so loosely call *'destiny'* are inextricably interwoven: sign is the key to the experience of vision which will reveal your ultimate 'becoming:' the wholly unique coalescence of meaning, change, awareness and life... that is to become to be *YOU.*

In the Realm of Consciousness,
Simply walking your Medicine Path,
By whatever name or ritual you would use
And falling Open in natural Wonder
At this endless Revelation of Becoming
IS your only need and your ultimate Destiny!

MAKING MEDICINE

To 'make medicine' all you have to do is to find a way in to your own *Free-Ritual Dance of Innocence...* and plunge into it in deep surrender. In whatever way you feel to, you can simply let your dance unfold. Again, the form and the content does not matter at all: trying to 'act out' a specific form or chant or ritual gesture, will only compromise your spontaneity and cloud your intuition. In free-ritual expression that takes you far beyond form and imitation, you can awaken and invoke all the powers and the protection of (the living archetypes of) Innocence, Openness, Surrender and Trust... just by *letting go...* and wholly believing... *whatever* comes through your Deep Surrender.

If you make a medicine prayer to your God, to the Great Spirit, to your Spirit Guides or 'all your ancestors'... you need ask *only* for help to be *clear* and *open* - for the clarity and openness to be a *living channel* - just as open as you can be at that moment (no more and no less), so that you may allow through your whole being whatever reflection-learning-service-healing-teaching can come to you this day.

Whenever you have accomplished this surrender, then *you* can evoke the Shamanic Powers of Intuition and Guidance -

Which all-ways awaken Revelation...
Which all-ways come as Sign...
Which all-ways evoke new Meaning...
Which all-ways illuminate and full-fill your Inner Vision.

To Make Medicine -
You need only sit in Stillness
Or stand or dance or crawl or leap
In this Medicine Way
To evoke the experience of Medicine
To evoke the experience of Guidance
To evoke New Awareness of the Living Mother Earth
To evoke the direct experience of Spirit
Of Spirit-knowing and knowing Spirit
In everything that you do.

And then you clear your Self to receive a Sign -
Through Openness - through Total Surrender -
Through Breathing Out - through Letting Go -
Through No-Mind emptiness beyond all Intention
By just being as Open as you can be
No more and no less:
Just as Open as you can be... Now.

And then you simply wait...
Breathing - Feeling - Sensing - Imagining -
Dreaming - Channeling - Intuiting - Playing
Until Sign comes
Until Meaning comes
Until Vision comes
Until you are filled with Vision
And Medicine be yours
And Medicine BE You
And then you will be ONE
And then You Are One With The Medicine Way.

There are other ways to find your Medicine -
As many Ways as there are Teachers-of-Ways.
But whatever Path you follow,
When Medicine comes to you
It will *only* come in this way:

Only through your own Innocence
Only through your own Open-ness
Only through your own Vision
Only through your own Revelation

And if only Open-ness and Surrender can awaken Revelation
Of all Medicine Sign and Meaning and Vision...
Then what else is there to do...

but Wait... and Dance... and Sing... and Play...
with Spirit...?

A MEDICINE JOURNEY: WALKING AND LISTENING

Today Father Sun sent a hot north-west wind surging through our valley, chattering the wide-leaf banana plants, trembling the wild rainforest and arousing a swirling, up-rushing *potpourri* of old leaf, husk, pod, twig, and feather. And as the great wind swept and tidied the forest, every living thing was inspired with the new-seed promise of Spring.

Today Father Sun was alive and dancing with the wind-spirits across the soft belly of the Mother River Valley. And today Ami and I set out to follow the wind together.

Today we walked along our dusty road casually in a free-talking way - not exactly a formal medicine walk, but not wanting to ignore any sign either, as we eagerly shared all of our little bits of unfinished business in preparation for separate travel in very different directions.

But even in a casual walk there are always new things to find... and new lessons to be learned. And today our Learning was about *Walking* and *Listening*... and *Knowing*.

Walking, talking, laughing, skipping, moving aside for the occasional vehicle, sometimes singing... totally lost and found in the daze of springtime. We skipped along in playful, light-hearted silliness as we children always do and our spring-dance traced a *Deep-Bonding Ritual* around our hearts... bringing us ever closer to the Mother Earth, to the deep medicine of this special valley... and to each other.

As we walked, talked, laughed, shared... I listened all around us. In between our words and laughter, I always 'listen out' - as far as my hearing will reach. From a childhood filled with a constant and insatiable passion to meet new animal spirits as I wandered alone in the then-empty hills of California and later, too, in the woods and swamplands of America's east, I was used to expanding my listening as I walked. And now (all these decades later) I so well understand that this kind of *'Deep Listening'* is a natural part of living as the Ancient Ones have always done... and an essential tool as we walk the medicine path.

Listening... listening... listening... no matter what else is happening. Hearing can be 'set' with an act of will and/or with an act of surrender, so that it is all-ways 'turned on' - always active and all-ways re-active to *whatever* is within the reach of the soft air-borne waves of energy which we know as sound.

Hearing is the only one of our primary senses which we cannot (easily) shut-off. Hearing is apparently meant to be continual. But, alas, so often we live in such total sound-chaos that we must allocate huge amounts of body-mind energy to shut out the unwanted barrage of noise. It takes an enormous amount of psycho-physical energy to manage our sound channels in the face of so much overblown noisiness. And once we succeed in getting things under some sort of self-control, then we become so conditioned to habitual sound-suppression that when we finally come to walk in peace in our most sacred places... well, then we are no longer even *able* to hear all the soft-sound which swirls and pulses around us... everywhere.

Listening in a receptive (*yin*-feminine) mode as we walk across the great body of the Living Earth is an energy-free process. It takes no energy from us because we do not have to send out (or project) energy to really hear all that is around us. We only have to *let in* whatever comes to us. And if there is no sound, there is no effort.

And then, when Sound comes, it brings its own energy to us. And then we have something new to feel-through, something new to discover, something new to be integrated into our whole-being awareness... or something which can be assessed and then totally released. And so, at last, we find we have a *choice* of how we use our sense of hearing... and how we use the *Power of Sound.*

Many of the most subtle and awakening messages of Nature come to us on the wind. And this mind-open kind of meditative listening is so often the only way to receive the news... the only way to hear the sound-wave medicine sign as it is offered out to us from under ancient rock, from the woven floor of seemingly empty grassland fields, from the rippled surface of the Mother River... and from the highest tree-top nests.

FEELING OUR WAVES OF EFFECT

As we walk through the world we move within an envelope of all the subtle energies that we are. We carry these multi-dimensional energies with us, everywhere we go: beating heart, swooshing breath, pulsing light and electric consciousness. And these energies broadcast outward in all directions around us, soaring into Father Sky and vibrating down through Mother Earth with each step, preceding and announcing us wherever we go. So the news of our arrival, often something of our intentions - and the feeling in our hearts - is common lore to every sentient being in every bush and on every blade of grass... everywhere around us.

To *'Walk in a Sacred Manner'* is to take full response-ability for all that we send out in this way. To 'own' the whole of what we project... and all that we feel... all that we do... and all that we *are* as we move through the Earth's living body.

As well as all the sounds of our living body-consciousness, every step we take sends out shock-waves through the earth and air and waters - energy-waves which inform and alarm millions of organisms that we never see.

Each step we take throughout the whole of our lives inevitably alters forever the subtle ecology underfoot: indeed, Life and Death attend our every move.

Every out-breath sends out a complete holographic image of our metabolic reality-of-the-moment.

Every movement that we make is at once the perfect *expression* and the complete *reflection* of the *'all and everything'* of us: our physical being, our emotional balance/imbalance, our whole-being experience, our state of consciousness... and our Spirit Heart.

'Who walks in Nature without care sees and hears nothing.
Who walks in reverence and in constant awe and wonder
Will be shown all the secrets of the Living Mother Earth
And all the mysteries of Life can be revealed.'

Animal beings of all sizes and all levels of awareness, see and hear and smell and feel and electro-image and thermal-image an endless stream of informational data-bits - our self-generated self-announcements to the living world-at-large - and continually process whatever frequencies of this broad-spectrum input their particular sensitivities will allow. Each life-form uses slightly different 'mixes' of these many channels (I would call them 'dimensions') of information input to know us as we move... and to 'choose' their re-actions to our presence accordingly.

By pre-programing ourselves for Deep Listening in purely receptive openness as we walk, we can learn to feed back our own out-bound signals as they are processed-through by other life-forms, thus creating a sort of bio-active sonar which is active across a very subtle and complex spectrum of energies... and which is active through the entire psychophysical totality of all of the energies (phenomena) which comprise our living selves.

Now these high-tech concepts are not essential to understanding the process we are exploring here... but this fundamental reality is:

No matter what we are doing and whether we notice it or not... every individual is continually projecting a highly complex energy-signal which we might come to know as our own, highly individualized *'waves of effect.'*

And perhaps the best (or only) way to become aware of these

expanded dimensions of self (and awareness) is to open up to feel our effect upon the world beyond. For however we might imagine ourselves to be... until we tune into the subtle energy returns (like sonar bounce-back signals) which come as free reflection from every sentient being around us, we simply cannot know how we are affecting the world-at-large.

Until we open to *deep sensing* on a whole-being level - feeling, seeing and listening well beyond the far horizons of our usual sensitivities - we will never know *who* or *what* we are in the living fabric of Nature... of the Earth... and of the cosmos-at-large.

It is a very subtle dialogue: our individual experience is the very hub-center of a wheel with nearly infinite spokes. How many of these separate dialogues-with-life can *you* allow to be active and alive within your awareness...? How much of your pure *effect* upon the living universe can you possibly bear to feel...?

To carry the analogy a little further... the outer rim of any Medicine Wheel that we might draw or envision is only a symbolic meeting place for the spokes of the wheel... which move outward-inward to sacred space - to Infinity - in *both* directions. When we begin to explore those dimensions of life which exist far beyond our usual planes of awareness, we often find ourselves at a spiritual doorway that opens into a *New Medicine Wheel*: a place where all living energies and consciousness meet in a Great Circle of Communion.

Aha! And perhaps you (and perhaps we, too) imagined that we were just strolling down a dusty country road in the warm daze of spring!

Well, once we start walking on *this* road - the path of medicine - it is likely to last forever! Ah well... Infinity is like that.

But today we want to expand our awareness just a little. Today we want to explore the animals' experience as they listen and dance with our sound-wave.

What are they feeling from us...? And what might they tell us, in return, of their secret worlds? And what might this reveal to us of Spirit and the inner soul of the Mother Earth Herself?

When we walk with medicine... when we learn to walk with the open-ears of the humble rabbit and the intense, un-processed, vibrational sensitivity of the common snail... then we can finally begin to hear the bounce-back re-actions to our own self-centered energy broadcasts... in very different and exciting ways!

Hidden away in their mini-worlds of stick or leaf or soil are many beings... most of them at first invisible to our eye-sight. By setting our hearing on its 'auto-receptive' mode of meditative openness (with a simple decision), then even as we talk, even as we laugh and even as we wave and call out greetings to passing friends, we can also be aware of all that is conscious (aware and feeling)... all around us.

As soon as we hear some hidden animal-being rustle a leaf or crackle a twig as it moves in response to our own out-ranging vibrations, we are immediately plunged into a bond of direct two-way communication with that little being.

Animals always know this. Humans seem to have to be reminded... that they already know this: all relationships with Nature are two-way energy flows. They hear us... we hear them... and *then* we can begin to dance together. And so we become 'as one being' for at least this one magical moment, bonded and conjoined in a Ritual Dance that will be wholly new to each of us....

The animals already know this. By the time they have made their first rustle in response to us... they already know us. From then on, it is entirely up to us to learn how to know them.

RITUAL MEETINGS: IN SEARCH OF UNKNOWN PRAY

As we've said... different beings detect us in different ways. And also, each being detects us at different times and at different distances from us as we move across the earth. So when we happen to hear a rustle somewhere nearby, how loud it is, how close it is, etc., will often tell us exactly what is near... *if* we know the code.

For example, birds meet us largely on visual cues. If you listen to their calls and the rustles they make as they take flight or hop around in the bushes near you, you can tell how far around you your own energies are projecting... to Bird. If you can feel where and when they begin to talk about you, to you, *with* you, you will be coming aware of your own *wave-of-effect*.

Once you can recognize that they are actually responding to *your* projected energy-presence (and not just randomly hopping around in the trees), then you might also begin to be able to feel them responding personally to you. [No, not 'personal' like saying "Hi there, Folks! We're out having a nice day today, how about you?"

Not that kind of personal. But personally *meaning-full* nevertheless.] And once this new opening occurs, then you enter into a new relationship to the archetype (and spirit) of Bird - and they are no longer just mindless beings flying about all willy-nilly and not just little sparks of 'bird-ness' which are momentarily lighting up your life as chance rustles in the bush or far-off calls from a high tree somewhere beyond your Vision.

No indeed: once you can *feel* your own *'wave of effect'* then it need never be like this again! Wherever you may go, Bird already knows you. Now it is up to you to hear and feel and come to know Bird through what Bird feeds back to you.

Yes, Bird meets you... meeting bird. But there is more: for once you understand this flow of energy-information-reaction, you can then *use* this pure bird-reflection loop to better understand *what* and *who* and *how* you are on this planet - just by feeling-through the medicine signs that come with every bird-dance that you share.

Next, you may also notice that the size of your 'circle-of-effect' is related to the size of the animals you are meeting. Medium sized, fast-moving animals, like wallabies, bandicoots, rabbits or martins often have a smaller radius-of-awareness than birds. They react to you when you are closer and you will often hear their tell-tale rustles from about fifteen to thirty yards away.

The slower moving, medium-large animals like wombats or raccoons may wait even longer before they begin their 'conversations' with you... while very small animals like fieldmice usually have a very small radius of awareness, sometimes as little as two to four yards away.

Of course it is not important to relate to these differences in awareness in number-terms as measurable distances. And anyway, the numbers will vary so widely from situation to situation as to be effectively meaningless. A robin on the ground may not see or feel you until you are thirty yards away... while an eagle in the sky may know all about you from a clear mile away.

What is important here, is the *relative difference* in the space that is inhabited by the awareness of different life-forms: if you know something about the animal life which may be around you as you walk, then you may be able to read the many little rustle sounds which your own energy field (or *aura*) evokes from animals all around you. And *this* is what I'd like to invite you to learn to feel.

So, let's look at a few more:

You can often tell the sound of a nearby animal which is at the top of its food chain by its sound: because they are not afraid to make noise! Big animals like bears who have little to fear in their natural habitat will often feel you while you are quite far away and let you know they are there, too - if they feel like it!

Snakes in the grass make a steady sound. Most of them will sense your presence by the vibrations of your footsteps and will move away. Well, most snakes, at least. In Australia there is a very poisonous, short snake with a very heavy and thick body who is an exception to this rule: the death adder (or 'deaf adder,' as it was originally called) will just lie there... in the grass... until you pass. And if you happen to step on it... it can jump as high as its length in a millisecond or so and... oops! *'Game Over!'*

The huge monitor lizards (like the local, Australian goannas) can be known by their nonchalant breaking of large sticks as they walk slowly through the thick undergrowth. They are very free to make noise because *nothing* in their environment will (or could) attack a five foot long lizard with the claws of a small leopard, the whipping tail of a crocodile and the well-toothed vise-like bite of a large python.

Small, grass-eating wallabies make a loud thumping sound on the Earth with their hind legs which can be scary at night... often about twenty to fifty yards away from you. Some say it is the sound they use to call their babies (their 'joeys') back to the mother's pouch. Anyway, a hefty thump in the dark can have many possible 'meanings' - I'm sure you get the idea.

The Great Whales have a *Circle of Awareness* which spans the entire Earth! They sing and communicate over tens of thousands of miles. What do they know of you... today... here and now...? And would you like to know...?

Today we walked along the dusty road, chattering and listening. We communicated heart to heart with each other... with nesting birds, with a frog or two... and, no doubt, with myriad unseen life-forms. It was a good afternoon's walk, to be sure!

A VISIT TO THE RIVER GANGES AFTER THE HOLY MELA

As the mighty, elemental Wind-Spirit slowed into quiet-mode, we stopped by the river for a rest... and just to feel its gentle flow through our lives... through our breath... and through our awareness.

Just beside us, the skin of the river looked troubled. It was scattered with bits of floating matter which was swirled into clumps along the edge of the shore beside us. I had never seen the river look 'dirty' and immediately went into mind-spin, wondering if it was too low and too slow for this time of year and so susceptible to overgrowths of algae and unable to flush itself of accumulated wash-down matter from farms, homesteads or from its own banks which were still flood-strewn in places with grass and sticks and debris from the deluge of rains of the winter just passed.

My attention was called away from this eco-musing when Ami found a dragonfly half-submerged and clinging to a leaf in the midst of a dense mat of this floating debris. We thought at first that it was a new adult being, crawling out of its larval shell. So we watched and waited, to see if we'd be able to witness its emergence and even, perhaps, its first-flight.

And then, as we watched this little drama with our faces looking downward, I heard that very distinctive crackling sound from about fifty yards away across the river.

It was a large goanna (lace monitor) lizard of four or five feet in length. And it was walking out of the forest and down toward the river with its usual care-less and noisy confidence. Ami and I were right out in the open, all visually ablaze with brightly colored clothing... and soon it saw us. But being so innately secure in its medicine power... it didn't really care. And as we watched in fascination, it stopped near a large fallen tree, looked at us from several positions by bending its long neck this way and that... and then settled down on a patch of warm, yellow sandy soil, for its afternoon nap.

I marked its presence in my consciousness. That is: I let it *in*. I acknowledged its being. I welcomed our meeting. And so I made a conscious bond - a mutual link-up with that huge reptile - so that it would know as much as it could of my peaceful intentions... and so that I would *know* intuitively if it moved from its resting place.

I showed Ami how to do it, too. And I showed her how we had just greatly extended our field-of-awareness through our link with the great goanna: now we had a *line of effect* which stretched all the way from where we were sitting to across the river and up the bank to the goanna... and even beyond the lizard in all directions, as far as *her* field-of-effect would reach. For now, any other animal-beings who encountered this goanna as she lay on the riverbank... would also be contacting her awareness of us! Because whatever she did - wherever she looked, however she might move, however she might respond to anything in any way - would all be done in *active relationship* to us for as long as we remained in this sense-link of mutual awareness of each other.

Now I know that Goanna was not lying there 'thinking' of us, of course. She was just having a nap. But still she was inexorably *connected* to us. And for as long as this deep bonding might last, she simply could not act in any way as though we just were not there. Simple as that. As long as we were within her awareness on any/every level she may inhabit... we were truly *one* with that great reptile. And this was great medicine, indeed!

This magical link well established and firmly in place... Ami and I could then turn our full attention once again to the life-to-life drama of the dragonfly which was re-birthing at our feet. My eyes scanned the busy surface of the waters, looking for that special dragonfly leaf. I had to effort to switch my tired, old-man vision from the long-range goanna contact to the microcosmic world of the dragonfly. The river-skin was such a mess of litter that I couldn't see it at first, and so I asked Ami to help me find it.

"I think it's just there... where all those flowers are floating in a little whirlpool around that big shiny red and green leaf." I looked where she was pointing... and was absolutely amazed: the river was not covered by accumulations of 'dirty' plant debris at all. How did I ever see it that way?

No, the slow-moving surface of the Mother-River where we stood was covered with a beautiful carpet of colored leaves, pine needles and myriad tiny lantana flowers... all blown from the forests and fields along her banks by the great spirit-wind which had first invited us to come out for a walk on this lovely first-spring day!

By now the wind had subsided and what was left on the surface of the river, shining in the bold afternoon sun was a mosaic of incredible delicacy and dazzling color. And as the waters moved, the mosaic moved also, rounding slowly, forming mandalas and streamings of many colors and ever-changing shapes.

But there was still more to this vision, because this mosaic existed in three dimensions: some of the heavier pieces of the picture (such as the half-floating pine needles) were actually suspended beneath the surface of the water - moving beneath flowing water, like smoke in the air moving in its freely three-dimensional world.

Looking downward into any water we usually see the swirls and eddies as two-dimensional movements... across the water's surface. And so the water-movements are visual-eyes'd as one, unified experience of flow.

On this most magical of days, however, the river waters had come alive with solid shapes and colors and objects, each finding its own special relationship to the surface, the depths, the current... and to each other, as they moved and dived and clung and slipped and writhed around each other.

And so the secret inner workings of the Living Water's dynamic flow were revealed by all these fairies, sprites and elementals as they danced in formal concert and infinite variety before our very eyes.

Just today, the elemental Water had come alive with beautiful miniature flowers, leaves and similar-sized bits and pieces of every kind of organic material which could be blown out of the forests and the fields by that strong mid-day wind: a beautiful air-born *potpourri* of seeds and seed-pods; small sticks, bits of tree bark and grasses; feathers and feathery floating seeds; small, whole flowers floating face-up and the single petals of larger flowers... all strewn across the Mother Waters like the aftermath of a grand, Indian *Mela* (Holy Celebration) on the banks of the *other* Ganges River.

In loving reverence - or so it felt - the river's flow had gathered and pocketed this rain of *puja* (offering) flowers into small groups of swirling colors along its leeward shore. Trailing veils of dancing *devas* (elemental plant spirits) moved and whirl-pooled and lightly rolled around in the gentle breath of the crystal clear shallows of this all-ways magical Mother-River.

And it was so beautiful... so tender... so subtle... and so fresh... that I would have missed it entirely if Ami had not told me what to see... and *how* to really *see* it with *Deep Vision* and with an open heart! Perhaps the whole event (as is so often true) needed that soft perception of young-girl wonder for it to be opened and revealed in my experience.

And the dragonfly nymph which was re-birthing before our very eyes into its new, majestic form on its own special red-green leaf...? "What about the Magic of the Dragonfly?" you might well ask.

Well, I'll tell you: Dragonfly was not emerging from its predatory larval form to soar on the Winds of Spring and make love and sex and more dragonfly nymphs. No, Dragonfly was already a mature adult... and with luck had already fathered/mothered hundreds of beautiful, new dragonflies. But as we came upon its wide-eyed face staring all around itself from a floating leaf, this dragonfly was dying.

Not that metamorphic re-birth and death are actually all that different for an insect... or for us, for that matter. But dying it certainly was. It had been a casualty of the Great Winds, and was also afloat on the river-carpet of *puja* flowers, moving through its last few breaths of life.

As we bent down in eager approach, it stopped dying for awhile. It dragged itself out of the primordial waters (once again)... just to catch our eyes and to say, "Hey there! Look at this! Check it out! Isn't this all incredibly beautiful today...?"

And then it slipped back in to the waters from whence it came... that its very body could be eaten by its own children, the dragonfly nymphs of the next generation... and it was simply and ever so gently... ever so magically... Dead.

In-focus on the peace-full dragonfly... sliding visual-eyes outward to the whole scenario of our own Spring-Dance *Maha Kumba Mela*...*

I just *had* to tell her this important message that only an elder could bring to her now:

"This, Ami... just this... just being here like this... together... is one of those experiences that you will probably never forget... one of the best kinds of experiences that Life can bring to us.

"You know... somewhere inside, *every* human being dreams of moments just like this: sitting with a beloved little daughter... or a beloved daddy... by a sparkling crystal-clear river on a warm spring afternoon, watching flower petals dance in the Sun-light on the Water... just like this.

"And all of those folks who stay in the cities everywhere... all of them would love to be able to do what we are doing now. It is such a little thing - so easy to overlook that I couldn't even see it all until

* The *'Maha Kumba Mela'* is a spiritual gathering of millions of people in India which takes place every twelve years. It is the largest spiritual gathering anywhere on the Earth!

you showed me. But sharing this Flower-Deva Dance with you is one of the most beautiful things I could ever imagine...."

"Me, too, Daddy... I feel so... peaceful... just being here...."

I smiled inside at my great fortune in life... to be here just at this moment, with this little, barely pubertal, child-blossom-of-my-heart... watching this Mela-Dance of Spring slide past us in the quiet waters.

But also I smiled from knowing what she cannot yet know: that someday when she is grandmother-wise and has 'walked in a sacred manner' through many decades to come... and through a world in which profound and one-way change is absolutely inevitable... she will have living in her Inner Heart, a memory of this day... of this path and this life-way... and of our time together... lazing and learning through long afternoons of pure and simple, Holy Medicine Magic!

And if only this can I give my children as seed-nurturance and centering for their adult life to come... and if there be only this time and this love and this moment to share with them... then I and they will have succeeded beyond all measure... and we will have full-filled my highest dreams and my most humble prayers for my time of fatherhood.

And so I smiled to myself... hugged my daughter to my heart... and we raised our eyes together to look far across the sparkling Magic River Waters... and rose to our next adventure: a meeting with the Great Goanna!

THE DREAMTIME SONG OF THE GREAT GOANNA

Across the ageless Waters... across the endless seas of Time... there was, still, a giant goanna sunning and napping on a warm-brown sandy place beside a bubbling river... no doubt dreaming in a lizard dreamtime never dreamed before by its kind... as it shared so intimately with Ami and I... and the dying dragonfly lying on a carpet of *mela* flowers on that special *'Day of the Great Wind.'*

We arose in silence... to offer human-meeting to this great and ancient totem being of this continent... one of the greatest of all living reptiles.

"Ahhh...! Look! It's *huge*!" said Ami, with obvious awe... and, of course, a little fear as well, as we seemed inevitably drawn to some sort of active encounter with the great beast.

And, after all, this five-foot long dinosaur was longer than Ami's ten-year-old body... and had a mouth as wide as Daddy's still-huge hand... and a body as big around as her own thigh. Such a thing must seem very formidable to a child, indeed! And even to a big-strong-daddy as well...? Absolutely! Deeply formidable, for sure!

Here is a little natural history: Goanna does not attack human beings. (Hey! It doesn't have to... any sensible person would run away!)

The Koori people of Australia - well, the still-tribal ones, at least - *eat* goannas: they rip them apart, raw, with their teeth, in fact, to extract the useful tendons and other essential recyclables. But after two hundred years of white settlement here - and twenty-some years of decided hippie-greenie influence - I suppose Goanna knows that *white* medicine persons (at least) don't eat goanna... and pose no real threat. Well, anyway, whatever its perceptions... Goanna just doesn't attack people. But there is this one troubling behavior....

What happens, and something which is every bit as bad as an outright mouth-attack in the end, is that when Goanna gets scared... Goanna simply bolts - a great headlong, care-less dash for safety. And Goanna is *very* fast!

But Goanna has a three-chambered heart that does not let it run fast for more than a hundred yards or so. So Goanna has another way of dealing with all-out fear: it simply stops 'thinking' and reverts to its very ancient natural programing (just like we do). And Goanna's fear-relief programing says it all in three simple lines of code:
"(1) Run up to the top of the tallest standing thing you can find!
(2) Do it as fast as you can! (3) And do it NOW!"

Probably just some simple coding error hiding in the very primitive programing of its operating system ROM ('repto-brain / ver1.o rev.A.' I believe it is) neglected to specify, *"...tree or rock!" "Be sure that you run up a* tree *or a* rock*!"*

And so the silly ol' thing can easily tend to run right up your leg... with a streaming flail of horrific, inch-long claws as it goes, each driven home by the awesome force of blind, reptilian terror.

So... it runs right up your leg, up over your (supposedly) private parts... and then carries on, charging right up your belly-back-torso and arms, all the while with feet, claws and massive tail flailing around all over the place... until it gets to your head... where it tends to either hang onto an assortment of face-eyes-lips-arms-neck-jugular veins-ears with its wild, frantic claws... or else it might bite hold of the top of your head (I have seen someone with actual scars!) where it then holds on for dear life.

Uhhh... for Goanna's life, that is... *not* for yours! Nothing personal, of course: at that very moment, repto-mind (any version, any revision) doesn't even know (or care) that 'you' even exist!

Now if you are at all like normal folks, this is not a behavior that you want to encourage... or incite. So when you approach Goanna... you have to be very ready to 'bite the dust'... as fast as you can and as flat on the dirt as you can get... and hope to be able to withstand the gross tissue destruction (your own) which can occur from being merely *run over* by a windmill of ripping claws... as Goanna desperately seeks to get past you... to find something *else* to climb which will not just fall down whimpering, blubbering and covering its head with its paws as you have probably already done.

Of course, far and away the best approach to Goanna is to be careful not to cross over its invisible 'threat-line' and so avoid triggering its terrible fear in the first place! But then... if you do it that way, you don't really get to *meet* Goanna body-to-body, or shake a claw together, feel its medicine power... or come to know the ancient magic of goanna through any direct, *Free-Ritual Initiation.*

So... if you want a face-to-face with a giant reptile, you summon all of your 'medicine cool' and try to project clear messages of greeting well ahead of you with every breath and on *every* available data-channel:

"Hail to thee, O Great Goanna! We come as friends... *please* believe me...! Uhh... pretty please...?"

REAL-TIME MEETING ACROSS EONS OF TIME

Ami and I slowly moved along the bank of the river - our side of the river, that is - and began to feel our way into the best position in relation to Goanna, the best place to try to wade cross the river while sending out the least alarming *wave-of-effect* to the great beast as it lounge-lizarded away the afternoon in the hot, damp sand.

Near the dozing giant there grew a few small, reedy sticks - perhaps only as large as my thumb - and a few tufts of grass below them. I will explain this surround for a reason: when you are intent upon minimizing your *Circle of Effect*, it is important to de-activate as many sensory channels as you can. Sight is the primary mode of contact-defense for Goanna... so we tried to diffuse this keen sense as we moved, by keeping our heads and eyes behind the stick-and-grass shields as much as possible. Just our eyes. And hiding our eyes, as it turned out, was concealment enough.

Now I am not a small-ly embodied being. And to imagine that I could hide behind a few sparse twigs and a few blades of grass is ridiculous, I know. These puny sticks would have to have been poking the lizard's eyes if they were to render me truly invisible! But there is a lurk, here, a special piece of medicine lore to be gleaned. And it goes like this:

The sense of eye-sight, for most animals, is largely a *relative* sense. It shows the movement of one object in relation to its surrounds. If an animal's sight-sense is binocular, it can also see whether something is moving toward or away from its position. Animal sight may also show something of color and size and other things, too... just like ours... only often much better.

But whatever species you might be, true visual contact - i.e., real visual *communication* - between any two sentient beings is always eye-to-eye. And that is the medicine trick-of-the-stick for today!

Without ever seeing our actual eyes, Goanna could only see a couple of enormous, shapeless, shifting blobs of pinky skin as we clambered, exposed and unsteady, across the rock-lined river.

It was fairly shallow here, but none of the main-streams of life are ever as shallow as they might seem from any shore, of course. All we could do is to remark upon this illusion and note it for future reference as we slipped about on the sharp rocks, laughing and falling and making pointless "Shooshh!" sounds to each other as we went... and always in between these outbursts, standing as tall as we could and swaying with the reeds with, undoubtedly, great medicine dignity.

I was surprised that we were able to reach the opposite shore without frightening Goanna away... sending her clawing frantically up the nearest tree/person/cow/etc. But Goanna stayed. Raised a great, long neck, flicked a half-inch wide purple-pink forked tongue-sensor our way from time to time... and just stayed where she was.

Now we were firmly on the solid river bank. About thirty feet from the beautiful monitor. She was just beginning to shed her dull and worn winterskin. And where the new skin shone through we could see delicate and intricate patterns on her black skin which looked like milk-white and golden bead-work tracings of star patterns in a clear, blue-black night sky.

But even as we watched in wonder at her beauty... an unsettling realization began to nibble away at our pure enjoyment of the moment: for now we were so close that all of a sudden *we* had become the highest 'trees' in Goanna's field of vision. And so it was time to take care!

I move ahead one step at a time. I move and Goanna hisses - a great steamy, slurppy, syrupy voiding of her constricted breath - raises her head, and cocks it to one side for an oblique angle view.

She looks as though she is thinking things over... but she don't fool me! Whenever she moves, I freeze for a moment and then very slowly re-position my head so that my eyes are once again hidden behind my two-twig veil of illusion. And, in time, Goanna goes back to her head-down, "Oh well... whatever...." lazy, resting position.

I wait. I take another step... she moves again, so I don't.... Then soon, she don't... so then I do.... Then she does, so then I don't... (etc.). And thus we slow-danced through this long-time ritual of non-meeting.

I was committed to success, however long it might take. Today it took a long hour. (Measured in gross, unfeeling, clock-time it might have been only about half that long).

I am very intent upon showing my children how to do this. I want to show them how it all falls into place when you don't rush meetings with wild things: when you respect their power and their space.

When I was a little one, I used to feel that *any* animal sighting was phenomenal: a bizarre accident of Nature... some sort of momentary mistake in the cosmos which opened a hole in the usually well-concealed Wild World Show for me... the unexpected opening of a window in the space-time continuum which had to be utilized *immediately*... or all would be lost.

So my usual *'Meeting Animal Medicine Ritual'* was either to freeze completely and just stare at them... or to charge headlong into these deep meetings with these most beloved animal-spirits-of-my-wildest-dreams in absolutely blind faith. In fact, a ten year old boy charging at the frog-of-all-dreams might be the original meaning of the notion of 'blind faith.' My passionate zeal to make contact - to actually touch them before they vanished - always immediately outweighed whatever I had read about how to get close to wild things by slowly and patiently stalking them and/or 'winning their trust.' Anyway... what *is* 'slow and careful' when you are ten (or fifty) and filled with the lust of Primal Desire?

For as long as I have been aware of anything, I have always been on the medicine path. And to me, then, (and now?) Snake *was* God and a doe *was* The Goddess and whenever divinity so appeared in the flesh... one simply *had* to get absolutely as close as one could... and in any way possible. Non-venomous or poisonous, scary or desperately scared... whatever and all of it: *I was immediately obliged and committed to act.*

A fleeting glimpse of a running-away deer-rump was a great, thumping sign of good fortune. And if the deer *actually looked at me* before turning to run, it was an even greater privilege... and always a power-full omen. If a snake paused to contract or move in direct relation to me before it slipped away from me, deep into the rocks, I was truly blessed. Finding two rare turtles locked in a mating embrace was a supreme Gift of Grace. So it was then... and *so it was!*

But subtle at age ten, I was not. No... the concept didn't even compute. Sure, I prided myself on being able to run on 'silent Indian feet' as best I could, as quiet as any excited kid could be as he crashed through the brush in pursuit of the ghost of a lizard's tail.

Sure, I'd hold my scrambling profile as low to the earth as I could, like a great tracker. In fact, I'd usually start out doing all the 'right' things. But in the end... I'd just lose it... and I'd bolt for it... and my meetings with Animal always came down to a mad-rush, down-on-all-fours, scrambling-race with Time... and a race with all of Animal's innate reflexes which were so many millions of years old... and a million times faster than those of even the very most desperately eager ten year old boy...!

Deep inside (and I never really shared this with anyone before) I used to feel that people who waited cowering in blinds to just look at birds or animals were people with no Medicine Heart: gutless and un-feeling wimps, un-caring, un-needy, un-loving and probably afraid as well!

I was, smugly, infinitely more passionate. I *needed* my Animal Time to be as wild and clawing and as ineffably soft and furry as it could possibly be. So I always preferred the more out-there approach of running right at whatever I most loved (and so most feared): snakes, frogs, turtles, butterflies, bunnies, raccoons, pheasants, ducks, porcupine, deer and even, on one bizarre occasion, the Great Bear itself.

It takes Great Warrior bravery (if not much shaman sense) to plunge into *'The Great Unknown'* in this way... but, alas, it does not often produce much result! The biography might read: "Boyhood daze spent in wild desire and pursuit... usually ending all alone and face down in the dust!"

Ah well, I am older now and slower, at least, if no wiser. And now I know that there is a different way. A gentler way. A more compassionate way. A Medicine Way: a way of blending into Nature to *be with* animal life more on its own terms. And this way really works!

And on this day... Goanna waited patiently there for me and we as the human delegation clambered inelegantly across the river and made our dodging way up the river bank. Goanna waited to meet me today. "Ahhh! Perhaps Goanna is getting older, too...?"

After our long approach this afternoon, there finally came a time when I was roughly within possible pounce-distance from the Great Mother Lizard. She was a little edgy, but she stayed put, and so did I. But now I had to wait longer between movements.

I wondered if she was staying close to some newly laid spring-time eggs (but later found by softly sifting my fingers through the sand there, that she was not). But being within 'pounce' distance did not mean that I felt all right to dive down on this beautiful and calm animal. What it did mean is that now I was empowered: now I could begin to *choose* something about what kind of meeting we might experience.

Up until this moment, my approach had been entirely dependent upon Goanna's whim: she could stay... or leave. There was always plenty of thick cover in the rainforest along the river escarpment. But she had stayed. And because of this, now I, too, held some power. And now I, too, was finally able to add some of my choices to this inter-species meeting-dance!

And I chose... just to wait. I chose not to prove myself by disrupting our tentative peace by pouncing down to 'catch' Goanna. I chose to try, even further, to win her whole-hearted trust. I chose to be better model for my ten-year old daughter than I ever was for myself at that age. I chose to find power in the rapport I felt with the great monitor... rather than the superficial power of mere physical skill - and its inevitable component of dominance.

By now I was so close that I was no longer able to hide my eyes behind the few sticks and grasses which lay between us. Now I could only hide one eye at a time. But I still used the twigs for cover: I kept feeling which of my eyes felt more aggressive* - which eye was tending to *look at* the goanna - and which seemed more content just to let her image come in... to receptively *see* her there before me.

And when I could feel any difference at all in the energy-emissions of my own eyes, I shielded the eager-aggressive eye by hiding it behind the sparse stickery which was between us... leaving only my 'softer,' (*yin*-receptive) *in*-lightened eye exposed.

Yes, it is getting very picky to be choosing eyes. But then... the further we move into the realm of medicine... the more subtle are the phenomena and energies that we must deal with. To move with respect for the natural polarity of the natural world is to embrace the principles of *Tantra* and the *Tao*. And the *Tao* is what moves it all along....

Consider this: Breath tends to flow in and out of only one nostril at a time... Mind tends to communicate *awareness* with only one hemisphere at a time... Sight tends to flow in-out of one or the other eye at a time. Polarity is in all things: the *Tao* is everywhere and all the time. If you can *feel* its dance... then you can use this *tantric awareness* to open the way before you... wherever you may go.**

And just as I was beginning to believe that Goanna was simply going to wait there in almost complete peace-fullness to feel my lover's touch... I happened to cross her spatial fear-line. Suddenly I was too close for her comfort. And she became unsettled and wary.

First she raised her great head to look at me and to tongue-flick the air around us. Then she cast her head sideways to check out Ami's position - laying low-down several yards behind me to watch and learn this medicine dance from a safer point of view. Then Goanna tried to give it all up and just sink into the sand once again.

---

* Wilhelm Reich has pointed out that the word, 'aggression,' comes from the Greek word *agresos*, which means "to reach out." And apparently, it has been only recently that we have come to associate the word aggressive with undesirable qualities such as anger or malice. In its original sense, aggression is the only word we have to denote this state of *positive*, power-full out-reach (while our language has many other words to denote outreaching actions of malice and hurtfulness)!

** For more in-depth exploration of Breath Magic, see: THE HEALING POWER OF BREATH - AN INTRODUCTION TO WHOLISTIC BREATH THERAPY - by the author, published in Europe by Prism Press (Dorset, U.K.) and available from Ajna Press. [See order form on page 400].

But something was still not right and try as she might, she just could not find her peace-state again.

Yep... Goanna was getting ever more restless and there was nothing I could do about it.

I watched her, helplessly, once again finding mys'elf in that familiar situation that I knew so well from my days as an over-eager ten-year-old. There was just nothing I could do!

She rose again, looked all around and then sank back, still trying not to see me as a threat. Then I could feel her deep inside, responding to the 'over-the-line closeness alarm' again. So she, too, seemed to have no choice! Human or reptile or computer: *programing is Programing*.

So, wearily, confusedly, she raised her head yet again, made a few short trial steps this way and then that way, settled down again, raised up again, etc. She was definitely readying herself to move off. And I knew that she was so well-warmed by the Sun and Earth that she could move off with great speed whenever she chose.

What could I possibly do to cut through this ancient ritual of habituated approach-avoidance? What could I do to become instantly trust-worthy?

How could I become so completely trust-worthy that she would even allow me to relate to her from inside her un-consciously pre-defined *Circle of Fear*? But try as I might - and try I did - I just could not *think* of anything.

Because Ami was there, I wanted to share this Ritual Meeting Process with her, however it came down... so that she could see-feel-breathe-through every nuance of this experience first-hand and as it occurred. And as I sensed that my time with Goanna was about to end... that Goanna was about to depart... I felt that I had little to lose by turning my head and speaking to Ami in a loud whisper. So I did.

Just to be safe, I told her to be ready for a great Goanna sprint directly at her and reminded Ami to keep low even if the lizard happened to run right across her body to get to the river. But I also assured her that I felt from the lizard's head gestures and the way she kept looking up at the trees on the hill behind her, that her movement would take her uphill and so away from both of us... and perhaps more deliberate (slow) than desperate (fast).

When I turned my head back toward the goanna, I was more than a little surprised that all of this activity had not spooked her into moving off... for she was just that close to leaving me. But she was really there! And so I decided to really try to show her my deeper heart. So I began to *sing* to her!

Open-syllable chanting: very soft. No hissing sounds! Just long 'Ahhh' sounds from my heart... with steady, even breaths. Goanna was calmed.

Was it my song...? Or was she (actually, merely, etc.) reacting to the calmness which came over me as I chanted to her...?

Which was it? Remember the Process: *it simply does not matter...* and... *you can never know for sure!*

She was - we were - being calmed by my gentle and loving chant. Reassured, re-centered, realigned in our closeness and recovered in our trust... and reaffirmed in our medicine dance... together.

My song continued... coming from somewhere far beyond my mind. And even as I chanted, mind laughed and wondered: "Let's see now, I know that snakes cannot hear... but they can feel vibrations very keenly. Maybe my sounding makes vibrations that can be heard... or air-borne waves of breath-taste which lizard-tongue can detect.... Or, perhaps lizards *can* hear even though snakes cannot...?" Mind chugged along with its usual chatter and I gave it free mouth. And all the while... *i-and-I* were somewhere else.

I began to trust this song more and more. The sound came louder and fuller. I felt an ancient beat begin. It was the same-and-always foot-step beat of the Old Ones shuffling in the sand. It is the rhythm of the beat of every heart. I laughed some more, inside, at being so silly... but I began to dance on the earth as I chanted. Very softly at first, then rising to a solid, in-place stamping step, matching the power of my *Goanna Heart Medicine-Song*.

I was so close to Goanna's head that she could probably feel the little puffs of dust which rose from my feet as I moved - and of course could feel the soft thud of my feet as they thumped in the sand.

I was so large as I towered over her that my swaying body was sending flashes of light and shadow across her visual-eyes as she lay in the late afternoon sun. And my song became so trusting and so full-voiced that even if Goanna could not hear me... every other being in the forest would... and Goanna would know all about me (inside and out) from their reactions alone.

As time rolled on... Goanna began to accept me. She raised her head less often when I moved out of rhythm to shoo the bothersome bush-fly or to steady myself on the sliding sandy hillside. And as I felt-intuited-channeled-imagined-dreamed (these are all the same: all one feeling) our trust-bond growing so strong and clear, I began to really celebrate this medicine:

I laughed aloud and called to Ami to come a bit closer. I thrust my head back and threw my chant upwards to Father Sun as it hovered, huge and golden-red just above the tree-lined rim of the Great Grandmother Mountain. I chanted special sounds to the Grandmother half-Moon which was floating like a white ghost in the Infinite Sky.

Thus I drew great medicine power from the Great Goanna and breathed and swirled it through every cell of my body-mind.

I had become as *one being* with this great and ancient reptile. And all of her power and all of her medicine and all of her magic and all of her spirit became mine... became me... became *us*. And for that instant I was truly *one* with all Nature in the Mother River Valley... just there... and just then.

Ami watched in silence, at first ignoring the goose-bumps and shivers which were chattering through her little body as she stood there in the chilling, sun-downing river, a little wet and almost naked - and so very exposed to the wind. She stood her space for awhile... but eventually she had to cry out for help and Daddy-care as that strangely eerie, damp evening chill moved upstream along the channel of the river... signaling the coming of the night... and urging all frail human beings to move homewards.

I began to wind-down my chanting celebration, to let go of this endless meditation... and to turn to nurture my Little One, my closest child-friend. And then, acting on a rash whim born of the reckless daring of that eternal ten-year-old's eagerness which seems to still attend all of my adult celebrations... I turned to Goanna and asked her if she'd like to come home with us... to meet the rest of the mini-shaman tribe!

And strange as it may seem... she said.... Well actually, of course, she said nothing at all! But I noted that she had not said "No!" So I just reached down very gently and took hold of her strong, sinewy tail.

Well, this was different than merely asking... so now she said, "Oh this. I know. You pull, I walk away. You pull some more and I either turn around and bite you or just pull away even harder. Anyway... I'm so strong that you can pull my tail all day and I'll just wait you out by hanging onto that log over there... until you get tired and go away...."

"No! Great Goanna...no! It needn't be this way this time. Come with me. That's all. I will not hurt you. You know that! You *know* me, Grandmother. You've heard my Heart Song. Come with me - I will carry you softly in my shirt."

And, believe it or... believe it (you might as well), with that she just *let go* of her claw-hold on the old fallen tree... and simply *allowed me* to pick her up. (It was 'allowed,' too, for remember, I have already told you how strong and fear-some she could have been in any other humor).

Yes... Goanna *allowed me* to pick her up, one hand softly holding her behind her head and one hand supporting her body at the base of her tail. I made a sling-support for her considerable weight out of my shirt. She held on to the button edge of the shirt with her lacerating, shirt-shredding, vice-grip teeth... and off we went to dazzle the family with our great medicine and to introduce them to a new and very awesome friend.

Once we were dried and dressed (sort of), Ami and I struggled up the hill to the dusty road that led to home, reeling under the weight of this huge reptile and singing to her all the while. We marveled at the fullness of our afternoon together... and what amazing medicine could happen just from going for a simple walk along a country road together... through our own, enchanted 'Hundred Acre Woods'... on what Winnie the Pooh would surely call, "a very blustery day."

COLLECTING THE GIFTS OF BELIEVING, FEELING & HEARING

As for the Grandmother Goanna... well, she was praised and admired and feared and loved by everyone. In a very short time she grew obviously tired of this new game of 'family' and made it abundantly clear that she wanted to return to her rainforest home. So we carried her once again, with great ceremony and child parade, to a clearing by the Ritual River.

I felt very trusting of her by this time - and hopefully she of me, too, to whatever extent reptilian mind has a 'trust' chipset installed.

When we set her softly on the ground and released her body to its own propulsion... she spent several minutes looking around, watched us all for awhile and then very slowly walked to the edge of a great eucalypt tree. Pausing there for another protracted moment, she then ran up the tree to a great height as effortlessly as she had walked on the earth. She spent the rest of the afternoon there, no doubt thinking about her strange meeting with a singing shaman and his laughing children on that fine spring day.

For the mini-shamans it was a great day of learning. Forever after, whenever they meet Goanna, they will approach her without fear, and with compassion, caring and great respect for her special medicine.

There is so much that we can fear in Nature. Whenever we can learn to meet even the biggest beasts in this gentle way... then we have succeeded in dissolving away yet another chunk of our armor and our fear... leaving us even more open to receive the great magic that the Earth so graciously unfolds - to all who will *Feel*... to all who will *Believe*... and to all who know how to *Listen!*

><><

CHAPTER 5

THE VISION QUEST

A VISION QUEST DEDICATION

"Tonight I am going back.
Tonight I am going Home...
Returning to my Inner Place...
To tap new wellspring Inspiration...
And to seek my Guidance there.

Tonight I have no Inner Knowing of Infinity.
Tonight all direction must come from without.

I can do nothing but prepare the soil,
Hope that the seeds are sown,
Carry water, bring nutrients and Love...
Clear away all obstructions of all kinds

And then there is naught to do but to wait...
To make Prayer... to make Sound...
To Dance with Breath
Through Fire and Water, Through Earth and Air
Through all the etheric realms

To simply hold in Stillness and endure....
That I may be Open to Receive

Whatever will come
Whatever is to be
Whatever will tonight full-fill."

THE VISION QUEST OF ALL TRIBES

The ritual of the Vision Quest is found in one form or another in almost every religious or spiritual tradition. Each tribe (or culture) finds its own language and mythology to describe and honor and evoke their own kind of vision quest experience. But despite all of these differences... the *process* is always essentially the same. And this sameness of process has evolved within so many separate cultures... simply because it really works!

In Buddhism the Quest takes the form of successive levels of understanding, leading to enlightenment' - and the process that is used includes many very specific forms of 'meditation' (stillness). As Buddhists progress in their understanding of the meditational process... meditation is taken out of the temple and into the experiences of everyday life. This is especially true in Zen Buddhism: *everything is the meditation.*

In the yogas of India, the vision quest process - the process of 'preparing for God' is called *'sadhana,'* and can include a vast range of fixed-ritual practices and many main streams or dimensions of spiritual pursuit. Those who follow the path of *bhakti yoga* base their practice upon pure devotion and (among other things) practice chanting 'Holy Name' - the 'infinite names of God.' *Pranayama yoga* is the yoga of Breath. *Hatha yoga* uses intricate postures, *mudras* and breathing with meditation, to open subtle energy channels which can connect the unified body-mind to the higher levels of spiritual being - to the *atman* (the 'overself') and hence to the Godhead. There are over a hundred other acknowledged kinds of traditional yoga - and all of them are path-ways to the one-and-same state of *one-ness*: oneness within the self and oneness with *'The All and Everything.'*

In our western cultural history of medieval Europe there were complex rituals of penitence, intoning, fasting and the keeping of 'vigils' in order to better commune with God. And psychotropic or psychedelic substances (which today are lumped into that catch-all negative concept of 'drugs') have been used through all ages and *every* culture in pursuit of heightened sensitivity and god-connection.

But the most familiar Vision Quest process in our culture today is that which has come to us from the Native American people: that special journey into a place of seclusion where the seeker prepares him/herself and then simply waits - for whatever revelation will come.

But however we proceed... the vision quest is not about the end result. No... the Vision Quest is about what we do... and how we are. It is about making ready to receive guidance and inspiration. It is all about *Process.*

So, wherever we look, and throughout all time... we find that the vision quest process is virtually the same for every tribe and every religion. It has nothing whatsoever to do with the specific religion or beliefs of those who seek the guidance and enlightenment of spiritual *Vision.* Only the trappings and the rituals change as we move from tribe to tribe, all around the planet.

The fixed ritual processes may differ... but by any name and whatever form, all the vision quests of all our tribes and cultures share a common purpose: every vision quest is simply the process of *'making ready.'* And this process seems all-ways to include these same elements of: *preparation, commitment, consecration...* and *deep surrender.*

In the end... there is only one state of being *'ready.'* And the vision quest (by any name, etc.) is the doorway that we pass through to enter that precious moment of special, rarefied *openness.*

Thus the vision quest involves the tilling of the emotional soil; the setting of the fire; the patience to be still; the trust to remain in openness to whatever is to come; and perhaps most important of all, the willingness to meet all of the inner fears and obstacles which will surely be summoned as the quest unwinds through (sometimes) several days... and nights.

In this sense, the vision quest is a formal *contract* between self and Spirit - at the highest and clearest level of self-awareness. The time of the vision quest is a special time - and so is vulnerable to every conceivable distraction (and many we could never, ever imagine). Therefore, most seekers of vision begin their quest by withdrawing from everyday life for awhile to make it easier to open to new discoveries.

Without our usual involvements (distractions), it is easier to feel ourselves and it is easier for other energies, beings and feelings (etc.) to find ways to slip past our usual expectations and ego-centered reality-views... to access our awareness and to illuminate new realms of possibility and direction for personal and spiritual growth.

But above all else... we retreat in to aloneness so that we can take full response-ability for dealing with *everything* that impedes our opening: the distractions and false promises of all of our mind-stuff, body-stuff and all else that we do to avoid inevitable meetings with *'The Great Unknown.'*

Every experience of medicine vision begins with a release of egoic posturing... with the humility of *Deep Surrender*: surrendering to open-ness... surrendering to new input... surrendering to new meaning... in such a way that new dimensions of awareness can be awakened within us... and new consciousness come through us.

And whatever else we might do, as *ritual accompaniment* to this primal process of Deep Surrender, the process comes alive only when we can open ourselves to 'let through' energies and spirit that we have never known before. In this state we truly become *channels* for energy, healing, consciousness, guidance... and Spirit. And as all of this passes through our awareness, we can be so suddenly and so profoundly changed that we feel refreshed, renewed... and sometimes even *rebirthed* in to wholly new dimensions of consciousness... and Spirit.

It does not always happen like this. We do not always arouse unknown entities or breakthrough into new dimensions of consciousness whenever we take ourselves away from our ordinary lives for awhile, wrap ourselves in our most special blanket and light a medicine fire with prayer and devotion in our hearts.... But it *does* happen. And, bottom line, there may be no faster-better-gentler method of awakening our re-union with our inner-outer selves, Nature and Spirit!

There are many ways of moving toward this 'altered state' of being, this privileged state of exceptional open-ness: we can do it through fasting, meditation, seclusion, chanting, walking, prayer, yoga, dancing, centering exercises, *tantric* sexuality, consciously clearing-through old feelings, etc.

The list is as long as the number of spiritual traditions and teachers that have ever been on the face of this planet... and then some! And it is so important to realize that *all of these different processes are effective*. They have all been through the test of time and experience of countless *yogis*. What is most important is to find the path that is right for you... and then stick to it until it flowers you into wholeness.

In the end (and as always), the particular path-way that we follow - how we walk, how we dress, what words we chant (etc.) - does not really matter at all. Because even though there are infinite path-ways that we might follow, somewhere they all merge together in to the common stream of our same-and-always desire for revelation, guidance, spiritual re-union... and profound, personal-spiritual wholeness.

But we are fickle folk and the grass always seems greener.... So we skip and hop from teacher to teacher, using our great cultural wealth and high technology to skip from lilypad to lotus all over the place. But try as we might to improve our odds by leaping from path to path as we meet new teachers and new inspiration, *every* master knows that all spiritual path-ways lead to exactly the same state of surrendered open-ness and the one-and-only state of union (one-ness) with all life, all consciousness and all Spirit. And that, simply put, is the very essence and the goal of *all* spiritual path.

Once we can see that the goals are the same... then we can be free to understand what every enlightened one knows beyond all doubt: that the particular path that we choose is never as unimportant as *how we walk* whatever path we have been given. And that is why Buddhist monks and Christian monks and Indian yogis and wild medicine people of all style and persuasion (and you yourself) *can* meet and share and learn from each other. For we are all on the same-and-only path. And we are *all* 'seeking Vision.'

We all seek, yes. But however we may choose to walk on our individual journeys in to Spirit, striving for that precious state of highly expanded sensitivity and openness that (alone) will *allow* Spirit to enter our awareness is like striving for deeper states of relaxation: this is something you cannot achieve by effort. Ultimately, you can only achieve it by *LETTING GO!*

And however (or whatever) you might try to do to help it along... Total Surrender and emotional-spiritual *openness* will come in its own good time. To invite its presence we can prepare ourselves. We consecrate (and re-consecrate) our space and time. We prepare to wait. We make *Vision Quest*... and in this process we *learn* to wait... just trying to be as open as we can... nothing more and nothing less. For *there is simply nothing else to do.*

And while we wait... all the esoteric forms of meditation, posture, dance and drama that you see 'spiritual people' do are nothing more (or less) than ways of stilling and quieting the ego, the mind-self... until the real magic of Spirit can be *allowed* to blossom... to be up-flaring and in-streaming within our whole-being, self-less consciousness.

In Time, because or in spite of all that we have done to try to make it welcome, this state of simple receptivity often finds a way to dissolve some weak place in our usually impenetrable (egoic) self-barriers and so finds a way to creep into our awareness like a cat on silent feet. The tiny crack or orifice is gently expanded... and then the miracle of real change flows in through that tiny opening and explodes within our consciousness, filling us with newness and re-birth... beyond all that we could have imagined.

This, then, is the Vision Quest
This is the Yoga - this is the Meditation
And this is our same and all-ways Path to Spirit

BEGINNING THE VISION QUEST: NON-DOING THE DANCE OF FEAR

If you know something about the possibility of medicine vision and understand at least a little of what it can do for you then you might choose to set out to 'meet your Vision.' And so you decide to 'go on a Vision Quest.'

The process of the vision quest is so very simple to relate: a vision quest is the adventure of creating a space of time and a safe place to settle down into your deepest thoughts and feelings, to meditate, to process-through any material plane blocks or worries... and then to open up to feel whatever sign may come your way. Nothing more... and nothing less.

It sounds so sweet and so very simple. But sometimes vision quests can be very painfully... boring! Usually boredom is a sign that we are afraid to *let go*. Usually boredom comes when change is very close. We are creatures who dearly love whatever is familiar. We are all addicted to maintaining the *status quo* - whatever it may be!

And as Change approaches ever so softly on its little cat feet - or comes crashing into our lives in its grandest blast of lightning strike - we all *unconsciously* try to maintain our *status quo* - we immediately try to defend our ego-selves against our deepest and only fear: the *Primal Fear of Letting Go*... (which is) the dreaded *Fear of Inevitable Change*... (which is) the *Fear of Becoming*... (which is) the endless *Fear of Death and Rebirth.*

Primal Fear runs deep within us all... and so great is its power that it causes us to lose faith and trust and even our own self-honesty. And when that occurs, we create from the stuff of Fear an unending stream of self-deception and unconscious defenses - defenses against meeting ourselves, each other... and Spirit. And as we make ritual to begin any vision quest, the yawning abyss of *'The Great Unknown'* is never far away. But even so... the whole purpose of making the time and space in your busy life to experience a real vision quest is precisely to *invite* this yearned-for and so-feared change to come... however it may walk... and however it may feel.

If you enter every vision quest with your eyes and heart as open as they can be... and bring to your experience all the sincerity and integrity that you can possibly muster... and if you try to hold faith in the old wisdom that says: "All the change that will come to you... is *your* Change to experience," well then... you simply cannot fail!

And beyond this... there is only (and always) the problem of Fear. In any vision quest process... Fear will appear. And simply said, Fear works like this:

INTENSE GROWTH AND POWERFUL CHANGE ALL-WAYS AWAKENS POWERFUL FEAR. The vision quest process works naturally to clear through fear on many levels. And freed of fear... we are free to change: to grow and deepen and expand on all dimensions of our beings. It is sometimes scary... but it works! We have all heard the fitness gurus say, "No pain, no gain!" But have you heard this one? *"No Fear... No Clear!"*

CLEARING FEAR IS WHAT IT'S ALL ABOUT. For there is *nothing* holding us away from health, fulfillment, enlightenment (whatever that may mean to you), or Spirit... except fear: fear of the past, fear of the future, fear of the present... and fear of becoming something new.

PRIMAL FEAR IS PRIMAL CAUSE. Primal Fear is at the root of all human dis-ease, all egoic obstruction, all confusion... and all suffering.

THE FEAR OF ALL OUR TOMORROWS IS ONLY THE FEAR OF CHANGE. Whenever we leave everything which is familiar to us... then we have already entered the realm of *'The Great Unknown:*

If you move from one school or city or country to another, your moment-by-moment awareness is pretty well taken up by making comparisons between your 'old' and 'new' situations... and by finding out how things work in the new environment. So when you are trying to understand supra-dimensional, whole-being change... Mind and Feeling will be kept very busy, indeed. Count on it!

But if you suddenly make a move from a bustling city... to the emptiness of a desert or the loneliness of a small tipi (or hut) on the top of a mountain... then you quickly discover that your *usual* lifestyle is full of defensive games: complex and devious ways of busying Mind and Feeling so that you simply 'do not have to' feel... all that you have to feel.

That is... we are conditioned from real experience to believe that if we can keep busy enough on all levels, we may not have to feel the abyss of emptiness or confusion which we all carry somewhere, deep inside.

This is the prime collusion of all modern culture. And what a good trick! Perhaps the best of all the famous tricks of Ego - that wily old master of tricks....

But there comes a time, for everyone, when maintaining the *status quo* (preserving the self-of-yesterday) is just not good enough anymore. And whenever this occurs... you may finally be game to *invite* Deep Change into your life. And when you do... there is no faster or more certain way to find new possibilities, growth and direction... than to just *let go* - to fall into opcnncss... to rcceive... whatever is to come. And in that surrender in to openness... you will have begun a true *Vision Quest*.

It sounds simple... and it is. The best ways are all-ways simple. But in its very simplicity also lies its challenge. Because, on a vision quest, there is nothing else to do *but* to feel... whatever is inside... whatever comes from outside... whatever sense-feeling-image-sound-memory comes along. And then there is nothing else to do but to live-through your every reaction... and to clear-through your every resistance... and so come to meet and clear-through all the fear that reaction and resistance have been born to serve.

When you are alone on a mountain with no diversions and no one else to play with... then there is nothing else to do but to let go... and *FEEL IT ALL!*

SURRENDER ONLY COMES WHEN THERE IS NOTHING ELSE TO DO

You are sitting alone in a gentle land. Just you and the Earth. Just you and the Sky. Just you and your Self. Just you and Spirit.

You want to seek vision but your mind is full of chatter. You want to be open to guidance but your body is restless and will not be at peace.

"Perhaps I should meditate!" you say aloud. "Maybe I should sing some Native American songs! Or maybe I should do some yoga!" And maybe you do... all of the above... but still no vision comes.

Just then the sun slips from behind a spirit-cloud and bathes your mountain in the soft red light of Father Sun's ritual "Goodbye!" Your heart surges, your breath draws in that warm radiance... and your mind leaps in excitement... and you are off and running! And...

"Ho! My Vision has finally begun!"

Many minutes later... you are still alone on the mountain... but the sun has gone. You are still alone with your Self... but the night is becoming cold. You are still alone with your fears... and whatever 'vision' was beginning to awaken in your awareness... long ago vaporized in an instant from your too-eager, too-egoic response!

When this happens - however it occurs - there is simply nothing else to do... but to begin all over again. *Re-Consecration:* the process of making sacred (once again), your process... and your vision quest: *Re-Committing - Re-Affirming - Re-Centering - Re-Awakening*... over and over again....

And for how long must we repeat these cycles of preparation? Well... most masters agree that enlightenment only takes a millisecond from any here-and-now moment. But getting to that particular millisecond... well, that is another story! And that is why it is called, spiritual 'practice.' For somewhere we all start as equally inept beginners in this craft of consciousness... and somehow we all must learn the *'practice.'*

And while we are waiting for Spirit to come... we prepare ourselves. And then we wait... for however long it takes And in this 'practice,' the vision quests of those warm, summer's nights and the vision quest of a thousand lifetimes are all-ways the same: the process can only succeed when we make total commitment to *DO IT--FEEL IT - BE IT*... for however long it takes!

FINDING AND LOSING SPIRIT

Weather provides some pretty good inspiration when you are alone in Nature... and some very welcome distractions, too. But sooner or later, every beautiful sun-set or thunder storm will pass... and you will be all alone, once again... with only your self-Self for company.

So... what will you do... now?

And now...? And now...?

Boredom... boredom... more boredom. Well, fear and boredom, actually... for boredom is all-ways a sign of fear. Fear and boredom, boredom and fear. An endless cycle. And there is no escape! You have made a commitment to do this vision quest... whatever it may entail. Yes! A commitment to yourself and to the Great Spirit, by God! And so you just have to sit it out... no matter how boring or meaningless it may seem... at least until you run out of cookies... plus an infinity longer. Again and again and again... boring and meaningless it will certainly become. Count on it!

But then comes that time when you have gotten completely fed up - long after you have gobbled up all the cookies (and everything else that you brought)... long-time since the great warmth and illumination of Father Sun ran away and left you all alone and nervous... that time when your spine(lessness) will no longer keep you upright and there are ants all over the ground... that moment when you realize that you really *might* have left something on the stove... or forgotten to refill the bird bath in your yard... or better change the bathroom light bulb in case it's about to blow... (etc., you know the drill) - when you are just about to pack it all in and come down the hillside, ready to admit that your Great Vision Quest was a Great Failure.

The little ego-mind-voice chatters on. You know, the one that is saying: "Perhaps Mercury's gone retrograde.... Perhaps I should not have brought that *whole* chocolate cake.... Probably 'medicine' is really for Native Americans and so maybe I should take up TV fitness classes instead!"

And then, all of a sudden, something changes. Something shifts a small fraction of a degree within your awareness... your spine tingles, your heart seems to stop (and your breath really does). And then... along comes a *Sign*!

Something very unusual, amazing, strange... whatever: *it is Sign!* You know it by your reactions - all those bodily-emotional things that happen even before you are fully aware of what is being revealed to (and through) you.

"Now... if I can only find out how to *read* this Sign... I just *know* that I will learn something really amazing from it!"

Aha! Self again! Ego again! That's it... stop surrendering for even an instant to celebrate how surrendered you are and... poof! *'GAME OVER!'*

So the sign slips away. The little shaft of spiritual light that seemed about to illuminate your inner universe-of-truth has fallen prey to a roving cloud within your inner sky. Whatever... Sign is gone!

And yet you will not be swayed from your spiritual path. Brave soul! You have read 'The Book.' You *know* that it is up to you to find the medicine meaning - if there is to be any meaning for you at all.

So... you hastily put down your hastily gathered possessions, abandoning all thoughts of that nice shower, warm pizza and friends waiting in the valley mists far below. In an instant and without any effort or mind-stuff at all... you *re-consecrate* your mind-space, you totally *re-commit* to the Vision Quest Process. And then you settle yourself to wait... to allow your clearer meditational self to host the working-through which will transmute *Sign* into *Meaning*... and meaning into *Revelation*... and revelation into *Guidance*. Ah! You have read the book very well, indeed!

Time passes. Sooner or later, even Slow-Time will pass. And as it does, your memory of that 'special sign' is becoming less and less clear. Actually fuzzy. Actually, pretty vague. But still you cling to memory's skeleton, still hoping to exchange it like a prisoner... for its intended meaning.

More time... perhaps the boredom... perhaps the fear. Perhaps memories of being all packed and ready to flee... perhaps a little chuckle at your own gullibility:

"Well... after all... it was only a ray of sun-light dancing on a leaf... or something like that. How important could *that* be...?"

What is important just here, is not to lose sight of the *Process* - the process that makes it all work: whenever meaning seems elusive... you can always turn back to the sign. For the sign *will* always bring with it the path-way to the meaning which it heralds. Somehow, your re-action to the sign will all-ways *work* as a catalyst for the meaning-to-come. And when you can no longer re-create the image of the sign on your inner vision-screen... you can still trace the sign by re-calling the *feeling* that it evoked within you.

That is... if you happen to self-distract, if you 'lose' any sign before its meaning is revealed... usually you need only re-mind yourself of how it felt when first it came... to awaken its medicine power once again.

If you have really read well, then you will know to ask yourself aloud: "What did that sign *bring* to me? What *happened* when that particular sliver of light filled my eyes?"

And even before you finish vibrating with the sound of those words... it suddenly comes to you! *IT* is suddenly there! All through you, all around you, as clear as anything you have ever experienced before... as obvious as anything has ever been: the meaning of that sign was the revelation of your re-commitment to re-consecrate your vision quest!

The sign brought you... *Sign*: sign of your commitment... of your readiness... of your openness... of your worthiness... of your power to receive *Guidance* and *Vision*. And is that not meaning enough?

Scratch your head in amazement... why not? Laugh aloud... dance... sing... cry. Why not? Take your time. Take all the time you need. And then, when time is just right for you... and *only* then... perhaps you will gently cease dancing-crying-laughing-celebrating... perhaps you will stop *pushing* energy out in any way at all.

In time... you just wear out and give up... and all pretense and acting out naturally subsides, like a post-orgasmic volcano winding down... and you sink downward in to your own infinite out-breath and in to the Mother Earth. With simple humility and deep surrender, you wrap your little-self in a warm blanket and sit upright in the Clear Night Mountain Sky.

For tonight you have *Medicine Work* to do. And tonight you have *Vision* to bear.

And *now*, Brother-Sister voyager... and *only* now...

Your Vision Quest can really begin!

VISION QUEST AFFIRMATION
- VISION QUEST PRAYER -

"I sit forever alone beside the Mother River
Open and amazed beyond all Mind
Here I am besought by no Other
Than the Shadow of my Dream
Here I am endowed beyond all Knowing
With a Heart of total Emptiness
Here I am beyond the pale of Wonder
Safely nurtured in the Trust of Innocence
As I move through realms that I have never known...."

FROM THE VISION QUEST TO LIVING THE VISION

However it comes through you... whatever you choose... however you proceed - however your own process unfolds and continually evolves within your unplanned, free-ritual experience: just to *be there*... just to have come to this moment of Ritual Dedication with all the *trust* and *surrender* and *commitment* and *openness* that you could muster... has *already* placed you within an instant's breakthrough discovery of what is perhaps the most profound life-changing realization of all. It is a discovery that can only come through direct experience... and it can only come when you are fully able to bear *'the all'* of its implication... and its intensity.

It is the incredibly simple realization that:

EVERYTHING IS MEDICINE!
And wherever you may go
And no matter what you are 'doing'
You are surrounded by Deep Medicine Sign.
And wherever there is Sign
You can Know there will be Meaning.
And wherever there is Meaning
Revelation will soon follow!

This is such a simple enlightenment... for those who can bear such simple truth. And as soon as it strikes, deep within you, like a lightning bolt hitting the heart-center of a mighty tree and bringing forth new and unimagined Life... you will ever after *know* your birth-right gift of *Direct Spiritual Guidance.*

In you, around you, far beyond you... however you feel it... there is an infinite promise within this Process and the promise is this:

However you meet the moment of your Awakening...
Once you have Opened to pure Medicine Vision...
You will never be alone again!

CONSECRATION & EVOCATION: LIVING THE REAL-TIME PROCESS

Ho! Great Spirit, I seek Vision!
I am Yours tonight!
Ho! Great Spirit, I seek Guidance!
Light my Way tonight!

"I now let go of all my Past.
I now let go of all Knowing.
I honor all my Teachers.
I honor All my Relations.
I Surrender all that I thought I was
To whatever I AM... to Become.
I let go of this very Gift of Life.
I let go of all Intention and all Illusion
As I open to be taken by Spirit tonight.

I clear my Head of all mind-dreams and thoughts -
I clear my Body of all needs and all doing -
I clear my Heart of all feeling -
I clear my Spirit of all attachment.

I open to your Teaching
O Mother Earth and Father Sky.
I open to the Word
Of Spirit in the Wind.

I open to the Vision
Of the Inner 'I.'
I open to the Guidance
Of all Spirit tonight."

Tonight a simple Vision is urging to bring Peace to fill my Heart. I can feel it. I am almost there... again... and again... and yet again.... I am (only) *almost* there....

But every time I feel myself beginning to be taken - yes, an actual physical sensation of being uplifted - I must be somehow recoiling within my inner fear. Somewhere Fear must be scaring away my trust and openness. For time after time, I find myself all alone again on the gentle bank of the Mother River... in a state of such mixed wonder and confusion... and very deeply bogged and stuck within my ego-self... and so very, very alone....

Feeling a time of Natural Stillness
Like a Healing Invitation from Spirit
I let Word trail away
And try to re-center my Self.

I move through whatever Free-Ritual comes to me
To re-Consecrate my Process and to re-Awaken Openness.
I Let Go to breathe-through the Meaning of Total Commitment.
I take Time to clear through whatever Feeling might arise.
And from this Deep Surrender...
I begin and begin, over and over again:

Seeking Stillness - Centering - endless Re-Consecration -
Seeking Openness - Meaning - Understanding -
Clearing Feeling - Thought - Distraction... and Fear.
The Process is a Circle - without beginning and without end.

And I must humbly re-enter the Sacred Circle
Wherever it is Open... and wherever I can.

RE-CONSECRATION: RETURNING TO SURRENDER

Ho! Great Spirit, I seek Vision!
I am Yours tonight!
Ho! Great Spirit, I seek Guidance!
Light my Way tonight!

Tonight I wait for my Vision
With open Heart and open Spirit -
I wait for New Direction.
I wait to be shown the Way.
I wait to be Cleansed - I wait to be Healed.
I wait for Wholeness - I wait for One-ness.
I wait for the Revelation of Awareness
I wait for the Clarity of direct Spirit Guidance.

Tonight I wait in Hope and in Trust....

Ho! Great Spirit, I seek Vision!
I am Yours tonight!
Ho! Great Spirit, I seek Guidance!
Light my Way tonight!

Tonight I am moving back in Time.
I am going back to the Home of my Soul.
Tonight I return to the Source of all Life.

I know and accept myself as I am.
I know that I have no knowledge.
I know that I have no path to walk.
I know that I am an empty vessel.
I will await the Guidance of Spirit.
Ho! Great Spirit, I seek Vision!
I am Yours tonight!
Ho! Great Spirit, I seek Guidance!
Light my Way tonight!

I can only work to prepare the soil
I can only hope that my seeds are well sown
I can only bring Breath, Trust, Hope and Love
I can only admit my Fears
I can only try to Let Go all Self-Distraction
I can only work to Clear the blindness from my eyes…
That I may be Open to The Vision *and* The Word.

Ho! Great Spirit, I seek Vision!
I am Yours tonight!
Ho! Great Spirit, I seek Guidance!
Light my Way tonight!

Now there is nothing more to Do…
But to offer this Prayer
To sing this Song
To Breathe… to Wait… to Hope
And to endure whatever may come.

If Vision is to come then LET IT COME NOW!
For I AM READY tonight for whatever will be!
Coming for - coming through - coming clear… TO ME.

Ho! Great Spirit, I seek Vision!
I am Yours tonight!
Ho! Great Spirit, I seek Guidance!
Light my Way tonight!

><><

CHAPTER 6

MEDICINE WALK VISION QUEST

THE DIFFERENT RHYTHMS OF CHILDHOOD

A Vision Quest can take many forms. But the inner experience (and the process) is usually the same:

I. You make yourself as ready as you can....

II. You withdraw from the ordinary 'commerce' of life and find a place where you can be deeply alone...

III. And then you wait: for *Sign*... for *Medicine*... for *Vision* to come.

It sounds very simple. And, on the outside, at least, it is. But *Living the Process* of being inwardly still and constantly trying to *let go* into ever deeper dimensions of openness is another matter entirely.

Stillness and waiting, preparation and surrender: this is the traditional recipe for a Vision Quest. Seeking self and Spirit in this way is great for adults - and can be a profoundly important Initiation Ritual into new dimensions of intentional personal and spiritual growth for adolescents. But things are different for kids.

Kid bodies are made for action. There is so much life energy pumping through them every minute that it is truly oppressive to ask them to be still at all, beyond their natural span of stillness - a wholly unpredictable length of time which is always changing, minute to minute and child to child.

For younger children, to enforce the strict self-control of the adult vision quest is wholly inappropriate... and impossible at that. I believe that it is actually *violent* to try to unnaturally suppress any child's always self-firing and ever-changing interest and feelings. Their attention naturally races all over the place... and their bodies eagerly follow!

It is saddening to recall how many times I have experienced ritual circles of all kinds being literally torn apart by children who have not been gently guided into the simple pleasure that can come from being a part of a magical circle.

Often these are the very children of those I would describe as the most sensitive and spiritually conscious parents. And yet these parents so often make the excuse that, "our children just haven't experienced any ritual circles before." Or, that "It is not fair to expect the children to be still" (or, apparently, to be *involved* in any way in the circle that is around them), "because the children's energy needs constant freedom and expression...."

Well now... this is a sad state indeed. Somehow even those children of parents who consciously seek deeper communication and some sort - maybe *any* sort - of spiritual process that they can share as a whole family, often lack the focus and the interest which would make this possible.

Over time, our family has struggled with this too. Overall, I believe that we have succeeded pretty well... *and* we have struggled to make it work.

There are so many path-ways to self-awareness and spirit, taught by so many other teachers and books. Here, we have come to celebrate the power of the Medicine Family Circle in all its forms and with all of its challenges. So let us explore this vital link between children and medicine; stillness and magic; between attention span and revelation.

Children, of course, *are* magic. Children *are* medicine. But children cannot be expected to hold meditational, one-pointed stillness for even long enough to feel what nice feelings (and other things) might eventually come to them. After all... keeping stillness is, in ways only meditators may understand, one of the most difficult of all things to do... for anyone!

As adults we can (usually) find ways to go off alone for our vision quests - even if it's only between breast feedings or child transport runs. But if we are to be families of the medicine way, then we need to be able to *make place* for our children in our most important Free-Ritual Family Circles.

My goal in learning how to share medicine with our children is based on one firm principal: I accept that we must find ways to include everyone: everyone's *experience* ... and everyone's input... in everything that we do.

And over time I have found that *there is all-ways a way* to include every child's experience... including their reactions of boredom or distraction. Yes, there is always a way... but the way usually involves changing adult expectations and devising new processes that can accommodate the different life-rhythms and awareness of the mini-shamans.

Children are more honest than adults in many ways: when a child resists letting go and sinking into softness and stillness, their defenses against surrender and opening tend to be expressed in active (and often disruptive) ways. Adults, on the other hand, tend to just shrink away into apparent complicity... and often into inward confusion, rebellious resentment... and, of course, that always looming free-range anxiety.

Be we children or adults, ultimately, of course, no form of defensive evasion is any better than any other... and (of course) *every* expression is a sign to be felt-through for its own meaning.

Children reflect the ambient energy of any circle in direct and very revealing ways: if we acknowledge that their whole-being experience is a vital and essential part of the family circle... then their potentially disruptive energies can be seen as mirrors of uncenteredness and unexpressed feelings of discomfort in the circle as a whole.

While adults sit still and inwardly use their minds to try to 'talk themselves into' meditation... children just vent their discomfort and re-channel their focus into something (anything) that will suit their expressive needs.

So we can use our children's restlessness and avoidance as Sign - often of our own uncenteredness and unfelt needs - and we can use it as a focus for healing and clearing. In this way what might have once been a disturbance... can often become a dynamic guide-dance. And if we learn how to read and follow this sign we can evolve processes that better include the whole-family's real-life energies and needs.

However your family comes to balance its internal differences during everyday life, times of Medicine Family Ritual are different.

For now it is time for everyone's every feeling and impulse to shine forth as sign... and as the Living Revelation of each family's medicine path.

In our tribe, we have all learned to follow the 'flow' of child-guidance. And we have watched many medicine-birds fly away when a less-than-aware child blurts out bird-scaring noise. But we have also followed 'unknowing' children into experiences of great magic and wonder. So who's to say where the next medicine experience will come from.... or what catalyst will bring it into our awareness?

In the end... the trick is to find ways to let the children lead us all in to new realms of Free-Ritual Magic... without 'giving up' all that adult guidance has to offer to the medicine process... and without letting the aimlessness of free-wandering child-mind dissipate the circle energy... and our circle experience.

THE RITUAL OF THE MEDICINE WALK

In our family we have found that even keeping attention open/focused in a very active circle can be difficult for the littlies among us - and especially for the little Beny Sky Virgo Bull. Silence, too, is a rare state of Grace which never lasts for long. And so often, as we delve into the shadows of the night, we find that any period of silence in our circle turns out to be merely a transition state: between eagerness... and some impending fear.

Given all of this, it obviously would not work to expect strict 'vision quest' commitment from those who cannot even remember what it is we committed to... or to expect 'vision quest' austerity from those who cannot even imagine the *Zen* state of *non-doing*... or to enforce 'vision quest' deprivations upon those whose natural yoga is the *whole-being celebration of all Life*.

But it would be a great loss to our family - to all our families - if we could not find a path-way in to medicine vision which even the children could follow. The notion of 'Vision' - the *power* of Vision, the *wonder* of Vision and the *experience* of Vision is just too good to miss... just because we are too young and *too free* to... remember... to be still... to meditate... to surrender... to feel the difference between inner and outer, self and Self, or between self and sign.

Through our family's deep explorations of medicine process together, we have found some ways to move through time and space -

to be one with the Mother Earth and still be free enough to move and feel and explore and to relate with child-fresh spontaneity to everything we experience and whatever we might feel, at any age, at any time... and in any way that we *must*.

And over time we have found a very exciting way to ritually integrate and celebrate the Deep Surrender and Open Wonder of the vision quest with the naturally distractible (and mutually distracting) consciousness of all children. And we have named this gentle process: *'THE MEDICINE WALK.'*

By walking into Nature together in silence (more or less) and being free to explore and share *whatever* comes to us, through us, in spite of us (etc.), we can engage the active child body-mind in a pursuit of Vision that does not compromise a child's energies or needs... and still honors our own.

So... whenever our family feels too young, too eager, too bored, too excited or just too impatient to sit around waiting for medicine to come to us... we just go out *looking* for it. We track *it* down, wherever it may be. We use our all-sized bodies to capture it with our enthusiasm and natural wonder. And then we look for its meaning together... and then: *Medicine is ours!*

As we move through our Medicine Walk Ritual Dance we are constantly integrating body-mind-feelings... adventure... and Spirit. And usually (as if they mattered not at all) all the more subtle dimensions of 'adult medicine' seem to tag along for the ride, perhaps to be seen by only a very few of us, from time to time, as we just walk along through Nature... together.

As we move together into 'The Great Unknown,' our relationships change continually. Each child is constantly moving around, within our Moving Circle: first in front of me... now beside me and clutching my hand... now behind me as I take 'point' as we move into the gloom... then in my arms when the wallaby thumps the earth to call its joey back into its pouch... or whenever the big owl sounds....

And each of these spatial-hierarchical relationships within the circle brings its own special experience... and so its own feeling... and so brings more for us to process-through. This is the grist for the mill of *Becoming*. This is the very stuff of medicine family sharing!

As we walk together we *are* a Living Circle. We all share (at least some) awareness of each other. We all respond (sooner or later) to whatever seems important to any one. And all the essential elements of the Living Circle: *breath* and *touch* and *healing* and *feeling* and *consecration* and *communion* and *channeling*... go on and on and on as the Medicine Walk Vision Quest Family Healing Circle moves through a darkening forest together like a great, amorphous 'spiritual amoeba' - tasting, sensing, subsuming (or fleeing) everything in its inexorable path!

We are not silent - and as we have said, *cannot* be silent when we are three... or six... or nine... or forty-some and responsible for all of the others. But we are 'quiet.'

The Littles have taught me that for children, 'quiet' is the state of *intended* silence. And it is almost as good - will have to be good enough - and has been a major breakthrough in the possibility of family-wildlife relations on our medicine walks.

The mini-shamans actually believe that if we all *intend* to be silent... then surely the fox and the wallaby and the wombat will just *know* that we are peaceful and so they will come out to 'be with us!'

To the Littles it is just as simple as that! Of course... we have yet to convince the fox... or the great ibis... or the cockroach... or maybe even GrandMother Moon... of this obvious 'medicine truth' of childhood. But we are working on it! In fact, already the very shy platypus has succumbed to our 'quiet' ritual maelstrom of splashes and giggles and sneezes and squeals... and has openly come to us for Deep-Time Medicine Sharing.

So, this is the process of the medicine walk. It is perhaps our family's most cherished shamanic ritual. It is open to infinite variation of form and place and mode... and content. And no matter how it unfolds... it is the *Process* that is special.... And it is the process that makes it all work.

Through sharing this Ritual Vision Quest Process with many families we have come to know that once any family finds its own ritual process... and once the process is really working, then all else follows naturally.

When we are 'making medicine' to clear a family's communication problems, to heal real-time dis-ease or to simply look to the wonders of Nature for some revelation of life's deepest secrets: it does not really matter what you say... or where you go... or what you wear (inside or out).

Once your medicine family has found its process and *whatever* rituals work for you... then you are truly on the path. And then... from sharing *Moving Circle Vision Quest Medicine Walk Ritual*

Expeditions of all kinds, it is just a short hop (and a true quantum leap of consciousness) to perhaps the most profound life-changing realization of all: the discovery through your own, very grounded, real-life experience that same-same revelation:

EVERYTHING IS MEDICINE!

And everywhere we go...
And no matter what we are 'doing'...
We can be Open to Medicine Sign.
And wherever there is Sign
There will surely be Meaning...
And from Meaning, Revelation too...
And so we will find Guidance on our Path.

And once this *Living Channel of Medicine Vision* is opened... it need never again be closed to our experience.

Ho! Great Spirit, I seek Vision!
I am Yours tonight!
Ho! Great Spirit, I seek Guidance!
Light my Way tonight!

SKIPPING STONES AND STEPPING STONES: THE PROCESS AND THE PATH

We have been evolving the Medicine Walk Process for many years now, as a kind of 'fast food vision quest' that seems ideally suited to the energies and attention-span of children (and adults) of all ages.

This process is a simple and non-structured path-way: we walk out into the world-at-large, feel the wealth of the ever-changing environment... and drink in whatever medicine might come our way. On the outside, that's about all there is to it. But there is more to the process than what we might *do*....

We have learned together that if we walk with care - if we *'Walk in a Sacred Manner'* - and if we pay close attention to our process... then the natural circle-magic of Sign and Meaning and Vision seems all-ways to be there for us.

Apart from sitting in circles... and making free-ritual in any situation... the medicine walk is our family's most precious sharing. And this is how it works:

IN THE BEGINNING...

We begin by opening our hearts. We begin with no specific direction. We trust that Direction will be revealed. Everything, in fact, will be revealed. And until it is, there is nothing to do but wait for Revelation to come. And so we begin as we would begin any vision quest.

But we do not have to wait in stillness - do not 'have to' and couldn't anyway! On our medicine walks we can walk, move, run, laugh, shout, dance... or whatever. But not all over the place. And not completely care-less-ly. If we are going to walk together in to deep wonder and amazing revelation, we know that there is but one requirement, just one essential 'rule' to follow. And that single guiding rule is this: we know that for the process to work, we must *try* to be in a surrendered and receptive mode. Nothing more is needed... and nothing else will do: we must wholly *intend* to be quiet. If we can but keep this one, precious discovery alive within our collective awareness... then Gaia-Nature-Mother-Earth will reveal Her deepest secrets and share Her magic with us, Her very most intimate friends.

We just need to *try* to be open - in ourselves... to and with each other... and with every entity... wherever our journey may take us. And as long as we are trying - each in our own way, within our very different inner worlds and very different abilities - then we know that we are doing all that we can. There can be no 'failure' (and so no guilt) when we walk together in this way. We need only to be just as centered and just as quiet and just as open as we can be: nothing more and nothing less. And we all try our best. With such earnestness do we all try!

We have learned that we can run and shout and dance while we wait for sign... or we can wait in a quieter space, which (not surprisingly) seems to help us be more open and sensitive in our feelings. And whatever we need to be at any one moment... is whatever we are. And we know that 'medicine' loves the child in us all... and 'medicine' will all-ways take us as it finds us!

At the very beginning of this shapeless, Free-Ritual Moving Circle, I usually say (with as much ritual solemnity as I can muster), "Shall we begin Now?" And with our collective agreement comes the commitment that from then onward, we will all try to *live* and *share* our medicine walk process.

We fall into silence (kid-silence, that is, 'intended silence,' that is, with all its natural clamor) and we walk out the garden gate and into the Magic Forest together, with open eyes and open hearts.

As with any vision quest, beginning a medicine walk is all about *Process*: opening, letting go, surrendering, allowing, sharing... with as much respect and peace and stillness as we can manage. We walk and we wait. And we usually do not have long to wait for the magic to begin....

We are out the gate and running once again! We are free-ranging in a magical realm. We are all of 'One Heart.' We have begun. From now on, whenever we speak, we will speak only of our Process: how we are sharing, where we are going, the basic mechanics of getting there, etc.

And we have found a way to ensure that even the littlest among us can hold to this firm commitment: we have always agreed that we will only 'talk process' when we are on medicine walks. So, of course, it only stands to reason: if we are committed to only share process... then *everything* that is said must be 'process' in some way or another. Just like *intending* to be quiet *must be* something like real 'quiet.' And it is up to us to find out how.

It is up to us (well, up to me) to follow the mind-mazes to reveal the process that we must re-discover and re-create, at every turn of the path. Like: who crossed the log first and why? Who coughed and giggled just when the night-bird sang? Why are we afraid to go into the dark bush right now? Or whatever: *IT IS ALL PROCESS.*

As our little process-ion moves through the forest, those who can understand anything at all try to help the moment become ever more magical by allowing each spoken word its full power of ritual medicine: every new idea and every word is Medicine Word... and so is known to be absolutely essential to our process... and to whatever magic is to come.

This is what it is like - on the *outside* of the experience - of 'talking-process' with the mini-shamans:

"Dad... why does Joah always have to be in front of everyone else on the path"

"Uh... Joah, isn't it all right for Kira to walk in front of you sometimes. Why don't you give her a chance to be our path-finder tonight?"

"Hmmm... I guess just never thought of it, Dad...!"

"Yes... I know...!" With clumsy shuffling, we struggle to rearrange ourselves under the eyes of Spirit... and we are off once again.

"And also, Joah..."

"Yes?"

"I was wondering... if maybe you're also feeling a little afraid to be the Last One...?"

"No... I just.... Well... yes. Maybe a bit...."

"You know, if you share your fear with us all... we may be able to help you with it. Do you think we could?"

"Maybe. Anyway... I guess I am a *little* bit afraid...."

So we stop for a cuddle, sharing the great and reassuring power of Father-Breath, Father-Touch and everyone's caring.

This sounds like what any family might be saying, as they do anything at all. Doesn't it? I mean... does this sound like 'medicine talk' to you? How is this different than 'everyday' sharing?

Well... it's like the notion of *intentional quiet* and 'real' quiet, once again. As a matter of absolute fact, *every* variable in our medicine process is like intentional quiet vs. real-time quiet: the difference *is* the Process.

Well... when you 'walk the walk' and 'talk the talk' with the mini-shamans... this is what you get. We can make it Ritual Process and we can allow it to be medicine just be choosing it to be so. And as soon as we make this collective commitment, then everything is Process.

Whatever happens on a medicine walk *is*... and so can be (and must be?) felt-through *in-process* until the medicine in the moment comes clear - until Sign, Meaning and Vision are revealed. Very simple. Very *Zen*. Very nice!

And so it goes on. On and on forever (as every parent knows), the care-full accessing and ritual revelation of all those feelings that lie just beneath whatever we are willing to admit. If there be any feeling among us, then I know that it will find its way out - directly or indirectly, we will all feel it all. So we might as well get into it whenever we sense that there is *anything* pressing for our acknowledgement... our acceptance... our release... and/or our amazement.

So our process is to 'follow the feeling.' And whatever feeling emerges always seems to lead us exactly to whatever medicine we are to find... and explore... that day. So being attentive to 'process' is not just about controlling our impulsive, disruptive selves: it is also about facilitating the Natural Revelation of all that we are... right there, right then.

This is a vision quest. We are in a state of preparation and surrender and waiting. We just do it on wheels to give Spirit a broader canvas on which to paint the clues... and so that Revelation can have a fair chance to keep up with our ever-scanning ever-swirling attention vortices. So... *Run for it, Spirit! And catch us if you can!*

For this medicine magic of Revelation to happen, *where* we walk really doesn't matter at all: for we are just walking to find out... *who* and *what* and *how* we are that night... as we move together in a sacred manner, birthed and re-birthed with every breath as we plunge into the Deep Magic of the Earth....

AND THE PROCESS IS THE PATH

Walking and talking. Sounds pretty simple, no doubt. What is different here - as we walk the medicine path in 'deep togetherness' - is that here we take *everything* as meaning-full.

Here, we can insist on (eventual) honesty and openness. And the pay-off or 'reward' for taking the risk to open up and share whatever lurks inside usually comes powerfully and at once:

We all give our full attention to *whatever* comes up for *anyone*... until that feeling-event-concern is *'processed-through'* (we call it) and leads us to a state of new-found clarity... until it has become another gem of medicine learning... and/or until it is fully dis-charged and becomes an emotional non-event. Completely finished. And *all* of us are at peace with the outcome.

But this is not the only difference between the Medicine Family Vision and more ordinary family sharing:

While we are in this *altered state* of highly responsible collective consciousness, everything that comes up in anyone's experience is also taken into our Ritual Circle as something very precious, very rare... and very worthy of our collective time, attention and effort... whatever it may need.

This is a state of *deep mutuality* that we can never maintain for very long without 'falling out' of the medicine process. So every one of us appreciates its 'specialness.' In this rarefied atmosphere, time, feelings, external phenomena, internal needs and *everything* else becomes very important to us all. And all the more because we know that every journey into someone's feelings is always a trip into the mystic - and all-ways a new adventure into 'The Great Unknown.'

As we head into processing-through anything which comes up within our circle... no one knows where the deep magic will begin... or where it will take us! We only know that somewhere within this process... truly amazing experience is likely to leap suddenly into our lives... because we have experienced it *every* time we follow this shamanic process of *'stopping the world'* and are willing to deal with anything and everything that might arise in anyone's feelings or experience.

So we have learned - and are always learning even more - that *everything* can be known as medicine sign: every thought-feeling-need-reaction-phenomenon-sound-etc. And we have learned through many such encounters that whatever comes to our family circle, never comes to just one of us, alone. *IT IS ALL US.* And from this shared flow of heightened feeling, we know that Guidance will soon come... for us all.

Thus we take the time to include everyone's dramas, needs and feelings in our medicine process. And as we process-through whatever comes up, we are actively *transmuting* all we can of the free-ranging interpersonal 'garbage' of life into new teaching, new lessons and greater personal clarity.

Whatever we cannot deal with on the spot, is (more or less) consciously put 'on hold' for the moment - ready to be *recycled* at some future time. Because we know that every little niggling unclarity in our consciousness will demand that we deal with it sooner or later.

Even if we find we cannot meet and deal with something here-and-now... we know that some other sign or situation will inevitably bring up every unresolved issue or pattern again and again... until they are all resolved and discharged. For this process of self-clearing is a natural healing process: this is how we all grow. And this growth is natural to life itself.

If our children can grow up secure in their understanding of this process, then our Medicine Family will have succeeded in its highest Vision.

So we walk the Path and we share the Process. And I know that ultimately, whatever is actually said as we walk along so full of everything - be it a few pithy monosyllables or great torrents of word - hardly matters at all! For it is not the content of the word... but the way of learning how to use Word to open new dimensions of direct Spirit Guidance and deep learning that is so essential to our process - and to our purpose here.

For even though our content ranges wide in scope and depth, still there is great medicine power in *every* word we share when we are *in-process*.

This is like no other kind of talk-talk. What will come of any moment of it is unpredictable in objective-specific terms. But what happens again and again on the *inside* of our feelings from all of this care-full and loving attention, is an amazing simplicity and heart-connected *Deep Mutuality*: a unique experience of personal and inter-personal effectiveness... a bonding with each other which we know will never be erased or over-written, no matter how hectic or intense our lives become - as they separate on the material plane and then re-merge over time, as we all grow older.

And I know that whatever is said from within the sacred space of our medicine rituals will be internally replayed and thought over, looked at and fondled, processed and re-processed... more completely, perhaps, than anything else that my family will ever share.

Well, up until now, at least, this has been our family's experience. And this is my immediate reward as for *taking the time* to move through these rituals of spiritual parenting with a degree of caring and wholeness which I hope honors the great privilege I feel in being the beloved father, friend and medicine teacher to these most worthy Children-of-Spirit... and through this Word, perhaps in some way, to you and yours.

And so we walk. And so we 'talk-process' as we go. And whatever comes up... whatever it is... whether it comes from inside or from without... that is our sign. And through our spontaneous *Free-Ritual Process of Meeting-Sign* we uncover its meaning. And through processing our individual meanings together, we can usually discover a collective meaning. And this is the meaning of *US*.

And as we move into this Deep Mutuality, shamanic vision is

awakened in us all and each. Some know it by its name and some drift within its nurturing enfoldment like sleepy babes in the woods of the night. Someday many years from now, I know that they'll look back on this time and suddenly 'awaken' with a start when they re-call my words of long ago and suddenly real-eyes the simple truth that they have carried through all their years:

'It is all Vision
It is all Real
It is all Medicine
And it is all Spirit.'

TALKING DREAMING - TALKING SIGN

Walking-walking, talking-talking... we move along our medicine path, hand in hand, heart in heart and mind all over the place. And for all our intentions of meditative silence, we end up talking almost continually. Talking 'medicine talk,' to be sure... but talk-talk nevertheless.... Fives and sixes do not go too long without words. They try... but true silence only comes with sleep... and by the next morning, they have forgotten that they ever stopped talking even to sleep! Nines... not much silence in there, either. To say nothing of father... himself known to love a Word or two....

We move through the tall grass carefully. In Australia, Brother Snake is always nearby. Anyway, children do not move easily through tall anything. We wait. We fall over. We cry. We get angry. No use. The stick which trips us doesn't even care.

"... but maybe it *does* care...."

"But I didn't *hear* it tell me it was sorry...!"

We each see something. We each see many things at once. We move through many talk-skill processes, mostly around who gets to share their sign first... who saw it first, who saw it best... or whatever.

While we are all telling our stories - touching into the special magic that comes from *'Talking Story'* - we feel into each other's real-time experience, inhabiting each other's scenarios if only for a brief, ritual moment.

We give attention to each show-and-tell magic object, each offered meaning and each stray memory of who-did-what some yesterday or another... and then move back on the track with some sincere feeling for the here-and-now... still another new ritual object... or whatever sign we think we might have found.

From and through this process, of all the Sign and Story and all the glimpses of Vision which we are trying to share with each other... one will always leap out at us with the power of its immediate and obvious significance... the irony of its precise appropriateness... and the most direct and clear meaning for us each and all... entwined together, woven and braided into a new entity: a medicine sign which will somehow re-awaken in real-time splendor the Guiding Vision of our medicine Family.

READING SIGN & FINDING MEANING

For an event to be sign, it must be imbued with its own energy-of-meaning. It must have Power. This energy comes through us as a feeling... the *feeling* of the power of the sign - the power of its rightness, the power of what it has awakened in us - and in this feeling we know we can dis-cover the special meaning-fullness of whatever has come to us as sign. And then we all know together: *this IS the Meaning of the Sign!*

This time the sign was a beam of sun-light wafting through the top of an eighty-foot high mountain ash tree... growing somewhere across the top of the hill. And the meaning of the sign evolved like this:

We could not see the trunk or branches of this great tree. We could not see the sun as it had already dropped behind the hill behind our garden. We would not have noticed that tree at all, this evening, except for the sun-light which danced through its leaf and its space.

So the sign was not so much *about* the tree... it was about the sun itself. We all agree on each step in the very circular flow of this intuitive sort of logic - the logic of synchronicity - the logic of feeling - the logic of medicine... the *special logic of Shamanic Meaning*.

A Sign of the Sun... but we could not even *see* the sun. The sun was just signaling to us that it was leaving - it was going out for the night. It had to get ready for Perth and the Indian Ocean... and to light the entrance to a sacred cave somewhere in the Himalayas. So

Sun was on its way out. So we all felt that perhaps the sign was not so much about sun-light as it was about sun-*dark*.

Darkness was coming. We would all be brave. No, no one had to walk across that dark log bridge (from last night's medicine walk) again if they did not want to. Agreed!

No, we will not walk too far from home this time. Agreed!

No, bears *still* don't live in these parts.

Yes. It was a doggy. Only a doggy. No, I don't think it was a very big doggy at all. Do you...? Really...? Listen again to his bark and we will find out just exactly how big that doggy is, ok? Just let his sound come all *through* you and see if you can *feel* just how big he actually is....

Somehow we are back on the Path again. It is darkening. We *are* brave. We're doing fine! And *everyone* is clamoring to find the log once again.... Everyone *wants* to walk across it once again! Or at least we remember feeling like we wanted to last night...

Aha! The log! "Hey, that was the magic of the *last* Walk. Tonight... ahhh! Something completely different is going to happen tonight...! Let's go find out what it might be, eh?"

Silence. We walk on. We are all 'in-process.' We are all waiting:

Waiting for a Sign....

TEACHING FOR THE FUTURE

As we move from drama to drama... I do not miss (or ignore) the programing I am writing into their future resources memory banks... and/or their 'basic life expectations' files. *I know* that I am programing them with process. And I know that this is precisely what I have to offer their very independent consciousness. Not facts or fixed truths (dogmas)... but the *process* through which their own truths will come to be revealed.

We know - they and I - that soon enough they may throw off all the forms and even the language that I offer them, like some grossly oppressive traditional native dress that the new-tribe kids don't want to wear anymore. Let them throw away whatever they want! *I know* that the Message and the Meaning will remain - in any dress and spoken in any tongue.

Still, while I know that rebellion will inevitably arise, I cannot actually know (and I believe that no parent really can imagine) how it will feel to become, one day, the archetypal opposition in their eyes: obviously someone and something to reckon with... but also something to compete with... even, perhaps, an oppressing force which they must overthrow.

Kids think like that. They won't *talk* to us like that... but I know that they can think like that. When I start talking to them about 'Medicine Path'... teaching them an ancient way of Knowing... I can see the rumblings of peer group ascendancy lurking just out of sight behind their openly agreeing eyes.

But for now, we are still learning to live in-process together as we 'walk in a sacred manner' along our wholly unpredicted path. And just for now... *I* still light the Way.

THE TEACHING OF THE GREAT UNKNOWN

Everyone was alert and alive, buzzing with expectations. What would we possibly find tonight? If you walk in the realm of natural magic that swirls all around us... and if you really *know* that sign will all-ways come... then every evening stroll becomes an exciting adventure into 'The Great Unknown!'

This evening we went to a new place. There was a small concrete dam and holding pool - originally made to water horses as they passed the small and fickle stream. I told the mini-shamans we were going to walk across the dam wall and that we would not be scared... and that if anyone got scared, we'd stop and deal with it right away, ok?

Yes. Agreed! That felt trustworthy enough. So we went on.

Fear did come up, now and then. But we would always stop, look over a few options - going home, going another way, waiting here - while everyone else crossed the (five-year-old's horrific projection of a raging) stream.

As the little Joah-Frog meditated on what he wanted to do, everyone else just *did*... walking far, far above big dark rocks and rushing water. And as we inched along, we were ever so slowly walking away from him. Suddenly he jumped out of his retractive, restrictive fear and plunged right into the positive excitement of trying to cross the Great Abyss with everyone else.

And so we walked across the dam, all together, little ones holding very close and hanging on each daddy-hand.

Aha! They think they're *safe* when I'm holding their hands...! In my experience, I feel that I am just as likely to take the Big Plunge as they are. But I won't warn them, tonight, about the folly of hanging onto a broken branch for support. And anyway... all feelings of physical safety are an illusion in one way or another! More sign. More process:

"Daddy... What if someone felled off the dam wall?"

"Well, that can happen. Sometimes we *do* fall. But it might not be too bad...

"Why?"

"Because, look at this: if *you* were to going to fall, maybe you'd have just enough time to choose which way you fell. So if that started to happen, which way would you like to fall?"

"I'd like to fall into the soft muddy pool of water above the dam... I don't want to fall onto those rocks way down there...!

"Me neither!"

"I don't want to fall down there at *all*!"

"Me too!"

"I don't want to fall either...!"

"Maybe we are going to fall...?"

"Me too...! I feel like I might fall now!"

"No, now I am holding you and you are safe."

"But if you ever felt you *were* going to fall... probably you'd be able to choose which *way* you were going to fall. Do you think you could? Do you believe you can choose your own Way...?"

"Well, sort of...."

"Isn't it nice to know that you might always have a choice whenever you *were* going to fall...?"

"Well... sort of nice...."

"Well, it's a good thing to remember, isn't it?"

"Well... sort of good...."

This moment's Ritual-of-Choice Initiation feeling complete - 'just as far as we can go at any moment and no further' - we can now get back to our Initiation Ritual-of-Trust: moving across the dam wall.

First we walked the wall together, holding hands. No sooner had we all exclaimed on how brave we were, than we changed the game and had to face walking the wall all alone, without touching hands - but still choosing who we wanted to have ahead and behind us as we each made that long walk into The Great Unknown all alone... and *practicing* choosing with each step, which way we'd try to fall in case we fell at all....

Next, we each did it all alone with no one else even on the wall... and with our eyes tightly closed (except for all the times when we just had to open them up). Then we compared how many times each one just *had* to peek: a test of honesty - which is, of course, yet another kind of courage.

Sometime shortly afterwards, we got tired of the dam. There was no more learning for us there... no more Sign, no more Fear... and so, no more Meaning. So we walked on to find other sign and to feel other things in the dark of that night.

Brave of heart, we tried a ceremonial act of walking under a canopy of trees and into total darkness... for many, many minutes we inched along... barely moving... barely breathing... everyone holding (everything) together as still and as tightly as tight can be... as you can well imagine. For after all... no matter what else is out there... darkness itself can be very... *dark*!

Ah! We made good progress - many good inches were covered by the Brave Family on that darkest of nights. And then all of a sudden we all spooked at once and leaped backwards into the safety of a blob of moonlight that was just lying casually around nearby.

"What scared us all?" No one knew. No one really cared to know.

"Uh... maybe it was an owl. Shall we use the light and try to look for an owl's eyes glowing in the tree?"

"No!"

"Want to stay very still and listen for whatever it could be?"

"No I don't want to..."

"Me too!"

"If we could find out what it was, I know we'd feel much better. Don't you think so?"

"Maybe... but I don't want to!"

"Neither do I...."

"...Daddy...?"

This was obviously not a time for medicine learning... or even for talking-process.... This was a time for retreat! Even so... from the safety of our moon-puddle I found an interesting bit of process:

"Why is it easier to move more quickly *backwards* to get out of the darkness... than it is to run ahead towards the light...?"

Silence. There were no takers for Zen games that night. Our time-to-be-brave had simply run out! Suddenly we were all 'too tired' or 'thirsty' or 'cold' - or whatever might work (you know how it goes). And so we were....

So the Rainbow Medicine Warriors went home (at last)... and told the Mother all about it.... And then we made a great pile of mattresses and blankets in front of the open fire... and curled up together to sleep our same and different dreams...

Yet even in the DreamTime...
The Medicine Circle
The Medicine Process
The Deep Learning
And the Medicine Walk itself
Go on... and on... and on...
Without Beginning...
And without End.

THREE STREAMS OF AWARENESS IN THE DARK OF NIGHT

It is a new time and we are leaving the house just before nightfall fully charged with Great Expectations... and new courage to match. This is our favorite time for medicine walks because this is the time of maximum change: Day is letting go into Night... and sunlit security is soon bound to be tested by fright!

Just at this moment of half-light, everything changes so fast. However a highly charged bush or tree might look as we pass it now... it will look very different if we happen to glance back over our shoulders for one last peek before moving on.

Nothing can be reconfirmed by our sense of sight or sound. Everything is in flux. What we could see just a moment ago, now we cannot. Where we thought we knew a shape as a rock and a tree stump... now we aren't so sure! This *is* the interface between the known and the unknown, between the mundane and the mystical. At every sunset comes *the Time of the Shaman.*

Just tonight, Joah is just five years old, Kira is seven, Ami is ten and I am... well... all of the above and more. We cover a wide range of ages tonight. We have many different levels and points of view. And now we are in the van and rolling... and now we are ready to meet the living entity of Night.

As soon as we were moving down the small road that led down the mountainside, I could feel the pure wonder rising in the mini-shamans as every new shadow loomed beside us. It was a moment to grasp. And so I said (with great ceremonial abruptness): "Let's begin... NOW!"

We all fell into silence... watching and waiting for whatever sign would come. And so our medicine walk was begun.

Driving further along the rough dirt road toward town, Kira said she'd like to find a medicine place in the treefern forest that was unfolding around us. I did not answer.

The forest near our house is on a hill and there is no running water. I was deep into thinking about water: we always seemed to head toward its certain magic for medicine walks. Something about the presence of elemental Water. Something about the interface between 'hard' reality and fluid awareness. Something about the deep-*yin* medicine of water....

As I flowed along with my water-mind... the van slipped out of second gear and, free-wheeling now, suddenly surged ahead, bouncing down the dirt road steep hill beneath us. It was the first unusual happening and so it our first sign!

Hard-stone reality becoming water-fluid: sure-wheeled traction becoming a sliding mystery: it was all good Sign.

Perhaps it was time to speak. So I began to talk about our process even as I moved to reclaim power over the metal beast: "Well, that was exciting, wasn't it? You know... this might be a sign about the van... or maybe a sign about what we are doing tonight. How do you feel it?"

No answer. Waiting for Daddy to reveal all once again, are we? Well, we'll see about that!

"Well, if it's just the van, I know why it slips out of gear sometimes.... It's because the transmission is wearing out... and that's all. It's not a good sign about the van... but I don't think it's a sign about the van anyway. What do you think?"

No answer: a real standoff was looming. "Hey! Maybe the van wants to go somewhere else!"

Everyone agreed, nodding and affirming my wisdom... and right there I had them! "Why are you all agreeing with me like this?" I asked with slightly affected incredulity.

"Do you think that *I* know what this sign means to you...? Well... I don't! I only know what it means to me. How can we know what it means to each other unless we tell each other what we feel...?"

A NOTE ON THE PROCESS OF NON-AUTHORITARIAN GUIDANCE

I believe that is very important that my children do not simply *follow* me. I can be their guide in these realms... but I am not a guide to be followed! I can be their teacher, but not just for them to recite *my* lessons. No! We have to learn together! I can be their leader... but only up to the doorway of their own discoveries... and to the breaking wave of their own self-revelation... *and my own.*

We are 'of one heart' when we are at our shamanic best. But we are never wholly of one mind: each person in our circle is a wholly unique individual. And every one sees with his/her own special vision. Each of us hears in our own special way. And no matter how tightly we merge and no matter how fully we agree (about anything at all)... if we all follow the perceptions of any one member of this medicine circle... then we must leave unnoticed and un-nourished, an infinity of other possibilities.

Feeling three pairs of very sincere eyes wide-open as if that would help to reveal what I meant... helped me to jump to a new level in our sharing as we drove through the night. Perhaps saying, "I don't know!" had popped me into 'knowing.' Who knows? In any case, I suddenly broke free of my familiar daddy-persona, leapt into bravery and spoke to them from another reality (that we also share). For maybe the first time I openly spoke to my children with the formality and detachment of an old tribal shaman-elder from any ancient culture, a medicine man who danced while the night-fire sparkled in eager child-eyes. Whatever I actually said, I cannot recall. But what I meant was this:

> *"Hear my* Meaning*! Hear and Feel my* Vision-Song*, Oh My Children, Oh My Family, Oh My Tribe. For my* Vision *feels pure and I invoke it with devotion to serve your Spirits. Hear me and feel me little Sister, little Brother... for it feels that my Heart beats now in my body only to spark and kindle your Holy Fires of Life!*
>
> *"Yes! Hear my* Dream-Song *well... but hear as well these*

words of Knowing. For the greatest thing that I know is this:

"The Song I sing for You, the Sign I read for You, the Teaching I reflect to You is only the sound of One Voice in the Great Circle of Us!"

"...and anyway, when I am alone, I don't know anything at all!"

A good round of laughter broke the tension (and perhaps the pretension) of my dramatic spin. But I went on... anyway: "You know I have medicine power, yes?" (all hasten to agree and affirm, and right on cue).

"Well, I hold power in our circle only *because* you have come to me to be my children. It is *you* who have given me the Power of Fatherhood. So the medicine power that comes through me has really come from you!

"So you see... *you* are more power-full than I am! And someday your medicine will grow to be stronger than mine. Your lives will last longer than mine and You can do more than I have done. For you are the children of the Future....

"Just now, when you are little, your spirits are *using* my love and my energy (my life-force) as a launching pad for journeys of your own. And as you grow older... your own medicine journeys will take you far beyond what you are learning from me. Just wait and see... just wait and see...!

"Come on, Kids... let me hear *your* Song. Share *your* vision with all of us. Let us all share the feelings and the medicine which can only come through *you!"*

Then I fell silent. I can wait for them to hear these words at the deepest levels of their consciousness. I can wait for their response. I can wait however long it may take for them to pick up the Talking Stick from wherever they happen to be... and to find their own way to share whatever they have to share.

And even if I get impatient and feel I cannot wait to make the point... I truly know that I *must.*

AS THE PROCESS-ION UNFOLDS

Wherever we go, wherever we turn to feel the magic and the signs... *I need them to know that they are self-complete and self-*

unfolding beings... with a father and mother to guide their first steps, to lick their first wounds... and to love them into maturity.

But they do not need me to read Sign... to open Vision... or to be One with Spirit. Ultimately, I am already an archaic artifact of their birth-rite Gift of Grace. I am the daddy-droid who is pre-programmed to care for them and to struggle through his own mass of unclarities, limitations and emotional garbage... right before their eyes. Ultimately, this brave self-revelation may be the best teaching of process that any parent can offer.

Along the way, children provide such great inspiration. I know that I *use* them - and my hopes for their own emergence into self-understanding - as the bait to draw me into (and so often the light to guide me through) my own struggles of healing and growth.

Just then, I was walking the father's path alone... hoping we would all come together somewhere further along: "...so listen to what *I* might feel the sign means... and what everyone else says it feels like to them... and then share *your* meaning with us, too. Ok?"

"What does the sign *mean*... to *you*?"

In a medicine walk we talk process and we talk medicine. Only thing is... I'm the only one who has any idea what these words mean. The mini-shamans *feel the essence* of 'medicine' but that concept of 'process'... well, that one still has them a bit mystified.

I am a teaser sometimes. I really believe in the effectiveness of a good absurdist *Zen* sense of humor! I 'talk process' with them - like talking about who should listen to who 'read sign'... and how to always look for your *own* meaning - and then I tell them that *this* is 'talking process!' And then they begin to grasp it:

Talking about *what - how - when - where - why*... and *why not*... is Process. And the *Zen* of it is that this is completely circular logic: talking about process is precisely the 'process' we have to talk about!

Now *that* is something to think about! Process turns out to be whatever we share... and whenever we talk about what we are sharing... we are 'in-process.'

The mind-set of the child is truly amazing! Children can grasp circular logic and circular abstraction better than most adults: they are at peace with wildly jumping dimensional shifts and conceptual downpours... because they live amidst endless maelstroms of change and are constantly plunging into the depths of 'The Great Unknown'... and because they are used to doing whatever they may need to do... to find out whatever they need to know... to become masters of their own universe of experience. Every child knows the power of dis-covery!

Exchanges of words carry energy and energy evokes meaning (feeling) and words express meaning and meaning is energy which evokes words which carry meaning. Yes, it *is* Circular (and also tautological as well). But it is also true. And the beauty of circularity in mind-logic is like the beauty of a circle of hands and hearts: You can enter anywhere. Any place you enter has meaning. Wherever there is meaning... there is reality. Grasp-feel-know any reality and you truly have direct access to *'The All and Everything.'*

And no matter how bizarre 'it all' may be... it is easy and natural to feel secure when everything around you... everything in your whole-being experience... feels so absolutely *real*!

SINGING THROUGH OUR FEARS

Our 'Medicine Wheels' van drove through the winding roads of the twilight forest without any lights, pulling on its own wheel to guide itself into the first road that headed toward a known stream.

Just before the van stopped, we passed a huge tree stump - the remains of a six-foot thick giant gum tree, original growth felled by eager settlers (like so many before and so many since). All heads turned as we slid past this gloomy giant... and without a word we all clicked on this symbol as our first real sign. Make what we might of a faulty second-gear downhill coast... *this* was 'real medicine' and *this* was our first real medicine sign of this night's pilgrimage into the subtle *Realm of Vision.*

But even though we all saw that tree stump and felt our insides jerk with the power of its immediate *feeling*... we carefully parked the van and moved well away from the vehicle before we began to breathe into the trees and the forest, to let go of our usual mind-stuff and to really open to feel whatever medicine was to come to us that night.

We always move away from the van before we begin this careful and conscious in-breath. But we do not move away from the van because it represents some gross level of materiality and mechanical-technological reality that we are trying to escape.... No, we *like* our technology!

We move away because the van is an extension of our home. It carries blankets, mattresses, food, water and extra clothes and weather-change gear. In fact, it carries so much of our worldly home-life within it at all times that we have found that we must make a formal 'leaving' of its familiarity each time we begin a medicine walk, if we are ever to feel really alone - or really *one* with the forest. As soon as we drive off in our van... it becomes Home. It is our haven. And when we go out into Nature for a medicine walk... we are seeking newness, surrender, adventure... and the pure Magic that only virgin Openness can bring.

So on this warm summer evening we left our home-base security capsule and headed bravely out into 'The Great Unknown!' We walked a few feet and then I asked if anyone had any strong feelings about anything around us. Each one of us is a channel for a different and endless song. No good asking the whole tribe - I have learned that I must ask each Little One in turn if we are ever to hear the whole choir sing our song. And so I did. And each one said, without a moment's hesitation: "I feel that big tree stump over there!"

We walked very slowly toward the huge monolith of streaked and eroded wood, with spears of wood-tissue still clinging to its most stubborn growth rings, still resisting inevitable change and collapse.

We were all eager to tell what it *meant* to us... what it *felt like*... what it would *say* to us... what we might *learn* from it.... After we had shared and shared all our projections, feelings and expectations...

I asked everyone to stop before we approached the tree to really feel what kinds of other energies or beings or spirits might be living there.

"Fairies!"

"Elves!"

"Tree Spirits!"

Or maybe... 'all of the above.' I shared their excitement. Sometimes such eagerness brings prickles up and down your spine... when you are close to something very meaning-full. It might be a medicine vision, a guided encounter with some other life-form... or merely your own child-like thrill of the fantasy of elfin lore and *The Magical Realm of Faerie* (that pagan, slightly scary kind of *Faerie* that is woven through all our ancient European anccstry).

But... fantasy or genuine 'close encounter:' *it matters not at all!* Live it! Feel It! BE IT! *It is all one experience*... and it may be the only Reality that we can ever know firsthand!

"And what do you think we should do when we come close to a

place where elves and fairies and devas might be living...?" I asked the little shamans. (No answer).

"What do you think we could do to let them know that we are coming to be with them in a peaceful and loving way and that we don't want to disturb their magic here...?"

Joah Froggy cleared his throat and assumed a very dignified pose. And then, half stating and half asking said, "We could sing them a song...?"

"What a good idea! And who knows a good song for sending our love to the elves and fairies?"

"*I* do," said Joah, eagerly, dropping his serious demeanor like the costume mask it was and lighting up like the inspired five-year-old that he is... "I know a really good song. Do you know 'Twinkle, Twinkle, Christmas Star?'"

I laughed inside. It was summer. Christmas seemed long, long ago, as south-of-the-equator season flip-flops made the notion of our just-past antipodean, strangely summer Christmas seem suddenly so distant and misplaced in time and space. But anyway, here we were about to sing his latest song to the elves. And why not? I'd never heard it before. Joah learned it at kindergarten. Now we all know it. I think you already know the tune. The words go like this:

"Twinkle, twinkle, Christmas Star
Tell me is it very far...
To the place where Jesus lay
Fast asleep upon the hay...?
Twinkle, twinkle Christmas Star
Tell me is it very far...?"

Sing on brave medicine families everywhere! The retro words really don't matter at all... and heart is everything!

And on this night our *One-Mind-One-Heart-Circle* was very, very strong and shining out all through that dark and magical forest!

We were all holding hands and walking up to the mighty elf-tree in a crescent moon-shaped line - a line that exactly mirrored the quarter-moon crescent above us.

The crescent moon is an important shape for medicine work, for it creates an *implied* circle. And this implied circle is also an *Open Circle.*

The very openness of this magical shape makes it a natural

sender-receiver of all kinds of energies. Its openness invites things to come in... and to pass out of the circle it suggests: energies, beings, spirits... or whatever.

It is also a vessel that holds whatever we *are* at any moment. As we walk it projects our energy outward in front of us like a softly curving dish-shaped antenna. And, at the same time it is a gentle scoop that collects and includes whatever we are to meet. It invites energy to come into its center (our center) and 'gathers' it up to enfold it in our trusting bond... to be with us... and to be within us.

Thus prepared and cleared and focused and open... we finally reached the base of the Great Tree. And as soon as we were there, we were immediately awed by the complexity of the world we discovered: little caves had been carved into the stump by the spirits of Wind and Water... and probably many other more purposeful life-forms as well. The opening of each little tunnel of darkness was festooned delicately with spider web silk, all luminescent in the light of Grandmother Moon. We could all sense at once that whatever might pass through *these* delicate doorways must be very sprightly... and very magical indeed!

Around the outside of the huge tree-skeleton life flowed in highly organized waves of orbiting mosquitoes and gnats and other light-winged beings. From every crack and cranny, the omni-present Australian Ant peeked, scurried and messaged its minions with news of our arrival and ant-mind's best guesses as to our intentions and capabilities... while always totally sure of its own.

The tree trunk was bleached white in those places where its softest wood still clung to the form of the harder rings, so huge and elegant moths were attracted to its reflectance and they flapped and furred the warm and damp night air with their delicate and delirious passage. It was a very power-full place to be!

We held hands and watched for a few seconds... and let those few seconds of clock-time stretch into an endless flow-by of real-time meditation... together. And in times like this... even our medicine family actually gets to taste natural stillness and real (beyond 'intended') silence.

I came up from my light trance state in good time to find a very warm and very sensitive boy-hand wrapped fully and firmly around just one of my probably massive-feeling fingers... and communicating a vast wealth of data with just a few twinges of a few unconscious muscles... squeezing Daddy's hand for security... instinctively clutching out to me, to find a little respite from a little touch of some fear which was sneaking in to the Froggy's world somewhere at the far corners of his awareness.

"Are you ok, Little One?"

"Yes." A long pause followed. I was expecting it. We all waited it out. It is a little ritual we are used to observing when talking with the Froggy Joah Jai. "Yes... *but*..." (squeeze)... (squirm)... "I think maybe there is something in those dark trees over there!"

"Hey! Fantastic! Let's go see, shall we?" It wasn't at all what he'd expected (or maybe it was). But how can anyone resist being reassured by the sheer absurdity of a big daddy who is so openly and shamelessly eager to plunge into what feels, just then, like the scariest place in all the known universe...?

The truth is... you cannot! No one could. That is one beauty of pinning your hopes on a still-infinite father. If he says, "Hey! Let's dive into it!" Well then... it just must be all right... somehow...?

We each and all *use* other's reactions to confirm or dissipate our fears. When it looks like everyone else can handle something, it can give us a strong camaraderie: "Oh well. If *they* can do it... so can I!"

Of course, it can also fill you with terror... but only if you let your self-self imagine that everyone else just doesn't understand... and only *you* have sense enough to be afraid.

It can go either way. But if you are five and you are out at night with Daddy and a few other bigger-littles... then it is probably better to try to keep up with the Old Warrior - *wherever* he might head - than to stand and face your fear-demons all alone. Because at five, and at night, even if he *is* really crazy... *he's driving!* And it's the only van going your way. So you might as well jump in for the ride-of-your-life! And so they do. And so he did.

And so we went to see what we could see. Wordless boy-hand clutched my own as we moved once again, O Dear Children-of-Trust, in to the mythic darkness of the tree fern rainforest on this special Night of Deep Magic.

Yes... it is time again: we must do it! We don't know what is in there. It is dark. It is scary. It is so incredibly breath-takingly exciting... we just *have* to go. For after all the fears and fantasies have played through our minds and pulled at our soft belly-centers... *there is simply nothing else to do!*

Night plies its same illusion after every sun-down. Night plays this game of now-you-see-it... now-you-don't... on every level of experience that it can possibly touch. But there is a way through the natural fear and trembling which comes up in all humans in the night:

GO GENTLY INTO YOUR FRIGHTENED PLACES! Give your Self the gift of patience. Take the time you need to feel right about each step... *but do it!* Move steadily ahead.... Walk with Fear and walk with Grace... but move right ahead in spite of 'It All' and dispel the darkness with your Trust and your Innocence... (and hold onto Daddy's hand just as tightly as you can).

And from *inside* the gloomy darkened thickets of your deepest fear... from inside the place of the most total darkness... there will be Light all around you and everything else will look bright and safe! It is such a short time that I will hold such *power of promise* of absolute safety for my little ones. I hope that we all use and learn from this Daddy-magic while it flows deep and strong and invincible... so that we may be safe within our whole-life experience, forever and ever....

In time the little hands loosen their grip and without a word, we all know that *Night-Fear has passed through us... and Fear is with us no more!*

On this occasion, what seemed to be the gloomiest, scariest, darkest place in the whole world opened up to reveal a gently grassed knoll. Trees swooned overhead and braced bare outlines of branch across the arc-mooned, dark blue Father Sky. And as we stood under (understood) their embracing arms... we began to hear a magical song of water devas (spirits) here and there as they glittered and played in the clear-night air.

THE GIFT AND THE SIGN OF WATER-SONG

Yes! It was Water. As I'd been feeling... and as I had wanted. We could hear the music of the unseen water-dance in special places with clear focus as it fluttered across rocks and pebble beds along its unseen course, between what must have been some deeper and more silent pools. (That I knew that this walk would take us near a stream made no difference to the freshness of our experience). We had found water by its sound!

The sounds of running water are always beautiful. Usually, though, we *see* the water flowing and so our experience is as much visual-eyes'd as it is an experience of sound. And when we hear the sound-melange of a large river (or the ocean surf) which is out of sight... everything is usually blended into a constant white-noise roar. But when we stand in the darkness and hear water rippling in a shallow stream nearby, tickling pebbles and leaves and sticks as it passes... each tinkle and each bubble becomes an exquisitely intimate and highly complex sound-event.

When sight falls away with the daylight, hearing leaps to a higher level of sensitivity, energy... and new meaning comes with every sound. When hearing is expanded by the darkness... every ripple and change in the water-flow brings new chimes and rhythms and melodies to our ears.

The sound of this water-music was immediately sign for us all. The sound attracted and pulled at our awareness. But we knew that the meaning of this sign was yet to be dis-covered... and must arise from within each one of us, as we each responded to the subtle music of the dancing waters in our own ways.

And so we stood in silence - yes, again, *true* silence - breathing in the darkness and breathing in the water sounds. From our hideaway under the spreading tree limbs we could see that all around us was a clearing, grass covered and safe for our sightless night-walking. So we closed our eyes and gently *walked in sound*, hearing and feeling the burbling brook as it arched slowly around our little, grassy safe-space.

We could not hear the entire stream, of course, only the parts that were singing the loudest: the little rapids and banks of shallow, pebble-paved, natural sluices. And as we walked in darkness and in wonder (and in silence, still) there came a point at which the water-music from the rapids to our right yielded to a louder and more distant water-song which began to reach out to our hearing from someplace ahead of us... a place that was cloaked in the mysteries of the impenetrable night... some yards (or perhaps miles) from where we stood within the easy security of touch.

This subtle change in the source of our sound-sign at first passed unnoticed by the mini-shamans. I guess this is what I am here for: to notice and to say, very softly, "Now let's stop here for a moment and just listen...."

"Where is the loudest stream-singing coming from right now?" (They pointed fingers ahead into the darkness, mostly still in silence).

"Now let's hold hands and just walk backwards about three steps. Now where is the clearest water-sound?" Hey! Now it was clearly coming from behind us.

Next we walked carefully ahead again, very quietly, without holding hands, listening intently to the water as we went. And eventually we came to a place of *perfect balance* - where the sounds from behind were exactly as present as the sounds that came from in front of us. And we found that we could rock back and forth on our heels and toes and actually 'adjust' the levels of each sound until we were completely *centered* between the two streams' water-songs.

It was a beautiful feeling to stand there together, rocking forward and backward as we breathed in the most delicate and musical night-sounds that we had ever heard!

And as we all had found our *own* sound-center places, the shape formed by our positions once again traced the graceful shape of the crescent-moon arc. And it is this kind of happening that seems so random... and yet so precisely coordinated... that awakens meaning inside us.

We were a crescent shape - that special kind of Open Circle that has such great gathering powers - and we were an antenna! And our shape began to reveal to us the line of the *'Path of Sameness'* - as it traced through space the balanced meeting point of *'The Sound of Two Streams Laughing'*... the *only* pathway that we could walk through that clearing along which the pure water-sounds would remain balanced and centered.

It was the way anyone might walk who did not want to give up the rich music of either sound-stream. I moved slowly to follow this line of centered sound. Now, for me, the line of balanced sound itself became the sign. I wondered how far we could move along this line of balance... and I wondered what meaning might arise if we followed this invisible path.

It seemed a clear direction. It seemed the only thing to do. But just as things began to feel (at least) this clear... we noticed that Kira Sanh was no longer on the same sound-path as the rest of us. As so often happens, Kira was hearing her own 'different drummer' and so had moved out of synch with the rest of her people. I am learning to trust her difference: she is inspired (guided and in-spirited) in ways that I have never met before.

I have been told very emphatically that she will always be (in the words of my own guidance) "strange and wonderful"... and that I must make safe place for her special ways and celebrate her special consciousness.

After this clear incoming message of guidance, I spent weeks telling her over and over that I found her to be "a very *strange* and very *wonderful* person." I celebrated her difference and shared this with the family circle again and again. I walked very carefully in this realm as I did not want (of course) to implant notions of 'strangeness' in her which might condition her to feel badly in (or about) herself.

And it was moving to see my caution *and* my risk-taking so rewarded! For Kira began to recognize that I was (and perhaps for the first time in her experience) truly beginning to empathize with the *difference* of her experience. And the further we explored... the more she felt free to open to her own special magic... and to share it with me.

Through this little *Ritual-of-Acknowledgement*, Kira seemed to discover that she had a true ally in me. Someone who may be willing (if not always able) to try to appreciate the world from her point of view and to see things from her different ways of being and feeling. And I (too) was excited by this awakening of such deep bonding and trust between us. Places in me which had been filled with reticent question and some resident perplexity were suddenly being infused with Wonder... and en-lightened with pure Kira-magic!

And Kira... well, she seemed to begin to feel stronger in her self... and seemed to feel more trusting of her own experience than she had ever been before. She was finally coming out to tell us up front and out loud what she felt and what she wanted. She began to feel more comfortable in herself, it seemed, now that her (obvious) difference-of-experience was being *recognized* and *reified* (i.e., 'made real' by my and our acknowledgment), and *accepted* and *affirmed* by her family. [Note: These are all discreet *and essential* steps in the process of *inclusion* of any attribute, any feeling... and any one].

Have you ever felt your self to be 'different' than other people? Perhaps even different than *all* other people? This is an experience often associated with adolescence. In a way it is (always) an illusion of the ego, striving to differentiate itself (your self) from everyone else. But in another way... it is also always true.

We are all different. We are each the elephant around which the proverbial ten 'visually challenged' people grope and cluster trying in vain to define the whole from their small slice of subjective experience.... And as well, in one way or another, we are all vision-impaired... and all groping to find the same truth... through our very different experiences. So whenever our own 'strange and wonderful' difference causes us despair, we can re-mind ourselves that, we may not be able to choose what we are, but we can choose a few good people to reflect back to us their own self-impressions - and in that sharing may find all the reassurance that we need.

Whoever can see and celebrate our individuality, our difference... our 'specialness'... *those* are every shaman's best friends!

Meanwhile, O Dear Reader, back in the glade of River-Song Darkness... I am still walking the line of purely balanced sound... and the strange-and-wonderful Kira Sanh had (once again) found a different place to stand.

I had to leave the path of balance to get to where she stood. And despite all our recent progress of intimacy and trust... somewhere way inside I still have a way to go: I felt mildly saddened that Kira might have (once again) missed out on the moving experience that seemed to flow so easily through everyone else.

(For, you see, I am still working on it: my joy in learning to share and celebrate her 'difference' does not yet fully offset my sense of uneasiness at some of her off-the-wall tendencies! The lesson is to learn to dance with both, I suppose, until they (and she) become an integrated, whole One-ness.

On this night, when I found that her attention/sensitivity/communion had apparently 'gone walkabout' (yet again), I think I said something really lame and probably irritatedly bitchy, like: "Oh look, Kira found some *other* place to stand. Is that *really* where the center-place is for you, Kira?"

But she did not respond to my half-veiled unclarity and simply said, with great firmness and surety: "Yes."

I stilled my own egoic attachment to the whole show always (or ever) going 'my way' as best I could, as I moved to share her 'different' experience of place.

And as I approached I moved into what this child already discovered... but hadn't yet realized that she'd found: there were *three* distinct sound-streams for us to bathe in... not just the two that I had been so proud to notice and share.

And only from the place where Kira was now standing, we could hear a new bubble-sound dancing out to us from behind the same large tree which had first been our medicine-place of Joy and Fear - and which had then become our place of safety and awakening into the sound-magic of the first two streams! And of all of us... only Kira had heard that third sound source. By drifting away from the guided experience which I was offering, she had once again discovered a new dimension of experience... far deeper and more complex than ours.

In the silence of the night I uttered a private little father-prayer which resolved my despair at my own ignorance and lack of faith...

> *"...and may it all-ways be like this for her.*
> *May she always be thus...*
> *And may I learn and learn to let her Be...*
> *And may it all-ways be so!"*

So, together we had found and formed a line of balanced water-song experience... and within this softly arcing meditative moment, lacing its way through linear Time and Space and Darkness, our sharing of the merging and balance of the sounds of two streams running had given birth to a third dimension of space: there were now *three* streams of water-sound to hear and to feel and to teach us... whatever it was that we had come here to learn.

And now, instead of a crescent-moon arcing line... we were a Medicine Circle once again!

Our meditative moment dissolved into worldliness with cascading peals of kid-laughter and all-at-once chatter and some 'show-and-tell' about what we had all experienced.

And when my turn came, I got to say and celebrate what I had learned from Kira, once again, yet again - *"...and may I learn and learn to let her BE... and may it all-ways be so!"*

Joah Jai got to recite his catechism of how he transmutes Night-Fear into bravery. Ami got to tell us how she had probably actually heard the third stream too... maybe even first... but had thought that we were supposed to listen to just the two *main* ones that Daddy had invited us all to hear.... And Kira restated exactly what I had said about her (and my own) experience, using great quantities of Word and Time to do it....

And then... following some unseen-unheard impulse... we all suddenly looked up!

Above our heads soared the tree-branch frames of our earth-plane visual universe... as I have already said. But now we noticed that the tree itself had chosen to grow in a perfectly centered place of balance exactly at the meeting place of the *Three Streams of River Song.*

And there was more... for over its long lifetime, this tree had generated three main branches. And each of these branches (of course) soared upward and outward from the tree-base to meet and to shelter exactly those places where the three streams were bubbling with excitement and singing out loud! And so the place where we stood began to take on even greater feeling of importance. And with that, of course, the possibility of even deeper meaning:

We had come into the primordial Darkness under a magical tree to meet the darkness of our fear. There we had come to realize that in the darkness of the night... the safest place to be may be exactly under the darkest tree!

And by coming into that special place - where visual-eyes simply did not work at all - we had opened our awareness to an amazing music, a sylvan song, a musical dance of water-sprites which helped us to find wonder and joy where there had once been dread and fear. And this profound *transmutation* of energy and feeling would have been medicine enough for us that night.

But as so often happens... once the medicine was found - once the magic had begun - the teaching just went on and on. For no sooner had we found the healing for our fear... than we discovered that there were two streams running... and that we could balance our body-minds exactly between these two streams of water-song, moving and floating between these two pure voices of what must surely be the only streams that ever were.

And then, even beyond these wonders, *Walking the Sound-Path of Two-Streams-Running* had caused us to form an Open Circle New-Moon Invitational Crescent that both reflected the shape of the Great Moon above... and also called out for other beings to come to us.

Next, and as if we had not already found meaning and magic enough... suddenly there were *three* streams of pure water-sound... and our universe-of-experience unfolded and expanded even further as we opened our awareness and moved from linearity to circle-consciousness once again... only to be moved still further when we found that all of this experience was clearly earthed and centered by a gracious tree which both sheltered us and pointed us to each magical nexus of pure water-sound along that gentle night-stream in that ancient land... and sounds which must have been bubbling around and through that little stream for at least as long as that lone tree had been growing there.

Stunned with pure Wonder, we just have to ask: "Who writes this stuff? Who thought up *that* one...?" And then all we can do is laugh. Inwardly sure, newly assured or implicitly reassured, all we can do is sink into the deep wonder of *'It All'* and laugh and hug and laugh some more....

Well, Tree had obviously *chosen* its Place... and its Purpose. And Tree and Stream must have chosen each other for this delicate *Dance-of-the-Tao*. But even beyond their mutual entwinement, and just at this place where our medicine family had been summoned... Tree and Water and Earth and Air and Sun and Wind and Time and Space... and Elementals and Devas and Faeries of all kind and feeling... had all somehow merged into an experience of perfect balance and wholeness.... And *we were there* to marvel at the all-and-everything in a rare and beautiful moment of perfect inward peace and such exquisite wonder... as we hugged each other close in silence (and for warmth) in the ever-deepening chill of night.

But even so... and with all of this feeling of great contentment and full-fillment... our discovery and our teaching was not yet finished. Still more new wonders were to enfold and enlighten our medicine walk on this special night!

THE SIGN OF THE CIRCLE

As we stood on the bank of the little stream and watched the sources of Kira's 'third stream of sound,' Joah began to feel pretty thirsty. And then Kira just had to have a drink... and then Ami, as that ol' Desire spread through our circle like any other good idea.

But even though we were standing by the very edge of a sweet brook, it was not drinkable water and there was nothing I could offer the mini-shamans then and there... except to "Wait and see what happens next!"

And as we sorted out whether we could wait, wanted to wait, would wait but only if Kira waited too, we suddenly became transfixed by a new Vision:

From the gloom on the edge of the far shore of the stream we began to be able to see a place where the bracken ferns almost touched the surface of the stream. And almost hidden in the ever darkening shelter of this cloak of ferns was a small pool of very still water.

The stream itself might have been about six feet wide herc - or perhaps much more vast, depending upon how old you might be, or how old you *felt* just at that moment. And the little pool we had just noticed was perhaps just one foot across in real-time size.

Then we noticed (and all at once) that within that sheltered pool, there were four or five floating leaves. Green, fresh, crisp, whole leaves... so fresh that they must have fallen into the water only minutes before... or so fresh that perhaps they were magic leaves which had been there forever and could never die! How were we to know? (And what would it matter anyway...?)

Anyway... whatever way... as this vision came to us, every leaf was curved upward, as though each were arching its back and floating with only its belly poking out from the black depths of the night-stream water and into the soft exposure of the pale moon light.

Each leaf was equally spaced from the others and all the leaves were *swimming* - yea, actually swimming, for it could not be seen as anything else. The leaves were swimming around in a perfect, clockwise circle!

It was the Medicine Wheel... it was our Family Circle... it was the Circle of the Mother Earth... it was the endless circling of the ocean currents... it was the Tibetan Wheel of Life.

We watched, entranced and amazed. It was so powerful to our so-open senses and feelings - already so finely attuned and expanded by what we had experienced up to that moment - that we were wide-eyed and wholly open to sign and meaning and vision, however such magic might appear...!

AND THE PROCESS IS ALL-WAYS THE SAME

Medicine Walks, Vision Quests, Meditations, Channeling Guidance, Conscious Conceptions, Tantric Lovemaking and *Free-Ritual Shamanic Healing Rituals* all have something in common:

> We must somehow begin by focusing our *Intention*... and yet we know that *'all intention is ego.'* But even so...
>
> We are *persona*-fied beings and so we must begin somewhere that our *personae* can go... and so...
>
> We begin as best we can... *looking for* Sign - Feeling - Meanings - Surrender - Magic - Presence... and Spirit.

We 'assume the position' - whatever position/practice we know... and whatever our inner cultural programs will allow.

We move through the *asanas*, the *mudras*, the *mantras* or the stylized breathing of our latest esoteric lore... whatever.

We Visualize, Affirm, Open and Hope... and all of these things are expressions of our Intention... our Desire.... (and all desire is an expression of *ego*).

But when any of these magical processes really begin to work... then all of our best intentions and well-rehearsed practices simply and completely fall away... as the pure power of the light of 'that-which-lies-beyond' - beyond the 'all and everything' which we can ever hope to imagine - comes floating or crashing into our awareness, takes full control of all of our senses, all our mind-processes and our highest vision... and invites and draws and propels us into the *Pure Revelation of Transcendental Experience'...*

And we are catapulted into those realms of consciousness where there is *no* doubt, *no* consideration... and, yes, not even the slightest remnant of any mind-self remaining which might be *able* to doubt or analyze or judge....

And there we meet Infinity
And so we are One with Spirit
And there we must become to BE
The Unified Circle of the Medicine Wheel
And so rediscover the One-ness that we all-ways were.

Sure... 'Do what thou wilt' is ok to get things *started* - and may be all that you can do. And of course, in the end (as in the beginning) it matters not at all which technique or practice you will follow. Anything that 'works' will take you to the same and only wholeness.

But no matter what you do to get things moving, when your process really begins to 'work'... then it will take you over so overwhelmingly and so completely that 'you' (your ego-self) will be lost... and found... and reborn... and reformed... in to pure Wonder and the Light of Revelation.

And whoever or *whatever* you thought that 'you' were... will simply cease to be.

WATER CIRCLE MEDICINE WHEEL RE-UNION

We watched those leaves swimming around and around for... ever... in that time-less space of intimate wonder.

Without saying a word, we all knew that if any single leaf so much as missed a beat, moved away from perfect symmetry in any way, or bobbed up and down in the water in response to some unseen force... that this moment of deep ritual medicine would be over and what had been 'magic' only a moment before would suddenly seem like nothing more than an eager illusion of our own collective fantasy.

If *anything* broke this powerful symmetry... the spell would have been broken for us all and we would have laughed (or sighed wistfully, perhaps) and moved on to other things.

But it did not. The apparition wavered not at all. The water changed things not at all. No wind or wave or bubble or transient floating debris dared to break this perfectly described Circle of Wonder.

And as we began to *believe in* what we were seeing, the medicine of this vision grew very strong and clear:

There were four leaves in the circle... and four of us standing in the light of their dancing spell on the bank of the stream.

The slowly circling leaves transcribed the path of the four cardinal points - the *Four Directions of the Medicine Wheel* - in a dynamic flux of becoming: north becoming east becoming south becoming west becoming north. And as with any circle, without beginning and without end. In time - over time - through time - *beyond* the living entity of Time itself.

And as the darkness settled in still further, with its usual sureness and absolute authority, the leaves became indistinguishable from each other. And so we experienced the *tantric* re-union of North and South, East and West... and the dynamic synergy of the *Circle of One-ness* which could enfold and dis-solve away all boundaries to total harmony and mutuality.

Once again we had found our medicine... through the ancient Elf-Tree... through the Water-Song... through the Secret Pool... through the Water-Leaf Circle... and through our Heart-felt Communion as we stood together in such reverent learning and wonder-full Celebration.

And we were all of One Mind and of One Heart.
And so we were All One with 'the All and Everything.'

And although these various symbols and shapes and coincide-ences were amazing, the real medicine, of course, lay in the *effect* that all of this experience had upon us - each alone, and all together. The real medicine is always the magical effect of any meaningful experience. And in our sharing of such gentle and perfect peace and quiet (!) and wonder... our separate faith in Nature and in the rightness of all things took a great leap... and we met at a higher and clearer level as a New Circle of Being. And so we were enlightened, each and all, and so we were also re-bonded, re-consecrated and ever so powerfully strengthened as a family... and as a medicine circle. And *that* is the 'real medicine' of it all!

THE RETURNING

There is a natural ending to all things... a time to turn away and move on to the next breath... or touch... or feeling. When there are no clocks ticking away in the background/foreground of your mind and no rules to follow, Time will sort itself out very concisely and clearly. And so we all could feel exactly when it was time to move on.

As though acting on an unseen signal, every one in our little *Circle of Wonder* suddenly drew in a long breath and raised or turned our heads to meet each other's here-and-now eyes and to see what was to happen next.

But just as we might have been about to speak for the first time in many (uncounted) minutes... we *all* startled at the sight of a wholly new apparition!

Some distance away from the stream, slightly behind us, and in the darkest darkness of the great tree's over-reaching stance... there were little fairy-lights dancing around on the ground. Not points of light. Not rays or shapes of light. Just amorphous little globlets of light where there should have been none at all.... And they were actually and undeniably *dancing*.

Our would-be-objective science-minds know all about visual

perception and night vision. In our science-heads even the little ones can understand that spending a long time in the dark allows us to see better - with our 'night eyes' they say. And when we are older we learn that the 'visual purple' (rhodopsin) that we need for low-light vision is bleached out of the retina by light... but begins to accumulate as soon as we are in darkness. And so forth and so on....

Now scientists know this... but scientists do not (have to) deal with the often overwhelming magical *experience* of seeing something where there was nothing at all, mere minutes before.... But right then and there... young and old... we did!

Suddenly, Breath caught in every one at once - as if we had to conserve everything which was *familiar* to us if we were to be able to look right into the face of such magical presence!

We held Breath, we let it slip away. We tried another, tentatively, carefully... and we waited. No, the Spirit-Light did not fade or go away. It did not metamorphose into fireflies or distant car headlights and move off in the way of those things. It simply stayed.

It danced. It beckoned. And we touched hands for stillness, for surety, for thank-fullness... as we walked toward the dancing lights on the most reverent and care-full feet we could find.

The magical lights did not stop as we approached. Nor did they run away. And nor did we! For by now we were clear as clear and we were all strong-hearted. And now we were ready to explore the phenomenon of this medicine vision on any plane whatsoever.

AND STILL MORE PROCESS...

For, you see... before we *could* walk toward the light without endangering the experience - or our circle (or perhaps even our selves) - we had to be completely clear in our selves *and* in the *Circle of Us*.

The sudden jolt which comes with any medicine happening (any phenomenon, vision, or whatever) is often experienced as a very real feeling of inner, physical impact which can be very powerful indeed. This sudden shock usually occurs with our first recognition of the implicit meaning of (whatever it is) and is usually dissipated as soon as we can fully *surrender*, to let the new *energy* and *power* and *message* come in to our awareness.

Once we have *Breathed-in the Sign* and heard its Voice, been touched by its Word and fully felt-through its Meaning - to each self and to the circle as a whole - then and only then are we free to begin to explore the material reality of 'what it is'... without fear of disturbing the circle flow or 'ripping off' the magical potential of the experience for any one (or all) of us.

As we slowly moved closer to our Vision of Light on that *'Night of Three Streams Sounding,'* we began to hear that the light was *also* related to a sound: and another water sound, at that. Well, at least one mystery had been solved: we had found the source of the strange lights, at last! But what material-plane happening was creating such dancing lights... and how the light made water-music... was a secret that had not yet been revealed....

Our eyes became accustomed to an even darker field and slowly, slowly, each mystery came to light: from an unseen place in the dense forest up on the hill that rose above the water on the far side of the night-stream clearing... there came a single shaft of rusted iron pipe. It crossed the stream very purposefully and came to rest upon a log which was mounted upright directly behind the dancing lights of our new medicine vision. A small stream of water flowed out of this pipe and cascaded into a very small, naturally formed basin-pool beneath it.

As the water hit the surface of this little puddle, some of it was formed into those amazing little water-balls - you know, those water-sprite beads which sometimes roll and dance upon the surface tension of water when you pour something into a vessel of calm water. And somehow these little, dancing water-globes were able to collect and reflect a few moonbeams from the moonlight which was barely dappling through the branches of our now-familiar little grotto.

So we had found out the 'secret' of the Dancing Lights.... explained in objective fact... but still not at all accounted for in the deeper realms of feeling. But there was still more revelation - and more gifting - to be ours. For painted in careful, free-hand lettering on the side of the pipe were the words, 'SPRING WATER.'

And so it was! And so we were given a drink of pure mountain water - probably a gift from some unknown park-worker who had long ago discovered the spring and then persevered to convince his/her foreman to requisition a length of pipe and a day's pay from the local Council so that s/he could tap the spring and make it available... to my Joah Jai who would happen along on a medicine walk night in the way-distant future... just happening to *need* a good long drink of fresh, pure Water as the perfect Gift of Grace to celebrate a wonderful vision-quest experience....

And so it came to be. And so we moved for Home... to tell Leia all about our multi-dimensional adventures... in our usual fast-talk and all-at-once way....

And Leia... well, she laughed and loved us all and tucked us all into our sleepy beds, sealing the teachings of our medicine walk forever with her mother's embrace and the deep medicine blessing of The Mother's good night kiss.

HIGH MEDICINE ON THE INFINITE RIVER

Moving through the endless dance of Medicine Spirit... we can seek Vision in stillness and aloneness... or through active Medicine Walks in the excited company of the children. But the process of the 'medicine walk' can be adapted to any environment... and any moment. The medicine walk can be a long roll down a grassy hillside... or a climb-and-fall from a too-high branch in a great fig tree... or the silent, stalking exploration of a soft meadow in the evening, just at 'wallaby time.'

In fact, any mode or medium will do. For any experience that involves physical movement tends to help the littlies into the (somewhat unnatural for children) state of Open Surrender... and so adds Deep Magic to our Family Process.

But of all the ways that we can find to move through Wonder, one of the most amazing experiences comes when we take our medicine walk to the great river that arcs and slides and roars and trickles through our every experience in this amazing valley. Sometimes we meet the River by wading and free-swimming. Sometimes we use air mattresses. But what we like most is to slip our (more or less) inflatable-deflatable boat into the River at any bridge-clearing that calls to us and feels just right. And then, just as soon as we cast off... we are suddenly free and clear of all our land-ties - alone together and free-falling in to certain magic and adventure in the realm of the Great Unknown!

There are those rare times when high energy levels, an actually air-tight boat, a slow-flowing river, soft weather and zero mosquitoes all combine to make this kind of medicine walk a most precious and unforgettable experience. And the medicine which comes to us in this way has *all-ways* been absolutely amazing!

We have made agreement for whenever we are floating - not a compromise as such, but an equal honoring of our two passions: our eagerness for *Play* and our need for *Vision*. And our agreement is this: we begin by paddling upriver as far as we can... with lots of noise. Laughing. Splashing. Free-falling in and out of the boat and the water until the two are one. We play and play and all the river plays with us.

We time this outward celebration with the sun's cycle so that after a good long play-time, little bodies and the sunset work together to wind down the energy of our gaudy, celebrational, upriver romp. Evening surrender begins to overtake our eager, up-thrusting 'push against the river' and whenever it feels right... we simply stop paddling... and *let go* of all intention.

And so the Medicine Walk Vision Quest has begun again. We cuddle into the boat and in to each other. We float downstream with only the barest of daddy-guidance of the craft and, of course, deep *in-process*. And so we open our's elves to... whatever Sign, Meaning and Medicine Vision is to come.

And medicine all-ways comes!

MEDICINE MINGLING WITH MONOTREMES

Powering upstream, floating downstream: our constant and beloved *Ritual of the River*. Laughing and playing as we force our wills against the currents and the winds... and then peace-full and receptive as we float back to base - back to whatever bridge or beach we'd started from - as the light falls into darkness.

In this clean Mother River lives a magical little being called Platypus. Most people know them from zoos or books. But alas, very few have met them in their natural state. And they are very different beings in the wild.

Now Platypus is not a very large being - about a two-handful body at most. Muskrat size. Platypus is a beauty: very soft, sleek brown fur and very large webbed feet; a large and flat tail section, darker brown than the body, that counter-balances both the small head with its black, beady eyes and its very wide, bill-shaped snout-mouth - which is packed with very sensitive electro-imaging equipment.

All of this makes Platypus a very unusual being. But the weird world of Platypus gets even stranger than all of this....

The males have an additional spur on their back legs that is not webbed... and carries a relatively mild poison. Perhaps this poisonous spur has only an *historic* function. That is, everything that lives in Platypus' world 'knows' the venomous spur is there... and so acts accordingly.

The platypus lives deep inside long and complex tunnel-houses that begin at the edge of the river and snake along under the forest above in intricate tunnel systems with built in flood control and winter nests. The baby platypus hatches from an egg... and then comes to its mother for breast-milk feeding. And this is a very unusual combination of modes.

Science-humans call animals that lay eggs (like reptiles) but also suckle their young (like mammals), *'monotremes.'* And there is only one other animal that does this. It is also an Australian and it is called *echidna* (or 'spiny ant eater').

Well... that's enough natural history for now. The real stuff to share about Platypus here, is about their heart, their spirit, their life-ways... and how they are as medicine friends and allies. And that is a tail to tell....

DEEP DADDY GRIEVING AND PLATYPUS DREAMING

There are only two times when Platypus can be seen in the open river: for about two hours just around dawn and another two hours at sunset. And that's it. Timed by the sun and absolutely regular. And for all the times we've floated in peace-full openness down the Medicine River, we have only seen them occasionally... and always from afar. A little brown hump just bobbles to the surface. No wave of movement, just a little 'pop' and then it's there. It stays awhile and then descends straight downward without a splash and without showing any more of its body.

If you are close enough and the light is just right, you can see their bills and tails. But usually it's just the hump of their backs that shows. Bloops into view... stays half a minute or so... and then bloops into the dark of the river... only to pop to the surface a few minutes later... and always somewhere else.

So this is what happens when you float through Platypus World in almost total stillness... or it does not. It seems that it is not at all up to us if we are to meet... or not. It is platypus' dance and Platypus calls the tune. Fair enough.

So even though we lived on the shores of a platypus river... and even though we spent so much time floating around and letting everything get to know us... most of what we knew about Platypus came from seeing them in the zoo... and then matching that information up with the bumps and bloops that we saw from our boat.

And so our sharing went on like that, month after month: we would watch platypus sign from afar as we floated down the river... or sometimes we would stop on the River Bridge at sunset to make a little river prayer and then we would see the sky reflections quiver and bulge far upstream - and from these little signs we knew that Platypus was there.

Then there came a special medicine day that needed a special medicine ritual. It was a warm, spring day in early October and it was the eleventh anniversary of the birth and death of my first daughter, Ewanee Shea.

Even all these years later, I always made pilgrimage of some sort or another on this special day. And always on this day I tried to share what I could of this amazing and terrible experience with my family - most of whom knew a different mother, and none of whom could (yet) even imagine Death... let alone all the dimensions of feeling that come from holding... and burying... your own, dead child.

Today we were floating down the Mother River in our usual, special Medicine Way. First in noisy effort... and then in silence for the down-drifting, Sunset Medicine Ritual. But today we were a little quieter. In some sadness we were, as we tried to feel-through - each in our own ways and such as our various ages would allow - the meaning of the sign of our family's First-Death experience.

I sat on the stern of the always-deflating boat and watched and dreamed of the beauty of all these children who faced me there. A snapshot for eternal remembrance of our Medicine River Journeys: one baby boy sleepily nestled and blanketed in big sister's loving enfoldment; a bigger little boy with shining face scanning all the universe for life-sign and his Destiny; middle child daughter lazing in the kitten-pile warmth as she dimpled a finger across the skin of the river, watching the patterns of light and droplets... and the eldest one watching even more closely for signs of her independent, adult life that always seemed was about to meet her around every next bend in the river....

Occasionally a water dragon (a two-foot long lizard) dropped clumsily from a nearby branch, making as big and scary a splash as s/he possibly could. Around another bend and we met the regular salute of the two-duck flap-flap as it honked and bleated itself into the sky, fleeing yet again from all possible meeting. Then the larger fish began their here-and-there evening bug-leap dance. And then all was very, very silent.

I was alone with my strange memories of all the dread and pain and urgency and horror of that death-day of so long ago.... I was alone with my inner joy and wonder at the beauty of the Little Ones that were so close in my heart that day... and especially I was, yet again, amazed at the 'happening' of my daughter, Ami... who never would have come through us and never would have been there to be the 'biggest sister' of this wonderful family, if Ewanee had not come and gone... and cleared so many of the obstacles that lay in her way.

Of course, it was not a literal 'trade' (then or now), one baby girl for another. But Ewanee and Ami were so linked... and the spirit of Ewanee so close at the moment of Ami's directly spiritually guided conception... that I always knew that I would never have met Ami - and so never have known all the joy and wonder and guidance that this best-friend-daughter keeps bringing to me - if Ewanee had not left us when she did. This realization never makes death 'right' (or wrong) but its truth is inescapable... and all of its many meanings are all-ways amazing!

And then, in the midst of all this multi-dimensional streaming of thought and feeling... 'Bloop!' It was Platypus. Right beside the boat, just beyond my arm's reach, Platypus suddenly popped into my Vision... and into our lives.

This was the closest I had ever been to the very cautious platypus. Somehow, this little being seemed to have found a brave place in its heart and had been very daring indeed! Or... perhaps s/he was just very careless and had popped up too close to our boat without intending to meet us at all. Either way... Platypus was here!

I motioned to the drowsing mini-shamans to turn their heads very slowly to see what was there... and just as the last one finally caught on to what was happening... 'Bloop!' Platypus was gone.

Well... we had had a meeting, of a sort, intentional or not. And no doubt we were just a little uncool to all crank our heads around so fast and point so excitedly at the platypus back that was bobbing there so unusually close to our boat. But our uncool was about normal for us... and so worth it to be sure that everyone was able to tune into the Platypus Sign before it popped out of sight.

Usually, when s/he is not terrified, Platypus dives to resume looking for food. Diving deep and moving its bill-mouth rapidly back and forth along the pebbles of the river bed, Platypus gets a 'scan' of what is there. If there is a little freshwater shrimp lurking there, Platypus gets a reading and even while the shrimp is being tumbled about by the platypus jiggle-wave, Platypus gulps it into its mouth. And *then*... Platypus comes to the surface... to eat! And that is why they surface at all... and that is why they never stay too long.

'Bloop!' they come. Munch munch crunch. And then, 'bloop!'... they leave.

We were so excited to actually see a platypus up close that we broke our (virtual) silence and chattered all about it for awhile, each one recounting the event at each one's verbal level. But the experience of that two-bloop Platypus Dance... now *that* was a rhythm and an encounter that we all could feel.

As we talked, I was looking ahead, for Platypus' next surfacing. And then, there it was... twenty yards away. But before I could summon all the fast- and slow-minded among us to follow the bouncing finger... well, of course... 'Bloop!' it was gone again.

I was happy enough to have seen it at all. I was open to whatever meaning this sign might bring... but at first only felt how gently and sweetly this visit had buoyed up our somewhat melancholy spirit: it gave us something new and real and beautiful and magical to appreciate. And that relief and uplift was meaning enough for me, just then.

And so we began to settle down again, into our respective arms, blankets and comfort - and I into the puddle that always seemed to 'come to me' wherever I staked out my turf at the inevitable low-point of our self-deflating boat (and hey, 'self-deflating' in more ways than one, it was, too).

And even as we 'cuddled in' (as the littles called it), my bright-eyed Joah said, "Hey, look! There's another one!"

And so there was. This was a different platypus - because I knew where the other one had gone. This one was not quite as close to the boat, but still close enough that we could see the bill and the tail just beneath the surface, and the little black eyes as the sole representatives of Platypus Mind that protruded from the surface of the water.

Another rush of interest and still more happiness saw this second friend come... and go. And then we were all very amazed, indeed. We had seen more than one platypus playing in this section of the water at the same time, before. Maybe as many as three individuals. But they always seemed to be separated by twenty to fifty yards, as they popped into and out of view during that short feeding-time just at dusk.

It was strange that today we had seen two in almost exactly the same place... and stranger still this place was right beside our boat!

And so we babbled and prattled and exclaimed and did all those 'great hunter' egoic things. Our somber Ewanee death-day mood was being lifted by having such a wholly new and remarkable meeting with these very beautiful furry beings - much loved symbols for all Australians of the natural wonders (and weird life-forms) of this very ancient and unique island continent.

We had met Platypus... and now we all knew that we were *real* Aussie bush-people, for sure!

And as we celebrated, by now having given up even any pretense of being 'still and quiet,' well... yes, you guessed it... yet *another* platypus surfaced. Only this time it was so close to the side of our noisy, bouncing, too-eager boat that I could have reached into the water and petted its back before it could have blooped away!

This was getting pretty amazing indeed! So we responded like the true medicine people that we were by - what else? - increasing our volume and our wild gesturing and our laughter, still further.

By now we were far and away the nosiest, crashiest things on all the river... probably making the most commotion since the Great Flood pounded her shores... and yet somehow (and against all principles of naturalist lore) ol' Platypus seemed to be wholly unafraid of us.

Yes... as though three 'comings' hadn't driven home the point that this was the Platypus Meeting Day... Platypus began coming from all directions, clearly to meet our tumultuous Medicine Family. Surfacing all around us, now, were more platypus than we could count. I tried to count by time, direction and any other objectifying mode that I could bring to bear... and my best calculation - or, well, my best *guess* - was that there were seven or eight individuals bobbing up and blooping down all around us... seemingly without any fear whatsoever.

Not apparently afraid of noise, or splashes, or our collective size, shape, color or erratic movements... Platypus seemed to be dancing all around us. The interface was so close, so intimate, that we were above and beyond any caring of the noise or commotion that we were making - beyond any need and beyond any ability to control ourselves at all.

Yes... we had become wild celebrants of the River Spirit and Platypus Medicine to be sure... and on that awfully aching Ewanee anniversary day, at that. On that very Day of Ritual-Celebrational Mourning we had been *met* by Platypus and we had been invited to feel such joy and such grand excitement... and we had been *accepted* in all our boisterous exuberance... by one of the most wary animal spirits of all.

Our Platypus Dance lasted maybe twenty or thirty minutes of linear time... but, of course, was much longer in terms of its feeling. And its effect has lasted... well... forever.

As we moved from cloud-concealed tears to such wild and ceremonial meeting-dance with our new, used-to-be-too-shy Platypus Medicine Allies, we had completed a great journey: yet another medicine journey from Darkness in to the Light.

Through this simple pilgrimage in to Platypus Celebration, I had been moved to yet another level in my long-range *Vision Quest Ritual Grieving*. Just before this magical experience, I had felt myself to be in a stuck-place of dry, sickly, unemptied Grief. I had felt that after eleven years of it, I was no longer free (or bound) to wallow in mourning my life's greatest loss. And yet I was still not free to fully celebrate 'the all' of Spirit's fleeting gift of such a momentary child. But through this gentle medicine of Platypus Dreaming I had been so gently urged to rekindle my capacity for joy by conjoining Joy and Grief on that very special day - and so gently invited to open yet again to my Deep Child Wonder.

But above all else, I had been shown again and again, as one after another of these gentle beings came to meet us with such mysterious and unusual Trust... and no matter what we did or how loudly we responded to each meeting... this so-simple and so-deep lesson that:

IT WAS ALL RIGHT once again, to be excited and celebrational and joy-full and childlike and awakened and amazed and full-breath eager... for the Wonder of Life itself... and for all the Wonders that were yet to come! Not just on every other day of the year... but through *every day* of *every year.*

It has taken me many years to get to the point where I could raise my hands to the Great Spirit and say in absolute openness and in whole-being Trust:

> *"Thank You, Great Spirit, for the Great Gift of 'The All' of this Experience - for the Whole Learning of this experience - for every Feeling of every dimension of this experience - for all of the Love and all the Sharing and all the Growth that has come through me in being 'The Father' to this beloved Daughter, Ewanee Shea!"*

...And then I wept for a long, long time. My children moved to hold me and stroke me and pat me with their all-sized hands and all-sized comprehensions. They knew I cried for Ewanee... and they just let me go through it within the deep-heart-space of their wholly focused embrace.

Ah yes... the Compassionate Ones: they knew that my tears came somehow from Ewanee dying, to be sure. But when I finally 'resurfaced' from my endless outbreath of release and surrender and sobs... I (finally) got to tell them that all my memories and all my pain and all my endless struggle with the life and death and burial and release of Ewanee Shea... now brought me new tears... for the very first time: *Spirit-Tears of Whole-Hearted Joy... and the Deepest Feeling of overwhelming Spiritual Thankfulness that I had ever known.*

When my eyes were somehow finally dry - when all our eyes were somehow finally dry - we were awakened from our embrace in timely Time, by the chill wind that slides up the river every night at just this time... and so we set our paddles to make for the distant bridge... and Home... brave warriors returning from far off realms of feeling... to bring all the lessons and the celebrations home so that we could feel-them-through when Time was right.

><><

CHAPTER 7

THE NEW FATHERS OF SPIRIT

LETTER TO THE SUN OF MY HEART

A Celebration for Joah, my Son…

I am bathed in your Love
As a boundless Gift of Grace
And my Heart opens in pure Wonder.
Not a sound passes your lips,
Nor a Vision fills your eyes
That does not resurge within me
And bring to me a Celebration
Of raging prideful passion
And the deepest Spiritual Peace
That I have ever known.

I AM YOUR FATHER.

I am your Guide and your Servant
And as I hold you in my arms,
Your little-body so trusting of my strength
I know inside that Time will move us onward

Until I am the Little One
And you loom large above me.
And I celebrate our exchange of Power
And all the Learning and the Growing
And all the Sharing of Heart
Which will bring us to that moment.

THE PROMISE AND THE BLESSING OF THE FATHER

For everyone in our family, moving along our medicine path is always an amazing adventure. But for me, the dance has a few added dimensions, which I must explore alone. These are the special realms of my fatherhood and my role as teacher-guide-facilitator to this family of my heart. For however close we can feel to and with our children... there is always the larger perspective of the Father/Mother which we must bear (and feel) alone.

For now - at least for now - if only for now - it is ultimately up to me to *teach* my children all that I can of this grand game of consciousness and to share with them some basic ways of being - some balancing motions, some tricks, some unusual skills - which will support and serve them as medicine tools through all their coming years as they develop their own powers and bring them to play in this art of awareness and the craft of living lightly on the Earth.

The experience which I must move through alone is the *Dance of the Father-Shaman*. It is an endless exploration of leadership in which I am forever re-balancing the primal polarities of *control* and *surrender* within our medicine process.

It is a dance of guidance which must steer a course for the vessel of our family circle through the infinity of all of our inner-outer energy inputs, distractions and illuminations.

It is a dance of committed self-exploration to find new ways of feeling-through each guiding impulse, each self-limiting idea and each expanding invitation which arises in me... and in everyone else.

My father-shaman-dance is also a dance of spiritual resourcing and provision which must facilitate our whole-family 'headlong pursuit... of medicine that (I know) simply cannot be chased.

It is a dance of path-finding to help us to search together for that which (I know) will only reveal itself when and how *'it'* will.

It is the dance of the tribal scout, who must be both guide and 'wagon-master' to a monumental mass-expedition of delightful crazies plunging through the endless maelstrom of 'growing up.'

And it is the dancc of the medicine man - the all-ways all-too-frail and almost blind and sometimes-only-maybe visionary shaman - who must try to chart a path-way through an endless vision quest parade of unpredictable happenings, always moving toward an endless horizon which is un-real to all our cultural programing... but of the very deepest intimacy and highest reality to the spiritual self... and which is the very essence of meaning for those who seek the spiritual wholeness of the path of the medicine wheel.

If I search for a name for all that I feel called upon to do and be and feel, I might call my role within my family that of Leader, Teacher, Guide, Facilitator, Spiritual Channel, Resource. For I am all of these... and still and all-ways the outrageously silly Daddy as well. But within my own experience, in my own quest for self-revelation and spiritual unfoldment I know my role here most clearly as the living archetype of *'THE FATHER.'*

From time to time the power and potential of this fixed-position suddenly fills me with amazement. Maybe I bump up against some new dimension or attribute or expectation of being a father and I am startled to realize that I have someone made a permanent commitment to 'always be' the father to my tribe. Yes... somehow it happened... and now I have become one of *'them:'*

I AM 'THE FATHER,' the living archetype of 'all of the above' for all of my family. It is a lot to imagine... and even more amazing to real-ize. But it is true! For all of us Fathers... it is all true! I hope that we never need to blind ourselves to the importance of this ritual position... or disregard the importance of its profound service.

And as I carry this archetypal medicine name - of *'The Father'* - I marvel to find myself surrounded by such amazing beings as these mini-shaman children who have come to be with us for this time of parenting.

In this state of absolute Wonder, I marvel at having realized such profound response-ability.

And in this state of enchanted awe and humility I realize that *I am learning so much* on so many levels of awareness... as I arise each day to learn how to better be... and fully committed to full-fill... as well as I can possibly do it... this Gift of Grace of being... a father.

While my children are young, my expertise, my judgment and whatever understanding of medicine path which I might be able to share with them, all loom large and marvelous in their eyes. Of course: this god-like power which is conferred upon all parents is a natural attribute of the very young child's perception. And I hope that parents everywhere appreciate the great meaning that attends such unasked-for power!

Nevertheless, for all their devotion to my every word and

gesture, so much of what I try to show 'us' falls away from comprehensibility at the lower end of our family's age-range - and/or is too often aimed at the low end and makes boredom in those who are at the top of the ageist hierarchy.

But this is also an important lesson to every one of us: what seems overly complicated today will someday pop into understanding in a flash (once again that experience of sudden revelation - or *satori* - in Zen Buddhism). And what may seem painfully simpleminded today can often contain the seeds of tomorrow's Deep Revelation. So we all try to learn to listen to *'It All,'* to all that comes from any source: from the spirits of the Wind, the Trees and the Night... and most especially, just now, to all that comes from (and through) from the Father-Guide.

I, too, listen to what I say when I am in teaching-mode and learn from it as it comes through me (as it *channels* through me - just like in this writing). We all listen to what is said in our Ritual Circles and casual family circles, by littles and biggers alike... and in every sharing, *we all learn from each other.* If families can just stay open to this constant unfoldment of meaning and the invocation of deep learning and profound change that comes from even the youngest of us... then the rigors of daily-life parenting can (also) become an uplifting time of endless discovery... and for the parents as well!

One of those popular beliefs that gets so much lip service from the very New Age among us tells us that: *'Our children are here to be our teachers.'* And we've all heard it - and endlessly repeated as well. But the truth behind this platitude goes deeper than it sometimes sounds: for we are all here to learn from each other *and* often that learning (theirs and ours) comes from the *synergy* of our interaction rather than anything that is directly and intentionally shared.

That is, we can approach every moment sharing with our children with the same openness that we might approach our most surrendered and sacred medicine... for this is the home-place of some of our deepest learning and most wondrous inspiration. We can just 'be there' without being or knowing anything at all. And then, if there is a need... then understanding, knowledge... and even wisdom... can come cascading through our awareness... illuminating many unspoken dimensions of awareness, far beyond the obvious elements of 'learning to care and learning to share and learning to serve.'

So the way I might express the platitude is a little different: our children are here to serve our mutual learning and to reveal our character at every turn. What they have to teach is often nothing more (or less) than their pure reaction-reflection of whatever we are with them. And in that gentle and terrible makeover of persons into parents... we all learn so much....

We learn of self and Spirit *together*. And as well as sharing vision and meaning and medicine and all other magical, wonder-full things... a wealth of *content* and *process* is revealed: physical-science facts and principles; Nature lore and Nature magic... new ways of communicating... new ways of teaching each other... new ways of sharing and allowing and encouraging... new ways of opening to *'The All and Everything'....*

And every parent-shaman learns as s/he teaches - the content and the process and all the *unhidden secrets* of the medicine way. And *this* is *'The Ritual Teaching of the Children.'*

As any-daddy sits with his very small child, trying to find a way in to the special experience of communion that often seems so much easier when they are asleep in our arms... it is so easy to lapse into adult thought: while goo goo goes dah dah with the wrinkled up paper and the belt we just drift away to the more pressing demands of our adult world. And try as we might... sometimes we are *us* and they are *them*.

But even while we muse on our present crises and future plans, we are still being 'The Father' to them. They feel us, hear our breath, smell our smells and *love us so much*. Watching Dad drift out into a long-space vision that we cannot yet possibly comprehend will be one of the juciest experiences of growing up....

Ami came to ask me something oncc, when she was six. I said, very casually, "I don't know about that.... I don't know why that is...." Her eyes looked up with shock and confusion. She teased me by say that she "thought I knew *everything*." And I said, "Well, I don't know the answer to than one." And we went on to other things.

Many years later - after Ami had about doubled her life's experience - we were talking about the powers of children... and fathers. She told me that she could remember the very first time when she first *found out* that I didn't know everything... and reminded me of that long ago moment. It took some patience on her part to get past my rather pedantic response of, "No... I certainly don't know everything," (etc.). And when she finally cracked it and broke through to my deeper self, I suddenly realized that she was being totally earnest: in that brief exchange so many years ago... Ami had abruptly learned that I was not God - *not* the absolute, omnipotent, all-knowing, all-powerful *G-O-D* she had always believed I was!

And so I learned that there are powers of 'The Father' that lie far beyond all that we human daddies ever imagine... that live within the experience and consciousness and dreams of our children. And now, when I speak to the very young... or even the very much older... I try to keep in mind that *being* 'The Father' - living the archetype of *'The Father'* - carries with it an enormous dignity and a literally unbelievable *power.* It is the power to affirm and encourage... or to deflate and destroy. It is the power to enfold and give the gift of father-safety... or the power to judge any child 'unworthy' of our great Medicine Gifting.

And whenever I am brave enough to carry this discovery of grandeur out of my family circle, out of my house and into the world-at-large... then I find that there is a whole world of un-fathered, father-needy and father-loving people out there... who respond to a smile, a kind word or a touch from any man who carries the father-grandfather look and depth.

And lo and behold it turns out to be just as real and just as natural to be seen and used as such a resource... as it is for men to find mother-nurturance when they lie on the breast and enfolded in the arms of their lovers/wives.

Just as natural and just as sweet... but something in our culture has formed our mass-mind consciousness - our feelings, expectations and self-image - in such a way that this deep need for Father-Love and the great powers that this archetype (and all the dads who live it out) brings forth. *Deep Fathering** is so little known in the recent past generations of our western culture that it can sometimes be hard to find anyone who feels well fathered!

This deep subject is medicine work for another day. For now I would like to invite every father to *believe* that he is just as powerful and as essential in his child's life as 'The Mother.' And it may be a gift to our children if we can all remember that: no matter how wonderful, powerful, scary, magical, mythical or divine we daddies

* The *'Deep Fathering'* adventure is the basis of other works by the author, including: FATHER-TIME and an in-process title: SPIRITUAL FATHERING.

may feel (or not feel)... our children feel us as Great and Awesome. May we all find ways to learn to support each other and help us all live up to *the father-promise that we most surely made with the very thrust of the urge toward conception.*

THE POWER OF THE FATHER

Some Fathers may know themselves as shamans on a conscious path of medicine and/or as spiritual seekers on the more traditional paths of yoga or meditation... while others may not (yet) have discovered that *every Father is a Medicine Man!*

Yes! Within the very essence of this magical state of being 'The Father' lies great Medicine Power. Great magic. Great love and great full-fill-ment. Just to look into the devoted, trusting and wholly open eyes of our Children... and to *accept* the Gift of Empowerment that shines out upon every Father is to *know* that however far your fantasies of glory and grandeur and magic and purpose may roam... whatever glimpse of frightening magnificence or incredible power may flash through your image-in-ation... whatever hint of mystical revelation may dance through your dreams....

It is ALL true!
And YOU ARE 'The All' of this.
YOU ARE 'THE FATHER!'

None of us can teach any other man to father... for we must each learn it for ourselves as we move through the course. But I want to invite all fathers to really *feel* the wondrous depth of the nearly absolute Power which comes with this ritual office... which is conferred upon us with every upraised child-eye and open child-heart... this boundless Gift of Grace and privilege. And then:

Feel the profound response-ability which comes
With every Man's spirit-born Gift of Fatherhood.

Through every Breath and every Touch and every Word:

Feel It - Accept It - Express It - Share It

And *let it flow* - through every Breath and every Touch and every Word.

Through the love of our children we are *given* the power to affirm... the power to encourage... the power to support... the power to evoke... the power to channel father-wisdom... the power to consecrate lives and process and every shared experience... and the power to guide our children through wondrous change and growth and in to new consciousness on every level of their being and experience (physical - mental - emotional - spiritual).

Laid out like this, in the full depth of Medicine Word, all of this - this Truth, this Reality, this Power - surges forth as an awesome privilege. And so it is! *Spiritual Fathering* is a gift of endless learning... and one of life's most amazing adventures!

And so I live and learn and write of and from this wonder. I offer Communication Circles and Free-Ritual Initiations and convene Family Celebrations to invite and urge all fathers to meet and share and cherish this great confer-ence of father-power: to hold it in our loving hands, with trusting hearts... and with *absolute respect* for the profound responsibility that comes with it. Responsibility to our children, of course... but also responsibility to all the Spirit that we are gifted to channel for all the mothers and all the children of the Earth.

And while I can struggle to try to become clear-channel enough to write medicine word - and while I can send out invitations of many kinds to invite Us to come together in *Father Circles* to share our deepest father-child experiences with Brother Man - it is not until we meet, father-eye to father-eye and brother-heart to heart that we can discover the essential liberation and affirmation and guidance that only brother-father-grandfather Man can provide for us, each and all.

There is simply no substitute for this kind of deep intimacy and spiritual resource that men feel when we open to share our intimate experiences of fathering together. And yet... our culture is so firmly based in traditions of self-denial and aloneness.... We have so very far to go before the deep experience of the Father-Circle can be awakened in our culture....

For now, maybe forever, we all feel it differently. And we hold fast to our right to feel it differently than our brothers. But however (or if) we can feel: every father-word that is empowered *by* our children becomes power-full, magic-all, *Shaman-Word* - and so has greater potential to affect our children... and all of their children to come... than we can ever imagine.

It is so important that every father somehow come to recognize this great power that we all carry. It is *The Natural Power of 'The Father'* and as well as learning to celebrate its wonders... we also need to learn to deploy it with great care and absolute integrity.

Brother-Father-Man: *BE The Shaman of your Medicine Family!* Trust the spiritual gift of your children's natural love... and the shamanic power they endlessly confer upon you, in such open love and trust.

The gift of fatherhood is like no other gift, a task like no other task and brings reward like no other commitment which a man might make. It is a spiritual path like no other and... let us always remember:

Every Man who is a Father
Has already Chosen this Path of Spirit!

Let us work together until we can all 'walk in a sacred manner' with our medicine families... and with each other's families... and then with *all* the mothers and all the children of the Earth. And may we learn to trust enough that we can openly release whatever Word will *consecrate* our every sharing:

"Let us Walk with Meaning
Let us Walk with Power
Let us Walk with Honor
Let us Walk with Softness
Let us Walk with Love
Let us Walk with Surrender
Let us Walk with Vision
Let us Walk with Wonder
Let us Walk with Medicine
Let us Walk with Spirit
Let us Walk with Magic
Let us Walk in One-ness"

><><

MEDICINE FATHERS

MEDICINE FATHERS know that they have been given their children as Gifts of Spirit: known or unknown... whether consciously sought or wholly unimagined... however they may come... Medicine Fathers know that gift is Gift.

MEDICINE FATHERS work very hard to discover what it is that they are here to share with their children... what it is that they have to teach their children... what it is that they must learn for their children... and what it is that they need to *be* for their children.

MEDICINE FATHERS are the first non-mother human beings in their children's universe. The first of the 'others.' The first to invite and entice each child to look beyond the mother-breast, to look beyond deep-trance fixation in the mother-eyes and to reach beyond the mother-child union to begin to taste in strong and safe embrace, the wonders of the world-at-large.

MEDICINE FATHERS stand in many doorways, holding obstacles away and holding stillness in space and time to let every new child crawl through to begin anew their timeless vision quest for wonder, enlightenment and fulfillment.

MEDICINE FATHERS are there to *initiate* the Children into new realms of magic and mystery... of feeling and mind... of sharing and surrendering with others... of personal empowerment... and spiritual unfoldment.

MEDICINE FATHERS are *living channels* for the transmission of the Living Culture - to bring the best of human resource to their children and to awaken in every child all the skills and knowing that will help their children be successful in whatever they have come here to do. And when culture begins to manifest in the child's experience... Medicine Fathers help their children see beyond its ignorance and all the limitations and false expectations that Culture inevitably imposes.

MEDICINE FATHERS stand in endless vigil on high ground, holding the *four directions* and acting as gatherers, conduits, receptors and living channels... for all the subtle energies of the elemental consciousness of Earth-Air-Fire-Water-Ether... for the consciousness of embodied and etheric beings of all kinds... for the sign and vision which will awaken gifts of consciousness within their beloved children and which will, in time, enlighten each child's special purpose on this earth-plane of mortal-immortal existence.

THE FLOW OF THE RIVER AMI

This is the Valley of the Mother-Waters. This is the Valley of the enfolding Mother River. All who live here seem to know and love this place as an embodiment on Earth of the spirit of *'The Mother.'*

And it is to this place that we have so carefully and deliberately brought our eldest daughter for an important time in her endless Initiation into Woman.

We shall stay in this valley and live by these magical waters and find our Sign and our Vision here until (at least) the time of her first menstruation.

We will let her lie in the soft mud-bath of the tropical earth, let the rains and the soft moist air fall into her open mouth... let the raindrops patter on her skin and gently knock against her womb to help awaken the sleeping Woman Spirit which has been growing deep inside her own soft belly center for so many eons. We will let her feel the clear Water Spirit of the rains run down her legs until it runs pink with her own upwelling fertility-sign.

We will let her seek her own vision in the cloud-mist of the rains and in the blazing sun-light of the warm, clear, winter days. We will help her to breathe in all the signs that come to her and help her learn to read them for herself, in her own way.

With - and beyond - whatever teaching and guidance we can offer, she will find her own meaning... and so begin to find her own place as woman in this world: as a *Woman of Fire*... as a *Woman of Air*... as a *Woman of Earth*... as a *Woman of Water*... as a *Woman of Power*... of *Medicine*... of *Vision*... of *Love*... of *Peace*... and as a *Woman of Spirit*.

All of this great potential (this great potency) is alive within her, even now, as a child of almost-ten years. If we can nurture her, encourage her, guide her and companion her through these times of passage and the trials and celebrations of the many initiations which lie ahead... we know that she will be helped to bring these qualities of magic and sensitivity and power and love into her adult life.

For now, this valley is to be our family's magic-place of medicine vision... and this river is our path-way. Ami must only come to know how to live in the valley and to be *one* with the River... and the Sun... and the Moon... and the Wind... and she will emerge into her womanhood intact and clear, conscious... and whole.

For me - and for all our family - there is a great feeling of *privilege* to be able to share this unfoldment with her. And I feel deeply honored to have been chosen as one of her guides through this brief moment - this *Vision-Quest of Becoming* that we usually speak of all too lightly, as 'childhood.'

As time passes, we will see - and Ami will *know* - what difference there is in the life of a child who has tasted the archetypes of power and clarity at such an early age.

Yes... here we will see revealed whatever difference there may be in the lives of *all* the children who grow into adulthood in harmonic one-ness with their natural grace and wholeness... who grow into their ultimate manifestation as living channels of great vision and powerful medicine.

AMI'S GOANNA-WARRIOR INITIATION

One day we found a very magical waterfall
At a narrow place in the river of our family.
Here, rockwalls formed a perfect spout.
And if we wanted to move upriver from here,
There was clear choice to be made:
To move up through the waterfall head-on and directly
Or to clamber unsteadily across the slippery rounded rocks
Which bedded the wide and shallow rapids.

Ami chose to 'Walk Circle' *around this waterfall*
To feel its power and drink it in.
And as she could not walk around.
She walked right in to the pounding torrent.

There she exalted at her own strength
And her newly up-surging independence.

And as the Waters pounded against her
She drew Power from this vast energy:
She became *the embodiment of the Water Spirits*
As she stood so surely amidst the swirling foam
Braving the torrent's driving, pounding, terrifying force.
And she held perfect stillness within herself... inside.

Ami passed through many minds as she stayed there
Stayed for so long... listening to Water
And hearing for the very first time
Her own Waterfall Medicine Song.

When the song was deep in her heart
And its teaching woven all through her being,
Through every image and feeling in her wide-eyed mind...
Then she opened her eyes to welcome dancing Water-Light.

And there riding high above the water
Was a very large reptilian head... swimming
Swooping over the surface of the river
Carried aloft by the mighty body of a giant lizard
A four-foot long lace monitor.
So once again we chance to meet
The ancient consciousness of GOANNA!

Ami was at once startled-afraid-excited-eager-hungry
To blast her thrill across the Water and through the open Air...
And through the bright Sun and its living insect veil...
To all her family... and then far beyond
To any of Earth or Spirit
Who would hear her New Woman-Warrior's call:

"GO-ANNAAH! GO-AHH-NAA! GO-AN-NAAH...!" she cried...

And she sparkled and shivered with the very power of her Sound.
Meeting obstacle... aloneness... and a fear-some ally...
And turning this in to empowered Celebration became
Her Free-Ritual Initiation as a Warrior of the River.
Her Medicine Song carried along the river channel
Heralding her becoming, upstream and down.

In time we all caught her feeling
And so we all came running...
Crashing along the riverbank
Splashing through the water
Where it met the Earth at river's edge.

And then all talking and all movement stopped.
We all fell into silence
All listening, all watching, all waiting...
For Goanna to come into our eyes.

And then, aloof from all our eagerness
The great beast slowly lumbered out of the river
And rose with certain majesty in to our view.

We have met Goanna many times before.
We know Goanna is a mighty being.
In its rainforest-river home it knows no natural enemy.
In this timeless land Goanna knows caution...
But Goanna is secure in its place and in its power:
Goanna needs no Fear.

As the great lizard emerged from the dark waters
We all could see and feel its size -
It was more than Ami's ten-year arms could span.
This was BIG GOANNA!

Goanna came ashore, hooked its mighty neck and stared aside at me as I approached with eager tenderness. Then Goanna chose a tree and moved slowly up the trunk, sliding away from my vision, embracing the tree, melting into the bark. Becoming *one* with Tree.

I slid through brush that was usually impassable to me, aware of using the hiding-tree's cover. Slowly. Carefully. Until I could see the tip of Goanna's great tail flicking gently like a tempting lure, just beyond my reach.

One more step and I had hold of the huge tail. I wrapped it slightly around the tree, while cowering away from the likely hail of thrashing claws and sharp teeth. None came. Goanna pulled gently, testing our relationship, then surrendered into my care.

With my free hand I grasped a large neck which my hand could not begin to encircle and in one swirling arc moved head and body, claws and tail away from the tree and onto the soft grass of the river's floodplain.

I kept myself safe from Goanna's claws and tail and teeth... but Goanna made no complaint. In time I motioned the mini-shamans that it felt safe to come near... and so came yet another wondrous meeting with one of Australia's largest carnivores, one of the world's largest lizards... and one of the Magic Valley's most amazing and prehistoric lifeforms.

When we had all made touch and talk and had felt our awe and wonder... I offered Goanna back to the safety of its river home and we watched the wake of the powerful tail as it arced its way through the water.

When Goanna reached the opposite shore it moved heavily and slowly out of the river... and then paused for a moment to look back at us. Raised, paused, met and held our gaze for a moment... and then moved off to find its own medicine in the darkening forest.

There is no way to tell another human being who has never held such a powerful being in frightened human arms... just how it feels to be so intimate with such a mighty animal... or how it feels to share this land with true *living dinosaurs*.

Whatever Goanna remembers of us as it now lies in the sand in the sun we will never really know - for who can know how archetypes experience their effects? But what we will never forget is the Warrior Ami's Initiation and her discovery. All alone at the waterfall, staring out across the primordial black-skinned river all alone... she saw an Ancient One... and raised her voice to call her people in an ancient way. And then everything changed: for suddenly this child-woman was being self-initiated into great, new warrior powers: *The Power to Watch... The Power to Find... The Power of Calling the Circle...* and the greatest prize of all:

Today Ami became the warrior-leader of her tribe.
Today she was the First and Only One!

THE STRANGELY KEPT SECRET OF PARENTAL BLISS

Each time I See my Children
Each time I Touch them, whatever we Share...

My connection with their Spirit
Breathes silent Prayer and Offering
In pure Celebration of all they bring to me.

And then I just fall Open
To simply real-eyes...
And I am enfolded in an Inner Peace
Beyond all that I ever imagined.

Now I know that all parents (at least inwardly) feel and praise their children's overwhelming beauty. Somewhere inside, *all* parents know just what I mean:

I know we all experience IT.
And yet we all bear such secret witness
To this Miracle of Intimacy
And we keep it all so private,
Holding our pure wonderment away
Even from the Children of our Hearts.

And yet we all live in this marvel together.
However difficult all other things may be,
Yes... deep inside each parent knows
This bliss-full state of Awe and Wonder.

And still we all go our separate ways,
Walking our so different paths,
Hiding even from our selves
That strangely mortal Fear of Ecstasy
Which always gnaws at our souls
And forbids the Celebration that Life is due.

Why do we hide the Joy and Wonder of parenting?
Why hide from each other this state of Magical Union?
Why pretend away this state of Holy Grace and Bliss?

If all the Medicine Families could sing it out -
Through all of life's pain and struggle and fear -
Sing out all the Grace and Wonder and full-fillment
Maybe this could serve as the catalyst we need
To begin the Change that surely must awaken us all.

Then we might all feel invited to meet as One -
Ecstatic eye to enchanted eye... to even I...
And 'The Great Secret' *of our Blessing would be out!*

A GOOD MORNING HUG IN THE HERE-AND-NOW

"What can we say? What can they hear?
And what can we hope to share?"

There is a deep vein of Question which always runs somewhere through the mind and heart of every parent: "What can we actually *teach* our children...? What do they actually *hear* when we speak...? What do they actually *feel* when we imagine that we are sharing some deep and poignant message, some amazingly joyful revelation... or even when we are just trying to grapple with our own mortal fear and trembling...?"

These questions are not new to parents of today. These questions are not new to the whole evolution of human experience (and consciousness). But they arise anew in every parent again and again, through all time. And each of us is committed to search anew for the answers.

Sometimes I feel my communication with my children is so clear, so precise and so elegantly complete. I speak a few words - or many. They listen. They respond in ways that I can understand.

Then I nod, or we hug and then I might say what instantly feels like unnecessary Word, perhaps to make token acknowledgement of the wonder I am feeling: "Well, it certainly feels good to share like this with each other, doesn't it?"

"Yes, Daddy. I like it too....

"But yesterday I saw a Big Doggie in the garden but he didn't bite me and I didn't run away this time...."

Sometimes everything seems to *work* - except their answers to me. When I tell them about things that even most adults don't share - beautiful things, but things that might be hard to understand - I feel so heard and I feel us feeling-each-other-feeling-together. And I know we are somehow merged into that state of one-ness, the most precious state of Deep Intimacy:

I Am. We are. It is working this time.... And so it must be! No matter what they might say when they finally speak... no matter what they say....

What 'works' must be judged and felt and *known* inside. Perhaps there will be no real-word process to confirm what is felt. Perhaps there will be no 'conscious attention' which even *can* respond to whatever offer.

But somewhere every parent can be assured that their every message is being imprinted on very receptive souls.

We can comprehend from our adult-outside place of (only) slightly greater objectivity - that all of our children's deep and fleeting responses are real and true and really *do* 'mean' that we have connected.

And we need not be disillusioned or saddened by what they might say *next*... because for them each moment is so ephemeral, so delicately fleeting that each moment is hardly even there... and the linear connection of moment-to-moment is even more etheric still.

Children's words follow their attention and attention follows feeling and what we get back is a stream of awareness that flows in many directions at once and in all directions sometimes. But even through this torrent of seemingly dis-associated word-streamings... there is 'The Father' coming in and out: father-word joining in the mind-dance, father-touch awakening the feelings and father-mind raising the subject of the gift of relation... wherever it may come from and wherever it may lead.

If we dare to really surrender in to the child-world... well, there we can feel how deeply we are met and honored. And deep in that place we can sometimes see that whatever we share is at once eagerly subsumed and so becomes a springboard for the ever up-reaching child-yearning awareness as it prepares for yet another quantum leap to a new dimension of discovery.

I pick up the baby Beny Sky in the morning. We run toward each other with outstretched hope and joy. My whole being aches to feel his warm, sweaty blond curls curving and tickling around my neck and my mouth. My whole life becomes that desire for re-union and re-re-union... which is our "Good-Morning!" hug.

And when we meet I reach for his outstretched striving body and fling him up to the lofty heights of my full arms' reach and then let him fall down and down into my beard and my breath and my loving embrace. And I hold him so close that I can feel my little boy self in his baby-body; I can feel my man self surrounding him; I can feel my all too aged, infirm self trying urgently to pass onto him my gift of spirit-seed and father-blessing and guidance and encouragement....

And for a fleeting second Beny Sky and I are lost and found in true one-ness. And then, perhaps, a veil-winged insect flies by on a one-way mission to meet the Sun. And with that new stimulus, perhaps the great physical height that we are sharing suddenly impresses his eyes: the new world-view across the top of the couch, the new cosmos atop the tables, the over-the-windowsill view looking across the high meadow grasses.

And maybe then his attention loses my face and eyes... maybe loses me in fact... but it never lets go of *us*.

IT IS US that sees the new-bird rise. And *IT IS US* that celebrates the morning skies. And *IT IS US* that knows the depth of love that we shine outward to the world-at-large from the private space of our embrace.

My presence, my commitment, my power, my love, my surrender - I bring *all* of this awake in his experience (and he awakens the same in me) just by picking him up! And how does he respond to my heart-song, my reverence or my deep-father prayer...?

I guess he reacts just as I'd have him react, if I were the mover of all beings: he pulls and stretches and strives to break free of my stolid, unmoving, uninspired ignorance. He urges with every cell of his body-mind to throw himself out of my arms and then I hear his message.

I hear his Message just as he must hear mine: with the ears of the billions of cells in my body-mind which are so attuned to this little person-sprout. I hear and feel his message call through every one of these cells, though it comes to me only in little infant squcaks and egoically driven fast-breaths and "sprggzzless" sounds and clutching hands wildly reaching all around.... I hear and feel his message and his great and urgent *need*:

"I want *that*! I Want to touch *that*! I Want to put *that* in my mouth! And right now, Daddy!" *"I WANT IT RIGHT NOW!"*

MOONWALK STORY

Sometimes - a few years back, now, when we were living in a very different forest in the hills outside Melbourne - I would come to the sleeping Kira child when my writing or music work was done, sometime during the last few hours of night-stillness before the time of dawning.

I'd wrap her in a special medicine blanket and carry her gently outside. She would hardly be awake - just enough to cuddle into to me and smile a little at being Chosen yet again.... And so we were off an another of our very special 'Possum Walks.'

On these short, night-time excursions, we would rarely venture outside our garden gate. Sometimes we seemed to scarcely move at all: just a slow dance through the night, through darkness and moon light and distant house-light. We would examine the play of a shadow-slung branch as it arced across the sky, then turn and see a whole new universe of winter-rain droplets dancing through a little apple tree, bared for winter's cold.

And sometimes... only sometimes... we would see Prickle Possum himself. Prickle Possum was actually a whole family of very beautiful, wide-eyed, Australian, brush-tailed possums who lived in the attic of our house and its out buildings. All the 'Prickles' came out at night to play in the trees and find whatever fruits were ripe enough to eat (before those humans had a chance to get them).

From high or low in the branches of the mountain ash (eucalypts) or the giant Moreton Bay fig trees they called out to each other with an other-worldly, eerie sound and stared peacefully down at us, with huge and glowing eyes that shined yellow when they were touched by any light.

When we were out at night, just Kira and me all cuddled together in the chill-winter air, perhaps we'd see Prickle... or perhaps we wouldn't. No matter. It was always, still, a 'possum walk.' But really the walks weren't about possums any more than sleep is about pillows or beds.

At first, usually, we said nothing. For many minutes we'd walk along very slowly in the dark, alone together. My only effort was to try to keep her so softly comfortable that she could waken gently or even stay asleep on my shoulder.

I would try to make her space so gently open-ended that she'd feel no pressure to relate to me in any particular way. I would enfold her in the deep luxury of daddy-love and give her time and comfort so she could freely muse and meander in her mid-sleep, dreamtime voyage... and feel the depth of *us*... and how we were sharing on that special night.

In this way I found that we could meet quite simply and naturally, without getting caught up in the myriad overlays of expectations and functional relating-patterns that so often fill the doings of the day.

After some time of silence had passed through us in that special closeness which only comes to people who hug together for a long time in the dark of the night without planning anything at all, I'd often find myself (of course) melting into a deep state of wonder and thankfulness and love for (and with) this child.

Sooner or later, I'd begin to speak, to try to share with her whatever I was feeling and whatever I could understand about our life together... and to begin to talk to this four-year old poppet about Life itself.

I'd talk a bit, offer her my father-blessing, maybe a song or a chant, maybe a cry or a laugh - often enough, 'all of the above' - and we'd dance around in the rain together as I held her to my heart.

Kira was almost always silent at these times. Sometimes my man-heart felt as though it would explode with the amazing love that I felt for this little being... and from the great joy I felt at being 'The Father.' And then all this feeling would gush out in words and blessings and thanks. And as my feeling flowed into her, her little body would soften in to even greater stillness in my arms, her breath slowing and deepening, as though she were fully *absorbing* this meditative moment.

She *felt* (as though she were feeling), but she did not speak. She never spoke, at first. As time passed, the flurry of my word-song-prayer would lessen slightly and sometimes there'd be pauses, time enough for her to speak... but she still remained still. Silent. Listening. Listening with such rapt attention that I have never felt so heard, before or since. And as she listened she never brokc her silence; never let out a single sound that might give away her inner experience. And this left me free to imagine... anything!

In time, my one-way devotional song would inevitably come to an end. And whenever this was about to happen, we'd both know it. And then we'd drop into even greater depth of communion in Deep Stillness. Meeting unspoken. Stillness unbroken. But very deep in love.

It is hard to endure too much poignance, ecstasy or spirit. It is hard for me to be still in the face of such intensity of feeling. So even as she remained still in my arms, without tension or movement, I would be racing through many states of fullness, emptiness, happiness and wonder - and feeling so rich with the special empowerment of the commitment and magic and the privilege of fatherhood.

And so I was very much at peace - believing that my father-word *must* have shared with Kira at least some of my joy... and my reverence... and my deep thanksgiving.

And then, as I gradually emerged from my own trance state of blissful daddy-song and the silence that followed, I would naturally begin to wonder what Kira was experiencing. What was *she* feeling... and what did *she* make of all this?

And then... and *then*... she'd finally take a deep breath and begin to speak, as though she'd been waiting for the perfect moment - *that* moment - for her perfect reply to all that I had shared with her:

"Yesterday I was playing with my ball and Joah wanted to have it too so I tried to let him play with it but he didn't care and he didn't give me a turn and I didn't want him to be like that but Mum came in and said that we were going to go to the shops and so I couldn't finish finding all of my pictures that I wanted to take with me and I really like my cat because she licked me yesterday.... Is it still 'today,' Daddy, or is it tomorrow...? Daddy...?"

"Yes, Kira. Yes my Dear, it is still 'today.' And it's 'tomorrow,' too.

Are we ready to go back in the house and I'll slip you back into your warm little bed now?"

"Yes, Daddy...."

"What can we say? What can they hear? And what can we really share?"

There is an answer which keeps coming up for me... I cannot find it in any memory of any real experience of actually back-and-forth connected conversation. But then, possum walks are not your usual back-and-forth situation. No, during our possum walks I share as deeply with Kira as I ever have - as deeply and as openly as I possible can.

I speak my heart. I speak from the far reaches of 'The Father' archetype that I am for her. And I leave nothing out. I understand that many of the concepts that I talk about, the feelings I sing from, the cultural messages that come with sanskrit or Native American chants... and all the medicine that I am... well, I know that much of this adult deep stuff simply overloads (or washes over) her four-year old mind-self.

But I *know*, too, that it cannot be bad to share myself so real-ly and so deeply and openly with her. And somewhere, I know, *she feels it all.* And that just can't be bad. No... that can't be bad at all!

And it is very strange: I have rarely met a woman - as friend, client, sister, mother or lover - who has told me that her relationship with her father was anything like the magical sharing which I experience with my daughters. And likewise, I have rarely met a man who has spoken to me of such deep fulfillment with his father as I have (so far) been gifted to experience with my sons. (And my own childhood experience was largely un-fathered as well).

So this is a great puzzle... and a very significant reality to me. Because if there are so few of us who have been really fulfilled in our father-connections... then there must be very few fathers who are getting full-filled in their relationships with their children!

And if we look around, if we look in to all the un-fathered child-eyes and un-fathered mother-eyes... and in to the sea of uncertain and lonely father-eyes as well... we can see that this is, sadly, all too true!

So many of us are missing 'The Father' in our hearts...
And so live out our lives, carrying a gnawing father-grief.
How is it that so many of us - children and fathers as well -
Seem to be missing out on sharing this magical experience
Of the living archetype of 'The Father' *?*
How is it that so many men who are completely dedicated
To their families' well-being and support...
Feel that they cannot access these deepest levels
Of Joy and Intimacy with their beloved children?
And above all... WHAT CAN WE DO to recover
Our birth-right heritage of Empowered Fatherhood?

One thing we can do - and beginning right now - is to *meet* with each other, Brother-to-Brother, Man-to-Man and Grandfather-to-Son.

We can work together to rediscover the beauty and softness and the power that is the essence and the heart of the living archetype of *'The Father.'*

And then... we can learn to share it with each other....

And *then* we can help each other to open to share all that we can of this newly empowered Father-Spirit with *all* of our children... *And then we can begin to offer ourselves to all the Mothers and all the Children of the Earth.*

Hey there, all you Dads of the Universe! This enchanted time of Fatherhood is so short... this moment of father-magic is so special. This potential to grow through the deepest mutual nourishment and care-giving of your lives is here-and-now *begging* you to notice and so yearning for your attention... and *so* worthy of your unconditional love and Father-devotion!

And so, Brother-Father-Man, I invite you to...

Clear whatever Fear you hold -
Whatever Fear that might be holding you back -
Then Open Your Heart to Celebrate this Wondrous
Gift of Father-Grace.
Find a way to Hear this Truth - and find a Way to Bear it!
And so find way to Believe in your own good fortune...
And then 'GO FOR IT!' with all your Heart

So that even through your darkest hours
And throughout all your joys,
You will all-ways have the Power
That comes with this Deep Assurance:

Your Children are born to Receive your Love -
And they have come here to Love You!
And if you can Open to their Endless Love...
You will never again be alone.

><><

CHAPTER 8

THE INITIATION OF GRANDFATHER SNAKE

A MEETING ON THE PATH

Nearing sunset on a warming spring evening we drove away slowly and in silence on a medicine journey to the Mother River, farther downstream than we usually ventured. Moving townward as we searched for a new place to slide into the water in our little puff-up boat, we experienced a strange sort of indecision. Unsure of where we wanted to be... perhaps even unsure of where we were.

On Vision Quests this sort of confusion is often a very *positive* sign: it can mean that there is something happening (or about to happen) which is still a mystery. Felt through in this way, indecision becomes a dynamic force which is often strong enough (in its energy) to de-stabilize our here-and-now reality... but perhaps too weak to be overwhelmingly obvious.

Such a moment as this is a great time to *let go* of ego-level, material plane structuring and planning. Such a feeling as this is clear Invitation to open... to whatever is to happen... and to whatever Revelation is about to come.

So, confusion is a transition state - an apprehension before entering a new dimension of experience. And whenever confusion appears on the horizon of your experience, there are many ways to respond. You can try to plow through 'it.' You can try to ignore 'it.' You can try to sidestep 'it'... but *IT* will elude your every effort and there will be nothing that you can *really* do to clear this feeling of unrest or discontent... except:

There is always Sign. If you can hold stillness amidst even your most disquieting *'confusion of place'* and just wait, watch, sense, feel... and *surrender*... there will always be a sign. And often it will come in the form of an impulse to do something strange... or maybe just to move or act in a way you just had not planned to do.

Something even more confusing might come to mind as a possible course of action... and by moving *toward* this still-greater disorientation you can often find the key to resolve your unclarity.

So it is that in feeling-through signs and following this medicine path - as is true in all personal growth or spiritual work - we soon discover the truth of that well known saying:

'The Way Out is the Way In.'

On this afternoon we drove further and further downstream, ritually counting every bridge as we always do. When we came to the one-stop general store, we continued even farther onward... downstream... moving toward the larger town which is about twenty minutes away by car. And as we drove we looked and looked for a good place to enter the soft and winding waters where the river was really deep.... But there was no 'right' place for us there.

We became more unsettled. Kid-noise became loud and strident. The special openness which we all agree to as we begin any medicine process was slowly but inexorably abandoned... by one and all.

Finally we found a place. But it was just a place... nothing special about it. And as we busied ourselves with boat and paddles and gear... all of a sudden it became clear that we were simply in the 'wrong' place!

Now this is a petty occurrence... and it happens millions of times a day to people all over the planet. This was not a great, earth-shaking kind of magical experience. No... just a feeling of 'not right-ness' which was, simply... *the only feeling* there was! And despite the fact that we had already driven far too long and the sun was far too close to the mountain tops to be changing our direction now... everyone could feel that this was *not* where we ought to be.

So we threw all our gear into the van, turned around and headed *up*stream... and back toward our home. When we got home, we all felt in a hurry... and still heat-hassled. So Mother and Babe decided to stay home this time... and four of us continued onward....

Few words. Had to hurry. Back on the road. Upstream... bridge counting ready. New choice of bridge as a launch place seemed imminent. All systems were on efficient auto-mode.

And so we headed out again with a new optimism, a new feeling of peace and excitement... and a renewed commitment to the care-full open-ness which is needed for a real medicine journey.

After we had driven around the first bend past our house, where the road dips down to the third bridge, I saw a glorious sight: a huge Aussie python was stretched right across the road, head raised, warming itself on the asphalt... and just waiting for us.

I stopped the van and said "There's a huge snake on the road and (hooray) it's not poisonous! Everyone come out of the van!"

One came, two stayed behind - unsure in that very human way: *afraid*.

This snake was special. And *this* snake and I were going to dance! I just *knew* it. And I had already committed to it absolutely, even before I had been able to stop the van.

This was a GrandFather Snake: yes, it radiated its old-male presence. It was the largest of this species I had ever seen.... And I knew that we would surely make some kind of Medicine Dance together... in celebration of our meeting!

What remained as a great yawning unknown... was whether we would dance in simple friendship... or with aggression and fear between us. For when you approach any large wild thing which is well equipped for survival... in the wild... it does not matter who is afraid or aggressive *first*. For everything flows in a Circle: once there is fear on either side, there will be fear on both. And as soon as there is fear... there will be aggression. And where there is any aggression expressed... fear will certainly follow!

Today, I was ready to impose my egoic will on GrandFather Snake. I would pursue him and 'catch' him (if I needed to) - and if I could - just to have a few moments to feel his beauty and his incredible Medicine Power!

As I left the van, my senses were firing on all points and I could feel that I was approaching a major milestone on my Medicine Path.

I approached the great Snake with great care, from an oblique angle, making certain that he could see me well, but still coming toward him from behind so that we both had ample space to avoid each other... if that seemed the thing to do. He lay still, head raised and 'tasting' me with his tongue. But he made no move to leave.

Suddenly, another car came swooping around the bend from behind us. Intent on trying to look ahead, around the upcoming corner, the driver would surely have been unable to avoid driving right over the snake. I motioned him to slow down and he stopped for a look. Husband and wife chattered about the size of the snake and was it poisonous (a fair question in these parts) and how we shouldn't take the risk of touching it and, "Here, let's take a picture of it!" Click! Click! Click!

I stood guard over 'my' snake, used the time to urge the shy ones from the safety of our van, said little but smiled at the tourists... and just waited for them to leave.

Now for the moment of our *First-Touch Ritual*. I was not a virgin to snake-touch... but had *he* experienced any closeness with humans before? No matter... it was time to act!

I reached out in total Trust... and then felt some fear come through me as my soft, pink hand approached his well-toothed and large, wedge-shaped head. Fear: one of the greatest of all our spiritual guides!

Big Snake recoiled a bit. Fair enough. And so did I (also fair enough). As I began to reach out again I knew that I just *had* to commit to 'going all the way' this time. To mask my sudden movement - frightening in itself to any wild thing - I gently draped my shirt across his head. Then I plunged down onto his neck with my hand as quickly and as gently and as surely as I could... and slowly lifted him toward my embrace.

His great body was very heavy to hold. He immediately used my firm grip on his neck for leverage - in the same way that he would use his locked jaws on a possible meal - and swung his long body around my arm, over and over again... until I was held so firmly in his slightly frightened embrace that my hand soon began to turn blue-white with the sheer force of his ever-tightening grip. I did not know it then, but this exact event - this primal snake reflex of 'grabbing-when-grabbed' - was soon going to become very important in my life!

We then paused for a moment, unmoving, as we each felt and acknowledged each other's physical strength and Medicine Power. It was one of those moments that stretches out into a great time-less spacc of perfect balance: no pressures from within or without to move, to change anything, to tamper with this state of subtly balanced Grace.

Together we hung in the infinite space of a starry sky and felt each other's medicine... and what we each could of love... across the eons of mutual inter-species terror.... It was not bad, for either of us. We held each other in tight regard and held ground, held honor, held power, held integrity and held balance... *together*.

I pledged my trust and showed my good faith by loosening my hold on his neck. He replied in kind by *immediately* loosening his hold on my arm. I began the sort of 'treadmill' movement of my arms which, I knew, would give him support and help him to feel free to move... without letting him slip too far from my arms. And so he began to move - very slowly at first, then faster and faster until he was up to gentle, 'slow ahead speed.'

After some time of this, I could feel his trust growing, calming his entire body and slowing his breath. I gently placed one of the main loops of his long body over my shoulder and he began to change in his orientation to me. Instead of moving steadily away from me, he began to settle *into* me, exploring my hair and face and neck with his soft tongue-touch... all the while flagging the air and flicking my skin with that big, blue forked tongue in perfectly rhythmical beats.

The mini-shamans gathered around, slowly at first, brave in exact proportion to their ages (and their body-size in relation to the size of the snake) and all had a powerful and magical Ritual First-Touch experience of the very clean and cool body of *a true master of reptilian consciousness*.

They felt his strength. They smelled his odorless skin. They all asked to "touch his tail" and tried to find their way through their very natural fear... in to the love-space dance of total appreciation *and* care-full respect that they could see and feel in me... and perhaps in Snake as well.

Still, they could not help shrieking and lurching to dodge his head every time Snake tried to come close to them. But, you see, that didn't really matter at all: Snake is always happy whenever potentially scary things move *away* from him... and Snake is stone deaf to the air-borne sound of voices. He operates in a world of sight, earth-borne *vibration-imaging* and infra-red heat-sensing. So a few shrill kid-cries floating around in the air near his head don't frighten him at all!

It is sometimes useful and reassuring to realize that you can *talk* about Snake right to his face... and he doesn't hear a word you say! You might want to remember this... in case *you* ever find yourself too close to Snake and just don't know what to say.... You can plan all your moves right out loud and talk it over with whoever is nearby... and that talk, in itself, will *not* change your relationship to any particular snake... or to your *karma* with the living archetype (the collective- or species-consciousness) of *Snake*.

Talk is free. In Snake-land, it's what you *do* and, above all, *how you move* that counts!

After introductions had been made all around our little impromptu Initiation Circle - and were then extended to another carload of friends and children who happened to pass by and stopped for some very appreciative "Ohhh's" and "Ahhh's" - we decided to invite this snake to come with us in our van as we moved forward in our plan to be floating on the water together as darkness fell.

Snake accepted the offer, curled up happily under a seat, and just waited there while we finished our River Medicine Journey. And as we moved upstream in our little boat that afternoon with our usual laughter and effort and splashes and spills... and as we floated down through the darkening, misting Valley together in wonder-full silence... we were all aglow and excited by the amazing Grace of having such a huge GrandFather Snake waiting so patiently on the road just to meet our Medicine Family with such intimacy... and waiting right then in our van to come with us to our home... to be our very honored totem-spirit-guest.

VISITATION OF AN ANCIENT BEING

Thus it was that GrandFather Snake came to be with us for a time. In our house, Snake was to be given no 'pet' name. It was not our need - nor our right - to 'name' him in that captive ownership way. This power-full being was not brought to our home to be our pet - to live under our control or to fulfill any of our needs for companionship (or dominance). If he was to have a name in our company, *he* would have to tell us what it was to be.

Even apart from this name-thing, we did not pretend any great intimacy with this great being... nor did we expect any in return. Instead, our relationship was one of profound and very formal respect: we honored the *spirit* of this animal-totem in our every sharing with this Ancient One.

He was what he was: whole, intact and perfect. Slightly aloof, slightly reserved... and very attentive. We knew that it would be up to us to dis-cover what our sharing might be... up to us to offer intimacy if there was to be intimacy between us... and up to us to read his every response to us as Medicine Signs. And so they were!

When he first entered our house and was set gently upon the floor, BigSnake simply found a hiding and peeking place under a large table and settled down to watch us for many days... hardly moving, tongue flicking now and then, saying nothing: *NO SIGN.*

He seemed to have had a small meal of some sort just before we met him... and for awhile he was content to lie around the house, looking out at us as the family lived and writhed and bubbled and danced all around him, with increasing openness and un-selfconsciousness, even though we were all acutely aware of his brooding presence... looking... looking... looking.

After a week or so of this inner stillness, he began to take advantage of the warming spring sunlight and would slide around the kitchen counter to rest in the window-sun every afternoon. And in a very short time, we all realized that he was so mellow that we needn't worry about him at all as we went about our kitchen work, unceremoniously lifting and shifting great coils of snake-body to get at whatever we needed.

Here we should note something little known about snakes: although they are subject to mites and internal parasites and infections - just like any other living thing - they are somehow unearthly, immaculately clean. Their skin is cool and soft and completely dry. They do not sweat or drool or urinate. When they eat - and they can easily go several months between meals - they digest their food slowly and then shit once or twice, from an opening between two scales on their underside which is located at the beginning of their (actual) tail. You will be able to see this place clearly if you ever look.

This opening is one of those double-purpose excretory-sexual outlets, something like the *cloaca* of a frog. In some species, the gender of the snake can sometimes be determined by the shape of the belly-scale right at this opening. But in pythons, it is necessary to either probe into the slit *or* just 'feel the vibe' and so *feel the sexual presence* of the animal. And very fortunately for those who invite a big snake into their homes... unless a snake has eaten fairly recently, they simply do not shit at all. Ah yes... very clean beings, to be sure!

But to return: outside it was September... early spring in the southern hemisphere. Snake had come to our Family Circle to celebrate the Vernal Equinox with us. When we met him he had probably just crawled out from a winter's sleep... and he was still moving very slowly.

"My, what a nice-s-s s-s-s-sunny day! I think I'll jus-s-s-t cross-s-s-s this-s-s road here and s-s-see what lies-s-s-s beyond...!" he might have thought to himself (if, indeed, he thought anything at all).

And then... whew! What a surprise he must have had! In almost no time at all, he was whisked away by a roving Mobile Medicine Family and soon found himself (if, again, you imagine that he could 'find himself' at all) in a totally new environment with wall-to-wall colors, lights, many new heat sources to explore... and a rotating crew of mini-shamans gleefully peeking at him and dancing around him as he lay coiled in serene dignity under his table... everyone trying in turns to seduce him into friendship. So, whatever he made of it... a lot of new energy and very stimulating experience came his way in a very short time!

Snake was also the center of several of our formal Circles and spontaneous free-rituals of all kinds. One of these was the standard naturalist's ritual of the weigh-in: he was measured at more than nine and a half feet in length and nine inches around and he weighed about fourteen pounds. [Australian pythons do not attain the heavy body-mass of constrictors from South America, Africa or the Far East. So they are more lithe and supple and move more easily than those other 'fatso' species.]

He was definitely a GrandFather of Snakes... and whatever he thought/didn't think, for us he carried an aura of great Medicine Power... and on many different levels of our experience. Of lessons there were also many: lessons for the little (and not-so-little) ones snaked through our Family Circle daily. We learned about meeting new life-forms, new beings, new fears... and learned how to move *with* him whenever we touched, so that he (and we) could feel safe.

We learned about how he was made, how he could move, what made him withdraw from us and what invited him out to play. But far and away the most phenomenal experiences - and hence the most powerful lessons - revolved around *fear* (his and ours) and *strength* (mostly his).

A large python is afraid of many things (which is, of course, how they survive long enough to *get* large). They are naturally afraid of unexpected movement, afraid of being touched by any other living being... and most especially afraid of being encircled by an eager (and/or frightened) hand.

When you handle a snake, if you make your hands and arms work like tree branches you can give support *without* ever completely wrapping your hands around the snake's body. Because just as soon as you completely encircle a snake... it will almost always feel immediately trapped and threatened... and so will react accordingly... with all of its awesome power!

If you grab any snake close to its head then it cannot bite you. But if you grab a large python (or boa constrictor) like this, it will suddenly throw coils all around you (usually just around your arm) which will produce an incredible *pulsing* sort of contraction which is pretty overwhelming in its raw intensity. This pulsing power cannot be maintained for long... just long enough to scare and quite literally squeeze the breath and shit out of anyone (or anything) stupid enough to have provoked such a deep-fear spontaneous reaction in this great, primordial being!

And here's another bit of snake-lore: whenever you first come toward any snake's head, it will tend to recoil back and arch its neck. This gives the snake a better visual fix on what's happening. It is also the first movement toward a 'flight or fright' response... and it greatly increases the snake's defensive-aggressive options. From this position it can move away more easily... and/or it can bite you, fair and square.

One of the most powerful demonstrations of the existence of true *'species memory'* (and/or past-life experience) is to see what happens inside yourself when a big snake which you *know* to be harmless, suddenly swoops its great head toward your face. At such times: we are *all* afraid.

The fear is so deeply ingrained that we respond reflexively before we can even think. And long after we learn in our mind-center that there is nothing to fear... that ancient, brooding, *primal fear* remains. And so we go on ducking, jumping or crying out whenever Snake suddenly looms closer to us... even when he comes in total openness and with absolute gentleness in his intent.

Now obviously, poisonous snakes will tend to bite when grabbed. Pythons are not venomous. But pythons bite too. And their bite can be a very painful and long-lasting, scarring experience! For when they do bite...they often will not (cannot) let go. Their short and very sharp teeth curve inward (to help them hold onto their prey). But they have no way to 'let go' of anything once their teeth have engaged.

So every bite is a one-way trip for both the snake... and whatever it has bitten. They (usually) don't have occasion to bite anything that they don't want to eat. So (usually) the system works very well. Thus it is that if a python takes a really big bite into anything... it must either wrench itself free at great cost to biter and bitee... or it must swallow whatever it has bitten whole and intact... or it will eventually die!

When pythons are frightened - as is true of most snakes - they tend move away first, then they hiss and fret for awhile... and then they bite. Once they strike, they commit totally and they hold on like a vise with their teeth while their huge bodies make circle upon circle - around a tree branch, around your arm, around your neck or whatever. It makes no difference at all to a frightened python: it will coil and hold onto whatever it can touch.

But for some unexplained reason (or non-reason) *this* snake never tried to bite any of us. And with at least one of the most ardent mini-shamans still in the 'heavy patting phase' (well, full-on bashing, really) of tactile communication, he had many opportunities to re-act with self-righteous indignation.

His first experience of my touch was when I grabbed him behind the head to protect myself from an anticipated bite when I first picked him up from the road. But he did not try to bite, even then, and so I was able to release him very soon to cradle in my arms. And right from that moment onward, I felt perfectly safe with that large being, whenever we met. Still, I didn't swoop down in front of his face and still, I would always pause after making first-touch to sense if he were tensing or is he was 'cool' with our connect. And cool he all-ways was!

After he came home with us he was touched by every one with great respect, but sometimes very abruptly by the two-year-old Beny Sky (especially). And he *never* tried to bite anyone. This has been a very important element in my relationship with this particular snake-being... and his with my children.

I have grown to trust that he will not react with bitey fear-aggression even when being wakened from the deep trance which serves snakes as sleep - a trance state, by the way, in which Snake can constantly monitor his surroundings through eyes that never sleep and subtle sensor imagery that never stops. Even while he *seems* to be fast asleep... he keeps a silent vigil, constantly scanning the light-waves and other electro-magnetic energy-waves all around.

Snake has lived in my converted bus (which is my music studio, computer and media center, medicine temple and primal nestspace), for several weeks, now. Even as I write these words to you today, he is sliding above my head on the long passenger hand-rails that still run the full length of the bus. Sometimes he appears out of nowhere and swoops down on my shoulder from above as I write or compose. Often he writhes up between curtain and window and gives me a real fright when I catch the primal fear-form out of the corner of my eye as I write. Sometimes, too, he positions himself directly behind my computer to be in the heat-stream of the power supply fan - just to 'keep in touch' with my work, I allow myself to imagine. And very occasionally he pushes tea cups and plants to the floor when he misjudges the effects of his great weight and girth... or the insubstantial techno-physical world in which I live.

Sometimes he even 'types' a few letters or plays a few notes as he passes over one of the keyboards. But writing and music are not his primary talents....

Time passed in our springtime snake-dance. I taught any who wanted the experience how to pick up Snake, how to hold him gently... and how to deal with any unwanted 'hugs' - which only occurred when Snake became off-balance or afraid... or when he was grabbed suddenly (a simple reflex, as I have said).

I taught Ami all that I could about Snake, and she was keen to learn. Kira was less brave and also less interested. And the Froggy Joah Jai, at first, wanted no part of snake-holding, "except for just holding his tail."

But the nearly-baby, Beny Sky, came to *love* that snake. I became suddenly aware of the depth of his connection with Snake late one night when I was carrying the over-tired and under-weaned 'Mr. Beans' into the house and he broke into tears because even in the completely darkened room (?) he could somehow tell that "Nake" was not under the table where Beny wanted him to be. Well, that was right: that night Nake was in daddy-bus and Beny needed several reassurances that everything was ok with Nake before he'd settle down into the real-time no-time infinity of the Mother-Breast... and the deep baby-sleep which always followed. And hey! Putting his snake-connection before his love of mother-breast is placing a very high level of importance on his new *medicine ally*, to be sure!

Even now, the first question Beny asks me every day, is, "Where Nake? In bus, Daddy?" Or, "Nake in house, Daddy?" *Every* day he asks!

It was because of Beny's great love for this being that we all began to call him, for awhile, in Beny-speak: 'NAKE.' Nake is a name which carries power for us all... Medicine Power which comes from this child's unusual power of *Deep Love*.

Sometimes we would speak together of the time when it would be right to let Nake go free... to let him return to his spring-time mission of getting some nice feed... and making more beautiful little nakes... and lying on some nice warm rocks... and arching great waves as he swam in the Mother River in the hot summer evenings soon to come.

But it was not yet time. I trusted that we would know when our season to be with Nake was complete. We would know... and Nake would know... and then we'd *make-circle* for him and let him slide into the Infinite River with all of our love and our blessings. Yes... we all knew that this moment of good-byes would come... but there was another great adventure ahead of us, before we were to come to the moment of our Separation Ritual.

INITIATION BY THE POWER OF SNAKE

Joah Jai decided to really *meet* Nake when a far-away friend visited him one afternoon. To be able to show his mate all about Nake, Joah would suddenly don an invisible ritual cloak of great bravery!

Yes! Today Joah could suddenly hold Nake's great length and weight and dodge his bobbing (and still scary) head without Daddy assistance.... Well, almost on his own, anyway.

Yes! Today Joah would use the strength of his Desire to become *Powang Ular* (a Balinese concept that means *'snake-power-man'*) for his friend... and then use this circuitous path to actually *become* a 'Snake-Power-Man' for himself. This was *good medicine!*

I stood by, proud of my Son as he met and overcame his Primal Fear....

> [No! Wait! Excuse me... but here it comes again... snaking across my desk! I will let Nake write whatever he came to write and I've promised him I'll include it in this book, unedited. Shhh...! Here he comes now....

"nnnnnnnnnnnnnnnnnnnnnnnnnnnnnnnnnnnnn09"

There! Like I told you, there it is. Nake came to add some of his own medicine to this tale and so I keep my word and save this actual line of snake-writing for you (the quotes and centering are my own)... whatever it may mean. (And if you can read *this* Sign... then you're way ahead of me). So I leave the meaning of this snake-write sign to you... to feel it as you will.]

But enough of this silliness (actually, Nake is not a very good writer anyway...). Let's go back to the past: on that day I stood by (in reserve), proud of my Medicine Son as he met and (sort-of) overcame his deep primal fear of the primordial Serpent. He handled everything well. He was cool. He was calm and he was very gentle with Nake. And thus did Joah pass through his *Big-Snake Holding Initiation on* this day.

Later that week, we were camped at a nearby Healing Festival where I was heavily involved in teaching, shamanic guiding and Free-Ritual Circle-making. One afternoon, because we lived so close to the festival site, we decided to go home to freshen up our food and clothes supplies. And once we were at home, Beny went right for Nake and held him for a long time. Joah was not to be outdone... so he asked me to put the big snake on his shoulders so he could hold him, too... and so I did.

A few minutes later, a little pain-crisis occurred with Beny and we fell to the task of applying love and medicine (and some medication as well) to his very sad penis which was hurting from the incursion of some festival riverbank dirt under his foreskin.

I was just about to move out of the main room with Leia, on some part of the Beny-penis-saving expedition... perhaps to move to where we would not be distracted by the usual kid-sounds and the small whimpers of complaint I had been hearing for awhile - probably from Joah creating a little jealousy-hurt by falling over a sharp toy or something like that.

Then Leia moved over to Joah, somewhere behind where I was bent over with Beny, and I suddenly heard her say, "Help him! Help him!"

I thought it was a call to Kira, who will often stand around in a sort of non-responsive cloud when there is a problem at hand.

I turned around, more expecting to prod Kira into acting than anything else... and there was Joah with the great snake wrapped three or four times around his throat, squeaking for help in small, pitifully sparse, airless cries.

At once I registered that these were the very same cries that I had been hearing in the background of my awareness for untold breaths-seconds-minutes and which I had been *deliberately ignoring* while I had my back to Joah and was so engrossed in helping Beny's sore dick, engulfed in the littler boy's loud screams of indignation and pain.

The very same cries...! *How long had this been going on?*

I leaped to Joah's throat and began to wrestle with the vice-like coils of the immensely powerful snake-body as best I could. But nothing would move! Joah was holding the snake's neck several inches behind the head and trying to pull it away from him. GrandFather Snake was looking at Joah and trying to free his own head from the boy's clutching grasp... and in his fear and confusion... inching his great coils ever tighter and tighter around my little son's soft neck.

There was a flurry of noise, voices, effort.... I tried to move steadily and firmly to free my little son without further terrifying the snake. For one thing, the snake could only respond to more fear by squeezing even tighter... or perhaps even by adding a savage bite to his already incredibly strong contractions!

I had already learned that I could not easily physically dislodge that snake from *wherever* he chose to be. And I had already learned how to trick him by dancing around his coil-circle backwards - dis-charging his compression energy. Nevertheless, I had always assumed that I *could* overpower the snake... but had never really tried, because I did not want to hurt him. We just had not had any sign in our relationship that it would ever come to flat out 'him-or-me' macho. Now... he felt even stronger than I had imagined. Precious seconds were passing and I simply wasn't succeeding.

"Could it be...? Right here in front of me...? Unable to get him free in time...? How long has it been choking him...?" was speeding through my left-brain, male-mind head at a gigabaud rate... ringing alarms on every level of my awareness. Still, I could only go on working as best I could.

"No... he's ok. Be calm. Don't panic!" ... said the frightened voice of my deepest inner panic!

I tried pulling the coils this way and that, still without success.

Still it had been only a few seconds... but of course it felt so much longer in the face of my own impotence. Failure at such a time of real crisis can undermine faith and shatter morale almost instantly!

Joah was beginning to become more afraid, too - his fear greatly accelerated when he realized that I seemed *unable* to free him. Family-sound began to raise to cries and screams. And as these sounds spontaneously rushed forth from increasingly fear-full hearts... the very sound itself began to flash us all back to our (other) child-death experience some three years before, when little Tiki Sky slipped away from our arms in the bizarre and unearthly death of S.I.D.S. - and left our Family Circle, never to be seen again.

I went further from Mind and all at once, I apparently recovered the right unwinding movement... and then I had freed Joah and he jumped into my arms and squeezed my neck so hard... and he cried and cried. He cried out his Fear... and he cried through his Rebirth... and he cried from such great Love for me. And I cried for his pain... and I cried for my fear... and our whole family's fear... and somewhere in all of that a few seconds opened up where I found myself crying for Tiki Sky....

Back 'on duty' in no time, I began to explore his neck and head... checking his pupil-responses, neck alignment, any painful places and his breathing, to make sure that nothing really serious had happened to him.

And then I saw that across both cheeks and on his lower lip there were bright red prickle-spots where capillaries had been broken inside his skin! Even in places which the snake had not even touched... small blood vessels had literally *exploded* from the enormous pressure exerted upon his fragile, little five-year-old boy-neck!

Joah said that the snake had been so tight on his neck that, "it was keeping my blood from circulating between my head and my body... so tight that my blood could not circulate in my head!" And how he knew anything at all about circulation... I'll never know. Leia said that perhaps he was feeling it all so vividly that he could actually *feel* his circulation as it became impeded... then blocked... and then stopped altogether. And so he could.

Our deep intimacy went on and on, as we gentled into the assurance of New Life. I held my son and soothed him and reassured him with words. I squeezed him and pressed him to me. I breathed in his pain and hovered near his face and softly stroked his neck and his face - to dis-charge his body of its burden of fear.

The good news of this terrible Ritual came very soon: Joah Jai was all right! He said he was just beginning to feel dizzy when I finally got the snake off his throat. And he said that he had just gotten to the place where he "couldn't have made any more sounds with his voice to talk to us and tell us to help him" when Leia's Mother-sense had suddenly noticed his plight - even over the desperately screaming pain and din of sore-dick, Beny Sky.

So it had been a close call... too close to the point at which hypoxia (lack of oxygen) causes unconsciousness... which occurs just a few silent minutes before brain damage... and then death. It is very true that if Joah *had* fainted... then Snake would have immediately and reflexively released his grip on Joah's neck. Maybe this would have saved him. But this was no consolation at all... for so many people in human *cellular memory* have come to death in great surprise with big-snake wrapped around their necks!

Joah was full of love for me for saving him. I was still very much caught up in that wholly efficient and objectively detached 'crisis mode' - which is certainly one of the very positive and useful attributes of *yang* (male) consciousness - and everything I was doing was still *other-oriented*: helping Joah Jai to clear-through his profound shock and crisis.

What feelings of my own that I entertained were allowed as luxuries, accompaniments to the 'real' crisis event. But I knew that the depth of my own feelings (and tears) would follow Joah's out - in Feelings' own time - and I would sometime be able to finishing clearing-through the death-fear and grief and feelings of profound impotence that had been awakened in me during this terrible crisis.

Joah said, "I was afraid that I would die. Like Tiki. Or I *felt* like maybe I would die from that big snake on my neck because it was so tight.... Do you think I could die from that snake, Daddy?"

"People *can* die from having snakes around their necks... but before you actually die, you'd get more dizzy and then you would faint - you'd just pass out like your frog did when Beny whapped it - and then you would just fall over... and maybe Nake would have let go then....

"But we got you free in time, didn't we? We got that snake away from you before you even fainted... didn't we? Joah - I am *so happy* that we got you free in time!"

Then Joah said again: "Just when you came over to help me I was almost ready to fall over because the snake was so tight and my blood could not move and it was getting very heavy to stand up."

We spoke about fainting - but only lightly. It seemed better to deal with what had actually happened, rather than to speed outwards to what *might* have happened... just then. Although, for me, of course, it was precisely what *could have* happened that was the source of all my own inner fear and astonishment!

Froggy said that he thought that, "Maybe fainting *is* like dying... only you can get up again afterwards. Do *you* think fainting is like dying, Daddy...? Like Tiki didn't faint because he could not get up again afterward, could he? Because Tiki *really* died, didn't he, Daddy?"

"Yes... Tiki Sky really died. And you did not...."

Still a partial prisoner in the patriarchal 'efficiency mode,' and despite the glaring voice-borne re-awakenings of our terrible remembrances of losing Tiki Sky... I was still not (yet) ready to fully feel how close Death had come to our family that day. So I reassured him that fainting is very different than dying... if only because "you *could* get up after it was over... *if* you only fainted...."

And we hugged each other in silence... loved each other in silence... grieved a little together in silence... and, too, we *celebrated* in silence - boy-to-man, man-to-boy, us-to-us... in one great, inseparable mass of muscle and sweat and tears and snot... and *absolutely humble thankfulness*.

CLEARING HEALING - FREEING FEELING

Within a few more minutes of *earth-time* (and an eon of *feeling-time*) we were deep into our *Fear-Clearing Medicine Ritual*: for the sooner Fear can be met and felt-through, in all of its forms, implications, content... and Meaning, then the sooner it can be dissolved away... and so be truly *cleared* forever.

I wanted to get Joah and Big-Snake reunited as soon as possible. I wanted to help Joah to meet and really feel-through the reality that Snake's reaction was just one of Fear... and had not carried any malicious *intent* to hurt Joah's neck. But in the great state of his inner love and purity... Joah already knew that Nake had felt no malice toward him... and would not have... even if Jaya had somehow lost life from that ritual exchange! He already knew... *'It All'*....

On a more practical level, we looked for what Joah called Nake's 'fearness' and found the scenario that caused the drama: Joah said he had wanted to hold "all of the snake" but had become unsteady holding its great weight while still trying to stay a little bit away from the big-snake mouth - which was "still sort-of-scary."

Snake had been pushed and pulled this way and that, had its head dropped once - "but only on the soft part of the rug, Daddy" - and had been, in a word, terrorized by the wee Froggy in his *Snake-Love-Fear Dance of Deep Passion.*

Snake had apparently remained as peace-full as he could. Snake had been entirely true to its nature and so had reacted to the unintentional mauling by... just holding on as tight as it could... to try to get some feeling of *control* over its own, wildly unstable, physical universe.

As it happened, Joah's neck turned out to be its treebranch-of-the-moment... and so it began to do what it can do better than any other animal: it tightened its body around that only available 'object,' muscle-strand by strand and cell-by-cell, until it was exerting a terrible pressure on Froggy's neck... and so throughout his entire head.

And that's all there was to the whole incident. Nothing more... and nothing less: mutual fear and mutual tension led to more fear... and more tension.

Joah could understand that Nake had been afraid... too. "But still," he said, "I don't really want to hold that Nake again *until it is not afraid of me anymore...."* (Isn't that an amazing level of understanding - and generosity - from such a wee boy)?

"Fair enough, Joah!" I said with an overdone, affected hearty laugh. Inside I was deeply touched by the over-riding power of this child's simple openness: even with a sore neck and a blotchy face he could *still* feel sorry for the fear which he felt *he* had "put into the snake." Absolutely incredible!

So we all gentled Big-Snake out from under its table hideaway and began to praise it and sing to it softly and cuddle it. Joah allowed me to put it around his neck and as it slipped across the nape of his neck he said, "Oh! It feels very nice now! It feels so cool on my neck, now!" And once again, I was astounded that he was able to use *Gentle-Snake* to heal the pains and fears that *Frightened-Snake* had caused!

As Joah's always-amazing Love blossomed outward once again, it shattered and dissolved away any fear-blocks which might otherwise have remained locked inside him... forever.

If he had not been able to re-connect with that snake right then and to feel its good-faith peacefulness toward him, his young, soft, body-mind would have no choice but to process the fear internally... and alone. And the associations would be locked into his body-mind on a cellular level.

I was aware that any of this trauma-fear which he could *not* spontaneously release would, in time, form chronic tension-patterns of (quite literally) *pure, crystallized Fear*. And once formed, this non-moving, un-feeling, fear-formed knot of muscle and connective tissue would then demand a lifetime of obeisance and servitude... as it enshrouded and concealed from Joah Jai the un-cleared content of all of his emotional memory of this shocking event... feeding ghost-feelings of raw, unprocessed fear into *all* of his experience-to-come.

No... *that* scenario I know all to well from the bodies of a thousand tortured souls that I have touched and tried to help themselves to heal. And of course I know it from the healing pains of my own un-resolved body-self as well. No... that scenario I just could not bear! For anyone who really cares about wholeness... a motto:

'The time to get Clear is while there is Fear!'

Clearing Fear is all we have to do. It is the only therapy, the only physical healing, the only personal growth process... and, ultimately, the only *yoga*.

Any process which liberates Fear naturally liberates the soul and invites ever greater flows of *feeling... energy... pleasure... hope... awareness...* and so directly feeds our evolving consciousness... and Spirit.

I sing *Medicine Song* aloud to my children when they are in Fear. I touch them often, sometimes with great, *inviting* softness - and sometimes with pointed, *provoking* firmness - to encourage Fear's release.

I talk to them, with them and *for* them - trying to find the voice they may not have to bring their feelings into word-mind awareness. And thus we learn to dance the fears away. We find new ways to act out its play (its drama) until release and wholeness come clear. We find a Sign and make Free-Ritual Medicine to learn the Meaning of Fear... and how to 'get the lesson' so we can be free of its otherwise endless grind.

In time we can usually evoke the great inner strength of happiness and self-trust. In time we come to a place of simple and power-full surrender - the sacred space of Deep Surrender .... And all the fear that ever there was inside us, each and all... melts into the simple primal sadness and anger and hurt that it always was... pervading all experience through all time... and so often without any essential relation to the here-and-now situation which we might have assumed to be its 'cause.'

And so we come clean and clear together - usually in a jumbled heap of hugging, sniffling, nose-blowing, grateful bodies. A long sigh from the erstwhile frightened one(s)... and then the long awaited 'all clear' and reconsecration report which often expresses itself with a sudden up-welling of: "Daddy...? I Love You so much!"

The Froggy Joah Jai moved completely through his Snake-Fear this day with all of us. He was brave from the beginning. He was that sure of himself... that he bore absolutely *NO BLAME* toward GrandFather Snake. Caution, yes, and deservedly and wisely so. But he entered his ritual with Nake with so little accumulation of irrational fear to meet... and such Deep Trust in our Process - the process *that he knew would free him* - that he was able to plunge right in to the very depth of all the *content* that he and we could find... and then he simply *let it all go* and so cleared it from every cell of his body-mind.

The Clearing Ritual that evolved was free-form and almost entirely his own orchestration: he tasted and smelled and licked and savored his Primal Fear. He formed it into various 'what-if' scenarios, shuffled and re-shuffled all the possibilities until he was clear and accepting of *every* aspect of his experience.

He rehearsed what to do if ever attacked again by a stray python-at-large. He thought about where it might occur. He explored the circumstances in which a python might attack him and... *he found none!* He planned out how he could call out before it got too tight next time. And so on and on he went, moving and healing and growing all the while.

Froggy danced *Snake-Fear Medicine* around the room, all through the house, laughing and shaking and gesturing and reciting the few basic snake-handling rules which can ensure the safety of anyone who hangs out around snakes as a sort of antidote to irrational fear... as a catechism of *Snake Magic*... until he was completely clear of Fear. At least... he was clear of all the fear that he felt that day....

I knew that it wasn't really over, finished and done. It would take some time for him to imagine a few more bizarre possibilities and to act-through these expanded scenarios in his Mind-Breath-Feeling Self. But I knew that he was open to deep change... that he was clear about the process he must follow... and that was accomplishment enough for that day. In fact, that was all that I could have ever wished for that day... or could wish for any other....

During our processing - the part where we try to put it all into some fairly normal context and perspective - I made some comment about "Joah pulling on the snake's neck to try to get it off...."

Joah interrupted me and then, with great solemnity (and deeply impressive inner sureness) said: "No, Daddy, I wasn't really trying to get it off... because I knew it was too strong for me. I was only trying to hold onto its head to get it to *look at me*... so that I could *tell it* to let go of my neck!"

And this was a very important piece in the puzzle of what had happened: Snake had become too tight, too passionate, somehow, and Joah had just grabbed him because he wanted Snake to pay attention to his request for Snake to let him go! In using physical force in trying to establish eye-to-eye communication with the great beast, Joah had apparently crossed over that subtle border which always exists somewhere in the reptilian mind-set: that thin line which separates feeling slightly off-balance-anxious from full-blown-have-to-save-myself terror.

Snake had clearly become terrified and had done one of those incredible sudden power-pulsing grabs at Joah's neck. I shuddered inside when I realized that at that instant... both Joah and Snake were wholly out of control... free-spinning in the hands of *karma*... and Grace!

Well now, on some levels, anyway, tensions were relaxing and the drama was resolving itself somewhat. And all of its multi-level experiences were finally beginning to find their place in the fabric of our family and our selves.

Integration was beginning. And yet, on may levels still, the whole experience was still full-on in its intensity... and in our fear-full-ness. And our little tribe had a long way to go before it would be wholly *clear* with all that had happened that day....

But we fumbled on as best we could. Next, we had to make a space for Leia to let down her parental-effective guard and to cry, too.... to cry out her relief... and to cry through the nameless fears and dreads and helplessness she had felt... until she, too, could cry in whole-hearted *celebration.*

In actual fact - though it is shocking to consider - if Leia had been alone with Joah when this dangerous thing occurred... she might not have had the physical strength to pull that snake from her son's neck... unless she had been able to *kill* it!

For Snake is unbelievably powerful. Yes... Snake is absolutely that strong! For all of our 'What if...?' fears - Joah's, Leia's, the other kids' and my own - I am so thankful that I was there!

Now we had passed through Froggy-Fear and Leia's release of her deep maternal pangs - Joah coming close (how close?) to death... and death-awareness bringing so many memories up inside The Mother of her little Tiki Sky going over the top so silently one day, all alone, long ago.

All related/unrelated fears and dreads, named and nameless, all cried-through, all cuddled out, all at peace at last. In time Leia emerged from the depths of the throbbing, pulsing Family Heap with a clear smile... with Love in her eyes... and with "a big special hug for her brave Froggy son! - And one for his brave Daddy, too!"

BREATHING-THROUGH THE SINS OF THE FATHER

And finally, as if from a ghostly place of great remove, attention began to come my way. I began to hear words of invitation... "And what about *Daddy's* feelings...? It must have been scary for him, too...? What are *you* feeling, Jai...? I'd like us to make a place for your feelings, too...."

And *then*... and only then... did my own reaction well up in me like some kind of anachronistic, displaced, past-life pain from some ancient war or disaster... with only one, clear message, which rocketed out in all directions and lit up my entire sky:

"I WAS NOT THERE FOR MY SON!
I DID NOT COME TO HELP HIM!
WHY HAD I NOT BEEN THERE?"

All of a sudden... my Son needed me *so* much... his very breath and life was oozing from his grasp... and *I had not been there for him.*

It was not that I was out, away, out of reach. No, worse: I had been across the space of one large room, listening to his muffled cries of desperation in the back of my mind while being overwhelmed with Beny's pain and noise... and I somehow *chose* to relegate Joah's needs (*whatever* they were) to the background of my awareness... while I sought to aid my other son's noisier but far less important Crisis of the Sore Willy. It felt so bizarre... so horrific... and so terrifying...!

Firstly, of course, I asked for *forgiveness*. Firstly from Joah... and then from Spirit. And then from Leia as 'The Mother'... and then from Leia as her persona-fied self. And my forgiveness came with their simple reassurance, acceptance and their ultimate judgment: *"No blame."*

Perhaps too easily, I was let off the hook and could not find any re-active judgment or blame from my family which I could have bounced back and forth between my own guilt and sorrow... as a kind of purging scourge. Whatever... I still had to forgive myself. I had to feel that I was, somehow, 'all right' in myself.... And that was the hardest of all.

So I, too, went through all of my wildest scenarios, breathing-feeling-touching-tasting and *wearing* all the implications of every possibility that I could imagine.

And then it hit me... with an enormous sobering shock and jolt. For all of a sudden I remembered that even while I was hearing Joah's constricted cries for help... I was actually beginning to prepare to summon Leia to accompany me to go down the hallway to the back room so that we could both better devote our full attention to ministering to Beny's sore parts... *without* the distracting 'background noise' which was getting in my way and distracting me in my deep attention to my fatherly 'healing work!' My mind spun wildly, round and round, probing for a grip on reality:

"Did that really happen...?
Did it really go that way...?
How could this ever have happened...?"

But you know...? *It almost did!* Leia found her son, beginning to expire. Leia first noticed his need. And Leia called me to him. And there was so much of my own behavior - choices, actions, feelings, ignorance - which now stuck in my throat and my heart. So much that amazed me, shocked me, terrified me, threatened me... frightened me... that I knew I'd be processing this fear and self-suspicion for a long, long time. And I was so thankful for the depth of Mother-Love... that could see Joah's need and feel the moment so much clearer than I, when we all needed it most.

Later that day we returned to the Healing Festival. I had Circles to do. You know: '*Medicine Path*' to teach.... I, the supposedly sensitive one... I, the supposedly intuitive one... I, perhaps even the occasionally supposedly wise one, from time to time... I the one who had been had been *totally blind and unaware* of my own little son's terror as he was locked in a mortal combat with a deadly, giant serpent, struggling for his very life... and calling out to his supposedly all-powerful all-loving Daddy to save him... just ten feet from where I was standing... while I was, somehow, *choosing* to ignore his cries!

Whatever else happened... whatever else it meant... I will never, ever be able to forget this strange irony. I was so humbled by this shocking reality that I felt totally impotent to preach or teach or believe that I could know... anything at all.

I reflected with friends at the Festival site about how I would feel if I had heard of another father being so insensitive, so care-less, so self-centered... with a deep primal shudder! Woe be unto any who would be so stupid in *my* presence! Truly, I would fear for my own reaction of pitiless judgment and inner rage in the face of such a man! And on that day... *I Was that Man*!

Perhaps I will gain understanding, tolerance, acceptance from this ordeal. Perhaps I will gain something in humility. Perhaps I will gain some greater depth of spiritual surrender. Perhaps all this good will come from our family's moment of trial. But I cannot decree such things. I can only make deep-ritual commitment to being open to receive whatever lessons may come.

As the Father, as the Teacher and the *Medicine Guide* for my children, I can only share some of my own inner wonderings and confusions with my children. Too often I alone have to decide what they can process - and what they cannot. In the end, however deeply we feel and however loudly we celebrate our one-ness... I know that I usually have to open to my Inner Guidance alone... and share with them what I can feel might be within their realm of understanding... and their need.

And yes, even despite these fond intentions, I all-ways seem to assume too much... and they all-ways try to *be* that much... for me...

and I for them. And so it goes, on and on. Sometimes it feels like we are riding through life together with an enormous driving thrust that races us all toward endless Change... and yet we are also gifted to be continually re-balanced, blessed and guided through our sharing of long out-breaths of great softness and long embraces of deep and mutual surrender.

Later that day, Joah overheard me tell a close brother at the festival that "A python almost killed my Son, today!"

When we were once again alone, he wanted to know if he had *really* been close to dying. A mistake that he should have overheard this said so dramatically! I have no need to plant those seeds in his five-year-old, open-trusting heart. I withdrew the careless statement carefully, smoothing over the terrain where it had been stated so bluntly before.

And in doing so I learned something else: in fact Joah had not 'almost died'... *because he did not die!*

Life and Death are a split second apart... fortunately, they (usually) remain mutually exclusive states of being.

Through that day... and still today... Joah is alive...!

And so am I... his Father... still....

><><

[This time of crisis so well met,
And after all had rested well -
And the Healing Festival ended (for me)
With an 'Ancient Earth' Jai-chant
Soaring out from a late nite stage...

We now move into the past, to explore some of our family's Clearing-Healing Rituals - and to reveal some more of the Healing Process which brought us so sweetly through this moment of such urgent danger... and Ritual Celebration.]

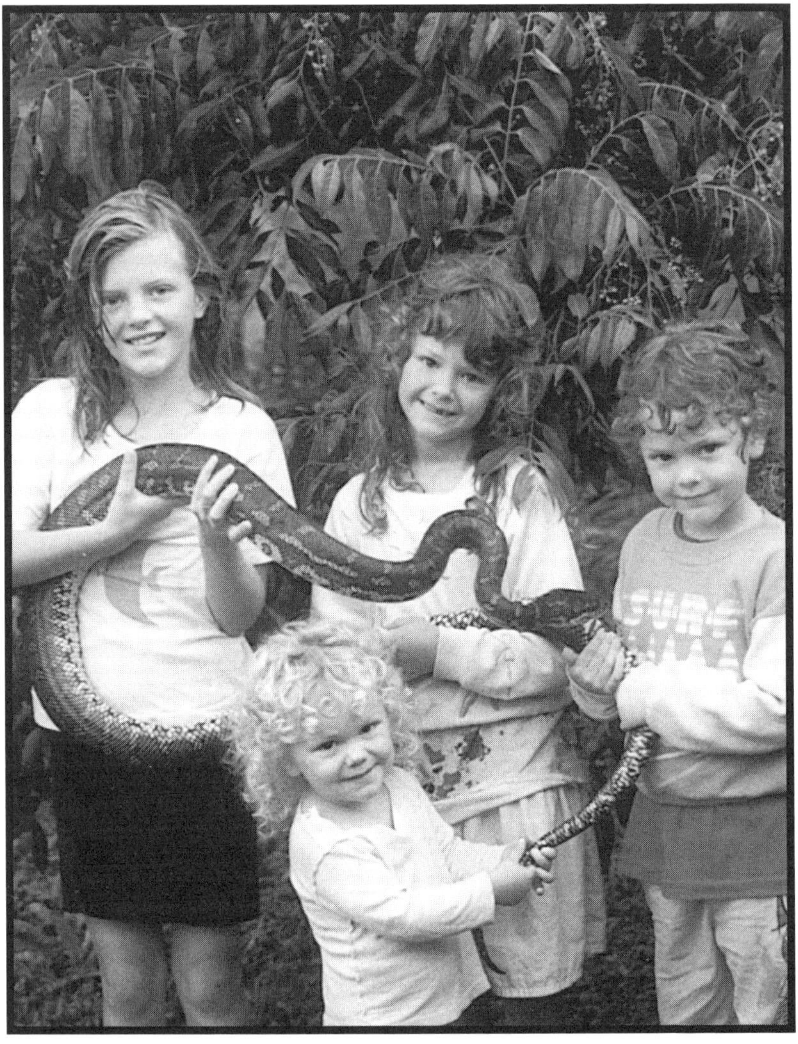

CHAPTER 9

HEALING THROUGH THE FEAR OF WHOLENESS

FEATHER HEALING AFFIRMATION

Joah Jai has just turned five. He looks like Christopher Robin, but he never liked the 'C.R.' image. Instead he long ago took on Winnie-the-Pooh as his totem-ally. We have been calling him 'Joah-Winnie' because he says he never wanted to be a bear... just a 'winnie.' But now, entering into that powerful new autonomy which comes with being five-years-old, 'Winnie' is no more. Now Joah has become a frog. Who knows why? But whatever it means, now he wants to be called by what he says is his 'new medicine name' of 'Froggy.' What a leap ahead!

Not unlike other little boys all over the planet, Froggy-Joah has a few problems with Desire. Not those terribly heavy guilt-ridden desire problems which are the bane of all adult yogis and meditators. No, just a healthy lust for, well, for whatever is coming along next. And, yogi or not, even this fresh and wonder-full desire of free-ranging eagerness can make you very sad if it constantly pushes your attention way ahead of the here-and-now action. And so it is making Joah sad, too. Day after day he is so eager to *become*... he cannot enjoy just *being*.

Froggy is not too spun out on material 'things.' He likes it all, but he is not attached to anything, much, in a lasting way... except everything with wheels... and of course his little bean-bag 'Froggy' doll (as all true frog lovers will surely understand). In fact, when

Froggy made a wish on his fifth birthday cake candles... his only wish was for "A tree with all different kind of fruits that I could climb anytime I wanted and pick different fruits off of it and eat them."

But for all his usual positivity and clarity, Joah Jai is becoming sorely stuck in *Future-Dreaming*: if we give him a toy, he asks if we have any more. If we take him on an adventure, he asks where we are going tomorrow. If you ask him how he liked something... you hear about what it wasn't. I think you get the picture, yes? A state of increasing dissatisfaction... amidst an abundance of natural life-wealth.

To understand the wee Frog's dilemma, it is important to realize that at its core, this is not a 'behavior problem.' It is not merely a matter of being impolite and ungrateful when people try to share nice things with him. No... this is a genuine problem of priorities and information handling routines that are (already) locked deep within his mind-game.

In time, if this little snag wasn't worked through, this way of feeling the world could lead to a lot of restlessness and discontent. A Joah like this could easily grow into one of those chronically dissatisfied, overly romantic persons who is always dreaming of something as yet unknown, something bigger and better and more 'perfect' than whatever fills the knowable world... and so, never happy with whatever *is*. Hmmmm... that feels like something we'd better keep a watch on for awhile!

In its most positive manifestation, this mind-set of continually reaching outward for 'more' is what often motivates those visionaries who illuminate the highest possibilities for all of us. So, of course, it wouldn't be helpful to guide Joah away from Vision. But it may be possible just to help him learn to separate the here-and-now joys of the world from the someday-sometime dreams of what the world might become... and how to find the pleasure in each and all.

And so we might well wonder how our Free-Ritual Healing Process may be put to use in a creative way to resolve this paradox.

My first contact with this little gremlin of the Froggy soul was very personal: I became aware that I felt personally squashed and hurt whenever I'd try to do something special for the little Joah. I was hurt that whatever I did - or anyone did - was never quite enough. I was sad to see the genuine disappointment on his face when he opened a present or when he discovered some magical token left for him by the two elves (Troika and T'rence) who live in the old hollow apple tree deep in the garden-forest.

I tried to clear my own feelings by sharing my hurt with him. I tried to elicit his empathy, to see what we could make of my problem once we were both on the same wave-length... but that didn't work too well. Since his distorted desire-mode was literally pulling him away from everything that was happening in the here-and-now, he could not really feel or understand how to deal with my real-time despair. (To say nothing about the built-in emotional-conceptual limitations of being only five years old).

No matter how I expressed my own feelings, it seemed only to make him sad that he was not responding in a way that was good for me. Thus I could tell that he could still very much feel others and so we knew that his deep compassion was alive and well.

Well that's our boy today: empathetic, no, but infinitely compassionate. Anyway, the problem became a self-feeding circle whenever I approached it by sharing my own feeling... and simply could not be processed in this way.

Affirmations are always good. Affirming the positive side of any situation gives us strength and hope... anytime. But when you are just breaking the horizon of five and always hungry for more from the out-there world, you have very little surrendered patience to reflect on subtle changes in the inner mindscape, to say the least! So the helpful reminders of his family to 'be in the present' and to 'find the good' in any presents... were just so much background noise - probably just more of that repetitive, preachy parent-blow that only cluttered up his clear streaming hunger for... *MORE!* And as time passed it became obvious: Joah Jai, Winnie or Froggy, was just not catching on!

The time of Joah's fifth birthday was the time for Ritual Initiation... it was *Time for Change*. We had all had enough! So one Sunday morning when we were all in our family circle cuddle-heap, we decided to make a Medicine Circle for Joah Jai. For we knew that when the chips are down a good Medicine Circle never fails.

We asked Froggy to come in to our center. We placed a large and very tickly feather in the Medicine Wheel and every one (each in their own way) consecrated this Initiation Circle by dedicating it to *'Joah-Finding- Happiness.'*

At first, Joah giggled and resisted a little, but eventually he fell into a peaceful mode of open surrender and waited to see what would happen - looking up into a the circle of our loving (and determined) eyes and cuddled and lulled by our *Circle of Breath.*

In time there was stillness and I began this new medicine 'work' by very formally wishing that Joah would find 'Great Pleasure' - so much pleasure that he would feel happy in his body, happy with his life and so much that his whole-life experience would be filled forever with great and magical things.

As I said these things, I moved the feather in a stroking sweeping way, upward from his deep-belly toward his face. The leading edge of the feather stroked his belly, his chest, his arms, his neck, his mouth and finally came to softly tickle his ears.

While I did this, Kira spontaneously began a softly droning song: "Everything is all right. Everything is good in your life. Everything is wonder-full..." she chanted, repeating this over and over in her shaky, little seven-voice.

"... and there is all-ways enough of everything!" I added, after some time of letting Kira's words float through our experience, weaving us all together, "...and enough love... and enough gifts... and enough magic... and enough time... and enough cuddles... and enough Mother... and enough Father... and enough sunlight... and enough rain...."

For what seemed a very long time, we all took turns stroking and reassuring him as he moved through many levels of his awareness: from big, soft, wide-open eyes eagerly searching outward for signs of what was to come, through eyes closed and wiggling and laughing softly as the feather flicked at his skin here and there, to a few sighs and shudders in his breath, to a gently needy and very small boy-baby, who finally rolled over and crawled into his mother's lap and cuddled into her belly to lie close upon the mother belly.

Then Joah reached up through a slightly self-conscious yawn and said "I feel a little sleepy now...." And before the last word left his lips he just closed his eyes and softly fell asleep. And so the circle and its free-ritual healing - was complete.

We all sat with him for awhile, watched him sleep in such open trust for several minutes, and then loved him forever more.

PROCESSING THE PROCESS

Only time will show us how this circle has affected him. Perhaps we have really met and re-solved this problem. Or perhaps we have just succeeded today in sharing the very beginning of the healing process: the part where we first *recognize the imbalance*, the dis-ease, the suffering... and then find way to *honor its rightness* (its appropriateness) as a perfect expression of this moment's needs and fears... and outreach.

And perhaps we have simply planted a small seed of hope in Joah Jai's inner repertoire of ways of dealing with whatever he is experiencing. But whatever comes to our family in a direct cause-and-effect way from this little feather-dance healing ritual, one thing feels certain: we know from this simple initiation circle that we have now been given a *form* for meeting this need... and a *process* for working on it... and a lovely affirmation-chant that seems to go so well with feather-stroking that probably, tomorrow, everyone in the family will decide that *they* need help with their needy hungers, too.

And why not...?

On a more intentional mind-body integration level, adding pleasurable sensations (the feather) to Deep Word messages has several knowable effects. For one thing, the word-experience becomes less abstract when it is naturally 'grounded' and integrated with body feeling... and so becomes more 'real' to whoever receives such caring.

Also, when it can be experienced on many levels at once, the message or the teaching is naturally *self-integrating* and so is felt as more meaning-full and profound than mind-messages that come to us only as Word.

Blending soft feather touches with affirmations provided Joah with such an intense sensation of delicious physical pleasure that our reassuring message was tickled in to every cell of his little body, and planted there like a tree, no doubt to fulfill his birthday wish and bear 'many kinds of fruit that he could pick whenever he wanted to' through all his life to come.

Time was also an important element in this magical mix: in the very midst of such a torrent of sensual - emotional - magical - loving - ritual experience, Joah's egoic body-mind had all the space and time he might need to run through anything he might need or want to explore.

Floated in the center of his family heart he could feel many things at once: he could play and laugh and resist and expect and desire and rejoice, even as we all played out our word-poem offerings and affirmations for him. And so he did. And perhaps it was the soft touch of the feather that finally broke through his outer 'act' of bravely defending against his inner needs to be babied and cuddled and loved - inner needs which were being masked by his constant outward striving for *"more!"* of everything... and also hidden from his own awareness by his very real love for the two little brothers who had so inadvertently crowded into his mother-love connection.

As Joah settled into his real pleasure, and as he let our words come into him... what do you know? Some hidden needs began to surface and all of a sudden he found himself feeling littler than he had imagined he was before... feeling needier than he had ever been able to admit to himself before... and now newly free to find the expression-fulfillment of his *real* needs.

Here he was in the circle of his family... and so close to that inviting mother-belly, the very first home of his five-years-plus-nine-month old little Froggy body. He just crawled right in to that ancient place of all Earthly Beginning in his mother's lap and fell into a deep sleep. No pills, no remedies, no great emotional catharsis: just the deep healing that comes when we discover true *Rightness-of-Place.*

As our free-ritual circle came to a natural melting away, the other (real) baby, Beny Sky, settled in to our collective enfoldment in an unusually peaceful way... thus giving Big Brother the ultimate Brother-Gift of open time and space to revel in deep baby-sleep in the mother-center place.

And I knew that in Joah's quiet dream-time, whatever this initiation circle might mean to him now (and whatever it could mean to his future) would be wholly integrated with his past and his present, mixed and re-mixed, filtered and refined, cell by cell throughout the whole of his body-mind...

And he would wake up Changed and New...
And he would wake up Healed.
And so he did!
AND SO WE WERE!

FIVE YEARS LATER: A RITUAL UPDATE

Joah Jai is now ten years old. And we are busy planning his first medicine trip to America. Shortly after we found out that we could actually do it, and after the first round of celebrations had us all bright-eyed and bubbling with excitement... we found out that we were many thousands of dollars short of what was needed for three of us to make the trip.

I don't have any way to teach economics to my children except by sharing the process of living with money with them. So when the shortfall was apparent, I shared it with the family, alerting them that 'the best laid plans...' might be about to go away.

Joah met this news with a clear-eyed (if un-breathing) braveness. He accepted the disappointment like, well, as we once would have said without our sick gender shame: 'like a real man.'

But as soon as he had collected his thoughts, he realized that since the other fares were covered by 'mileage' points, it was *his* ticket which was the most immediate problem. With proud chin raised and clear Vision shining through his up-welling tears, he offered to stay behind, "so that Kira and Dad might be able to go anyway!"

Fathers melt in such open showers of love and personal integrity. In the face of such spirit, Fathers commit to do 'whatever is needed' to ensure that everyone could go. And so I made promise that we would find a Way... and that we would make it work for everyone.

For those who live in trust that there is all-ways enough - sometimes *just* barely enough - this will not sound surprising, I know. For those who believe in the standard TV sitcom version of moral reality, this will seem like any other story. But within one week of Joah's Ritual Offer, some music studio gear sold that had been begging for new owners for over two years, a workshop was offered to me... and more money came from overseas.

I am not so romantically foolish as to say that Joah's Feather Ritual of long ago evoked all of this test-affirmation-success. But I would be foolish, indeed, to imagine that it had no effect on *'The All'* that my son is becoming... or that his feather-ritual did *not* open him still further to the inner guidance of the Deep Spirit that has always accompanied him and beamed outward to us all from his pure heart.

FROGGY MEETS HIS FEAR-NESS IN THE PRIMEVAL FOREST

Healing Ritual works in many ways: with talk, with feathers... with anything that comes to serve us as a Tool. We have already seen how Joah met the Great Fear that was evoked when the Grandfather Snake hugged him too tightly. And we have also now seen something of how our Ritual Healing Process works.

So now we must once again venture back to the early years of Joah's Froggy-hood. And here we will learn how the Little Frog came to be so brave!

Now it is high summer and the long days stretch into late twilight nights as the kids celebrate the longer non-school nights and gradually return to the real-time life-rhythms that best suit their own needs.

Given a free-time mode, any body will naturally respond to tiredness... with sleep. This is even true for children. They may deny their fatigue, but they cannot deny sleep: it just comes when it will... no matter what.

So when there are no artificially scheduled social rituals like work or school to conform to... children can stay up as late as they want to at night without any fears for their health. If they misjudge one night, they'll just pass right out the next afternoon and recover their rhythm with a good nap.

In the perma-hot weather of tropical lands, a natural surge of awakening and revivifying occurs around sunset and all the little neuro-mechanisms within the body-mind can begin to open to other adventures than merely trying to keep the organism cool (and sane).

So these days... our family is awake and active together until far into the night. It is a very special time.

On one such evening I invited Joah-the-Frog and Kira Sanh to come out for a special *Medicine Walk* adventure. We drove awhile until we came to a small picnic area by a small stream in the midst of a eucalypt and tree-fern forest. It was not yet dark, so we all felt day-light brave as we headed off across the neat and official little wooden bridge and made our way along the well organized and totally environmentally controlled public walking-trail-of-no-surprises. It was, after all, just a little tourist park by the side of a tourist road. But in the dark, even a park....

Yes. Darkness was beginning to collect in the shadows which pool around the base of trees... but we scarcely noticed it at first, since the tree tops ahead of us were still actively alight in the evening sky. Elemental Darkness. Primordial Darkness. Darkness with character... and maybe even *intent*!

But as dusk continued its inexorable spread, the Darkness became more obvious than the waning Light... especially to Joah Jai. Because when you are four years old (and even if you will be five next week), you walk very close to the Earth and even fairly small things can loom up and appear quite large and scary from this humble perspective. And the darkness was beginning to feel pretty large and very scary to Joah as we walked together in silence along the forest path that night.

I could feel Joah's caution... and then that caution turn to fear... as his body began its natural fear-contraction, pulling inward toward his belly-center. I could feel his hands tighten into fetal positions and spontaneously pull toward his mouth. With all of this reflexive busyness filling up the inside of his experience, Froggy held my hand... tighter and tighter and tighter as every shadow under every bush inhaled the night and swallowed up more and more of the last puffs of cloud-light.

Joah Jai was afraid. Clearly, Joah's fear would be the stopper... or his fear would be the focus of whatever magic was to meet us there. For whatever medicine was to be ours that night... would either have to pass through his growing fear... or bring help to this child so that he could *walk through* his fear and emerge into a more peaceful openness. And as we walked along, I wondered which it would be....

Just then we noticed something very special: on a tree nearby, there was a small smear of some sort of creamy-white powder which seemed somehow luminescent in the rising darkness. And then, beyond that patch of light and just where the pathway melted into the obscurity of real darkness, there was another patch of the same substance, glowing in the center of the trail.

After carefully examining the strange powdery stuff on the tree, we walked to the blotch of light on the trail... and, sure enough, from there saw yet another spot further along the path. One patch led to another and soon we were excitedly following this magical trail.

What this substance was seemed less important than where it might lead us. And maybe most important of all, why it was there for us on that night. Some being - perhaps human, perhaps not - had obviously made same-sized spots of this powder stuff along the path. The spots which were furthest away were always just out of sight in the gloom which was fast claiming everything under the fern-tree mandala canopy above.

While I was feeling the fun of sharing the mystery of who left it, where did it lead (and why), Joah-Froggy was becoming evermore frightened. His hand felt as though it was of two minds... wanting to pull away from me and run away from wherever that trail might lead... and at the same time wanting to hold on even more tightly to be sure that I didn't pull away from him.

He tried to bury himself in my legs somehow... perhaps so he would be less of a target to whatever he imagined was out there... but only managed to keep tripping us all as we walked along... very quietly and very carefully... into the primordial darkness of *'The Great Unknown.'*

Then, when I felt that it might be time to get into Joah's fear with him, the old Gestalt therapist rose up inside me and I wanted to play 'worst case-best case possibility' with him.

"*Listen* Boy.... Listen inside. What are you actually afraid of here?" (He said he didn't know). "I mean... what is the very scariest thing that you imagine could possibly be out there...?"

His answer was perfectly clear and matter-of-fact: "I'm afraid that there is a tiger in those dark places."

"But there are no tigers in Australia," I said. And then a great flatness of tone descended on my speech as I quickly remembered the many well-documented sightings of black panthers which regularly appear in the local 'Mountain Free Press.' But these sightings are as yet unknown to our littlest ones, so only I had to fear their fact! We walked a little further and I just waited for his response.

Meanwhile, Kira was being brave. After all... she is six and a half. And feels very big, of course. But also, she is less afraid by nature - and less afraid *of* Nature - than my first son. Kira has a deeply centered trust in her own rightness and well-being. It feels as though it is located deep in her belly-center and proceeds up her spine to continually bathe her mind in calmness... at least on this primal (first-*chakra*) level of basic survival. From this great calm of maturity, Kira assured Jai that there were no lions in our woods.

"NO!" said Joah Jai, firmly and deliberately: "Not lions... TIGERS!"

"Well, there aren't any tigers either. Not here," she said. And somehow this assurance really seemed to work for Jai. It completely washed away his fear of lurking tigers - a magical act of very effective expert reassurance which perhaps only this very caring older sister could have provided just then. Well, it washed away his fear of tigers once and for all... but then, of course, there are the Bears...!

Now bears can be very scary, too. Especially to a little Aussie who has never been much exposed to all the good kinds of bears that fill American children's early years: Care Bears, Cuddly Bears, Yogi bears, teddy bears, etc. We get all that stuff here in Australia as media imports. But it simply doesn't have any cultural relevance... and so the friendly-bear message just doesn't seem to stick. And, for my Froggy Joah... these days (and especially just now), bears are pretty scary things to imagine.

"Joah," I began, thinking I could just ride along on Kira's gift of calming reassurance, "there are no bears in Australia either. You know that. No bears at all!"

We had stopped on the trail to sort this out. But even though we had stopped, the nightfall did not and I could feel the little Jai trying to press deeper and deeper into my clothes, my body, my mass, my safety... even as we talked.

"No, Jai, there are no bears here because bears don't live anywhere in Australia. Does that help you feel any better now?"

"Where *do* bears live, Daddy...?"

"Bears live in Europe and in America and in Russia and in Asia.... Bears live in many places, actually. But bears do not live in Australia. They just don't ever come here! Australia is a huge island and they just don't ever come.... Now what do you think of that?"

"I think that they were bringing a bear from America in a helicopter on a long rope and the rope broke and... maybe the bear got here like that, by accident. Maybe it's the *only* bear that is loose in Australia and nobody knows about it yet..." he said, staring even more intently at the next spot of white powder which seemed to glow from the bushes ahead. "And maybe bears eat this kind of white powder-food...?"

Ultimately, of course, it is impossible to really clear through Fear by trying to logically dis-charge every object of fear: *Mind will generate a thousand objective excuses to account for every un-named and un-met fear*!

I felt that we were not really *clearing* fear here... but merely hanging out in Fear's domain, generating endless new possibilities to account for it - with at least some sort of rationality, however meager and however distorted it might be.

If we could find a way to help Joah to really *meet* his fear - and then *own* it, *accept* it, *feel* it through , *express* it, *share* it... and *let go* of it - and so finally come *open* to let some new feeling rise up inside himself... well, then I knew that his fear would be healed: re-solved, dis-charged and released - and he would once again be as fresh and whole-hearted as ever!*

And unless/until we could find the Way, unless we could *feel* our way into whatever Free-Ritual Process might effect such magical release... then there was nothing to do there and then except to merely keep the child as safe as I could and hope that he could trust me (at least), until we were back in the familiar world of car, headlights and home, once again.

And so the *scanning process* began....

I asked Joah if he felt that he could trust *me* to keep him safe, and he said he trusted me, but he was also still afraid.

Then I asked Joah if he believed that his elf friends - 'T'rence' and 'Troika' (who lived in our garden) - might be able to help him with his fear. He said he did, so we made a trembling Circle-of-Three and asked Troika and T'rence to come there right away, to be with Joah (and all of us) and to keep us safe from any tigers or bears or whatever else might be there.

A LITTLE NOTE ON PROCESS

In moments like this, where time is short and the goals are pretty specific... and where the littlies might be at a loss as to know how to proceed, I often find myself using guided imagery as a process... and as a deliberate tool.
I offer a medicine-prayer or an invocation in very simple terms, one phrase at a time and we all repeat the phrases - wishes, images, prayers, etc. - as they come out. I repeat my own words with them, and the power of our circle-prayer is felt more strongly when we all speak together. That I say things first is merely an invitation - *like writing something on a wall. The real Medicine is always in the Process of the Sharing.*

---

* These are the very specific steps that we all move through during any emotional clearing. We can get stuck anywhere... and we always have to go back to ask: 'What am I feeling...now?" I have developed this process as: *'THE EMOTIONAL CONTINUUM,'* - and it is a mainstay and guiding inspiration in my Integrative Therapy work.

> *In time, the others also find things to add to the image-dance - and we all taste and repeat these words together as well.*
>
> *I feel that it is very important, when assuming such a direct leadership role, to keep the messages as simple and as general (or 'generic') as I can. In this way I hope to lessen the possibility that I will be 'putting words in their mouths' -* programing *them through the intrinsic power of the circle (and the power of The Father) to recite something which they may not actually believe.*
>
> *And of course this must sometimes still occur. And even so, of course, there is still clear learning and 'shaping' value in reciting any good Medicine Word.*
>
> *With these few considerations in mind... this process is a very ancient and effective way to teach, to invite the child shamans to take an active role in making every ritual circle happen... and also a very simple and positive way to introduce them to the lore or content of my own medicine as we learn to 'walk in a sacred manner' together.*

As we finished our little *Elf-Magic Invocation Circle Ritual*, I asked Joah if he was feeling any better. "I feel good..." he said. "But I am still afraid!"

"Whaaat?" I cried. "Don't you trust your elf friends - and me - to keep you very safe...?"

"I *trust* them... and I trust *you*, Daddy.... But it's just my *fear-ness* is too strong and it still makes me feel scared!"

Without thinking about it too much, I broke off a sprig of two white flowers from a native flower-tree and asked the two elves to come into those flowers and to be with Joah and Kira on their adventure... and to protect them from anything that was scary.

Joah held his flower for a long moment, just looking at it in silence.... When he finally raised his eyes to meet me, he said that he felt much better!

Had we somehow really already succeeded... with such an impulsive and easy gesture? As often happens, I couldn't tell whether Joah was really feeling better... or just trying to 'say the right thing' to help *me* feel better about his feeling afraid.... So I said, "Well come up in my arms anyway, Little Frog, and I will carry you. But my back is still a bit sore and so I may not be able to carry you all the way to the van...."

We walked on in silence once again, the only-slightly-braver Joah clutching me like a small monkey, and Kira's grasp on my hand beginning to tighten, too, now, as she found herself all alone down there at kid-eye level... as we walked on and on, always following the mysterious patches of white powder on the trail that led us through the brooding Darkness.

Well, it was a tame path to be sure, from where I stood. But for the mini-shamans, it was a wild and desolate trail without beginning or end. And now it was leading up a frighteningly steep incline and now disappearing over a great, rocky ridge, with a sheer precipice on one side, a (very poisonous) snake-infested forest on the high side... and falling into impenetrable darkness all around. And whenever you cannot see ahead (or beside), if you are four or six, you can easily imagine an infinite abyss below... and certain flat-earth fall-off ahead! Very scary and very powerful stuff, indeed!

Now all of this sounds like a great ordeal, I'm sure. And to the little ones, it was one of the major expeditions of their lives. But in that boring linear way in which adults measure space and time, we had been away from the house for less than an hour... and had walked no more than two hundred yards along this very predictable (and ultimately circular) path. And all the while, our security-base of the van-with-lights was waiting patiently for us... and never more than fifty actual yards away.

All at once, the white-spot trail abruptly stopped.... We looked all around and there, in the 'Great Unknown' of the infinite depths of darkness (and all those lions and tigers and bears) to our left, was a great fallen tree. The trunk of this fallen giant arched downward in a long and sloping curve, as it strained to sink into the hill and meet the stream down below with the whole of its barren, ash-white body.

It was a beautiful log making a natural bridge across the stream. There was no bark on this mountain ash eucalypt and it seemed to glow with its own inviting light. Aha! Now here was a sure pathway home at last!

We sized it up. It was a very steep descent. And there was a very muddy patch between our path and the beginning of thc log. But we were game to try it. I asked Jai to wait on the path - gave him no time to say no - and carefully ferried Kira onto the log, where she flapped her arms and tried to come to balance while I went back for Joah.

He was up on the path, looking *very* carefully all around him -

probably scanning for that "only bear in Australia" and very happy to come into my arms... even if we were about to descend into the ominous darkness of the ravine... and toward the crashing gurgling sounds of the hidden torrents of the Great Black Waters below.

We began to walk along the great log. Slowly, inching our way down the slope of the log sideways. Joah was in front, holding my left hand and Kira was holding my right. All that we could see was the log we walked on... as the terrible sounds of the water crashing across the jagged rocks and the swirling, foaming, whirlpool rapids grew closer... and closer... and closer.

Somehow, each of these little ones were being very brave as they walked sideways along that fallen tree in almost total darkness. But *I* was scared! I was not all that steady on the log myself... and as we began to cross the river I really felt the bad faith of having conned them into making my assumedly infinite strength and prowess the very mainstay of their physical security!

I could have slipped off at any instant. But our leader, Joah-the-Frog just moved steadily, step after step, with each step being the exact width of one of his shoes plus two inches - the two inches as an obviously willful expression of his new bravery! I don't know how he did it. But then we got an unexpected surprise: there on the log beside us suddenly appeared a definite white-powder spot! At once we realized that we hadn't 'bailed out' - and that we were still on the trail of our Medicine Walk pilgrimage!

We paused there and looked down into the raging torrents below. True, the water-sound was quite loud. And it is true that we could only see the barest glint of light on the surface of the bubbling river as is hissed and gurgled so far below our shaky and bouncing log.

Joah said he thought that if we fell, the river would carry him away and he would go all the way to the ocean and drown in it! I again lied and reassured him that I could keep him safe.

Kira was scared, too, but not too much. She was just *doing it*, scared or not, and not talking much as she went. Her hand felt fairly relaxed in mine, and her step seemed confident. Clearly we were all involved in Joah's Initiation Ritual that night... and not hers.

And as we stood there teetering on a too-small giant log above the primal sounds of rushing waters, only I, as the sole adult-of-the-moment, had the benefit (and the limitation) of any kind of objective awareness of where we were. I knew that the raging river was only about four feet beneath our log, that it was only about four inches deep, that it was only about fourteen feet wide, and that even as we perched so precariously there, our van was parked about forty feet away from us through a small grove of forty trees....

For the little shamans, though, we were all deep in a primal life struggle to meet and overcome our primal terrors... *and we were succeeding!*

Surely and steadily, Joah was walking into the primordial Darkness one step at a time, with Daddy in tow and leading his Medicine Family out of the forest and toward the warmth of Home.

One step at a time, *Joah was walking out of Fear.* One step at a time he was walking toward his own transformation from a quivering and contracted being-of-fear in to a future life as a Medicine Warrior of great calmness and self-assurance. And ah, the great beauty of that was fine nourishment for the Father, to be sure!

We moved through many dimensions of feeling and experience... each of us seeing many different aspects of our selves in many different lights. And this was a timeless experience, beyond all order or design: a Ritual Crossing-of-the-Darkness and a Ritual Coming-Into-the-Light.

After many ages of ritual metamorphosis (and of course a very few minutes of clock-time) we came to the other side of the log. And just as we prepared for the short jump from the log bridge down to the waiting, green and mossy Earth... there, on the ground, was a very carefully written letter 'F' formed in the same white powder on the bank of the stream.

And all at once we knew: it was the end of the trail. We knew immediately that this was the end of our Medicine Walk Ritual and must somehow also be the end of our pilgrimage through the Gates of Fear.

Yes! Joah had come through! And right there before us, written on the Earth at our feet, was the Froggy's initial, 'F' just as clear as clear could be... to welcome him into his new bravery. 'F' for Froggy; 'F' for Fear... 'F' for Finish... and 'F' for Free!

As we rested on the end of the log-bridge, smelling the river and the log and the trees, fully comfortable now, with the white van peeking clearly out of the bushes and promising safety and Home whenever we might need it... I asked Joah how it was that he had been too afraid to walk on the wide, clear path, but brave enough to walk down that great long fallen tree into the Darkness... and to cross the river when it was so noisy and so deep and so frightening.

And what he replied touched my heart so deeply that I have recounted the whole adventure here, for you:

"I put all of my *fear-ness* into the flower you gave me and so I could do it. And now I will keep this flower forever and ever because they have all of my fear-ness in them. And now I don't have to be scared anymore!"

We drove along the winding road to home, and made a plan ('talking-process') that Joah would get to tell the whole story of our adventure to Leia without Kira or I "talking over him" and ripping off her attention. And so he did.

Barely through the door, Joah began to tell Leia the whole story in one fast and breathy flow of word-images. Out from his tired, relieved and very proud kid-mouth flowed the most incredible one-sentence poem about enormous bridges and thundering rivers and Infinite Darkness and lurking tigers who might eat white-powder tiger-food and helicopters and accidents and ropes and the only-Australian-bear and Daddy carrying him-but-not-Kira and Troika and T'rence coming to him and all of us following the magic powder trail and crossing the log that went down the hill and over the river that didn't carry him to the ocean and drown him and the big white letter 'F' at the end of the log... and how "I put all of my fear-ness into this flower and I am going to keep it forever and now I will always be Brave!"

And so he is. The flower, of course, has long since melted into the pile of pillows on the living room floor and is long forgotten in its physical form.

But the *Flower-Medicine that Heals all Fear*... well, that we shall certainly keep... forever.

DEEP HEALING RITUAL STORY

This is a medicine story of a free-ritual healing that occurred between Kira and me... and her Guidance... and mine.

This is the most complete and detailed account of an actual healing experience (and the way it comes to me) that we will share in this book. I hope that this story does not become too long or too complex to serve as a simple revelation of the power of *Letting Go* and *'The Healing Power of Breath'*... and as the heart-felt story of one of our family's most frightening ordeals... and one of our most powerful Rituals of Bonding and Rituals of Trust... and that this tale will flow from the Deep Wonder in our Family Heart... to awaken the Wonder in yours....

AND ALONG CAME A SPIDER...

There was once a little redback spider - the Australian version of the American black widow - which lived under an old general store, in a (truly) sleepy town, simmering in the heat of the South Pacific Sun.

And one steamy day around our (southern hemisphere) summer Christmas time, we decided to drive from our home in the Mother Valley to visit the Mother Ocean... to move from rainforest green to the whitesand shores... and to cool our hot bodies in the dazzling azure-blue waters. And so... off we went, all loaded into our big van... and ready for a day of adventure (but perhaps not ready enough)!

Just fixed yet again and full of new hope (mine, at least), the tired old 'Medicine Wheels' beast trundled down the road... for awhile... before being rudely stopped by billows of steam and that all-too familiar smell of deep fried engine rings.

Unloading the van before we abandoned it - reclaiming its mass of swimming-diving-surfboard-sun-and-camera-gear, plus all the loose food, clothes and general mess, followed by a long, slow and arduous time of sun-high hitchhiking back to town left us all in a daze of tropical torpor.

Leia and I had simply had it. The mini-shamans had had it. The Medicine Family was totally collapsed into a pool of sweat!

As the small ones sat down on the sidewalk in the shade, the head honcho Medicine Daddy went off to find another kind of vision - a 'medicine mechanic' - one who would basically work for Spirit and love, of course. One who would take our trouble in capable hands... and make everything 'all right' again.

An impossible dream? Of course. And who was I really looking for? Well... in that broken down space of helplessness... I can see now that I was looking for 'The Father,' of course. I was out on the streets looking for 'Daddy' to somehow make it all right once again!

While I wandered the streets on this quest for fatherly enlightenment of my new burden of metal (and money)... the small redback spider crawled out of a vent in the wall of her store... probably coming out in peace to meet the Medicine Family she had heard so much about, up close. But Kira, alas, had not noticed this little offer of silent friendship... and leaned back hard against the poor spider.

It could not call out... and she didn't notice... and so it bit her. And who wouldn't, about to be squashed and all? Right behind her heart it bit her, exactly on her spine.

Kira squirmed in irritated pain. Thinking it was just a mosquito, she leaned back again against the wall - and then she was bitten for real! Kira cried out in sudden pain. These bites really hurt! Leia was with her. She saw the spider crawl away and then she knew exactly what had happened. So she stilled her own fears for a moment, committed the other kids to care for Kira and then pulled herself away to race around the little town looking for me. And soon enough I was found.

There were others, too, on the street that day. But from the moment that our family began this journey through *Redback Spider Medicine*, all who were around us seemed strangely detached and oddly disinterested. Everyone seemed to just mill around, watching us with a kind of vague emptiness as we moved to meet our sudden emergency.

Amidst this odd assortment of un-feeling bystanders, our family flew into a scurry of effort: we needed a place for the great pile of things which had been removed from the dead van. We needed help with transport to get Kira to the hospital high on the hill above town. We needed to figure out who could take the other kids and who should go with Kira.... And then there was Kira herself, urgency and fear welling up in her eyes with already great intensity.

Kira's first reaction to knowing what had bitten her was to flash into Fear - the fear that she was going to die! For every Australian child knows all about the dreaded Redback Spider - the sorry subject of many playground myths and late night scary stories... and not without good reason!

The Aussie redback accounts for more deaths here than snakebite. But now it is (now) only very rarely fatal, since the discovery of an antivenin. But, fatal or not, its poison is a powerful heart-toxin. And within a few minutes of a bite, a strange and intense internal pain and a localized swelling occurs somewhere between the bite-site and the heart. The suffering is intense and can go on for more than a day. But to be bitten *at* the very heart-center (the *anahata chakra*) by a heart-poisonous *anything* can be something else altogether!

So... Yes! This felt like a time of real, mortal crisis. And even if we'd known them, merely hopeful statistics of survival rates simply wouldn't help! We knew that we were facing a very real threat to Life itself.

To me, the location of the bite felt instantly meaningful. It was Sign.. and sign that demanded immediate understanding, immediate resolution. But what did it *Mean*...?

I believed that somehow, as always, the answer to this question would also contain the seeds of the healing that we so urgently needed now.

A TIME FOR HEALING

Some healings take place in idyllic glens, in Medicine Wheel Circles of loving friends, while we savor precious moments of being totally 'at effect' - having all the time we need to surrender into whatever is inside us and time to clear it through and be healed.

But this was a different scene: we were all fatigued, short on patience and off-balance in the soggy heat and blazing sun. We were all un-focused, out of 'medicine' and heart-deep in the muck of our other real-world, mechanical crisis. All of the other kids were out of phase and bitchy with their own reactions to all of this.

And then, very suddenly, amidst all of this personal-collective confusion, Kira *needed us*... to be focused, alert, sensitive and magical... in a way that she never had before.

How Time does this, I do not know for sure. But there are times when Time itself becomes very malleable. We have all experienced it - the seemingly endless fall from a high place, the slow-motion rolling and crunch of a long-time traffic accident, the fast and slow moment of birth... and the infinite timelessness of a deep meditation. Time is a very fluid medium in which we swim. Without watching the clock, no two breaths would ever fill exactly the same time-space.

Well, just at that moment, everything colluded with everything else: Time made Space for us and all the people on the street just fell away from us so that we could do what we needed to do. Amidst all the flurry of family feeling, our ragged energies flying everywhere and the all-ways casual Aussies going about their business-as-usual around us... Kira and I were somehow left completely alone.

FEAR & MEANING & THE SIGN OF GRIEF

Alone we were, in a swirling vortex of feeling-breathing-loving-energy. Kira was afraid. And *I* was afraid.

I have been doing healing work - psychotherapy, shamanic ritual healing, breathwork, etc. - for as long as I can recall. And I have seen many truly amazing things. But I had never treated a spider bite like this, or even read much about them. So I did not feel that I had even an informed *medical* perspective to guide me, let alone any experienced medicine. And as burned out and un-centered as I felt that day, I could not feel confident that my intuitive sense (my Guidance) would keep pace with whatever was needed from me... or maybe even be there at all to help me feel a way to proceed... whatever it was that I was to do....

So I was afraid, too. And yet, I did not want my own fear to start ping-ponging back and forth with Kira's already rampant terror - reinforcing her own fear and further clouding us both when we so needed all the resource of all the clarity, trust and openness that we could possibly achieve.

In any situation, whenever we encounter the *Dance of Mortal Fear* in any of its varieties, it is so important to remember that whenever Death presents itself - as primal fear, or memory, or even through some unlikely fantasy: *Mortal Fear (Fear of Death) is Life threatened from the inside out.* And however it comes, once this special dread arises... no one can know what the outcome will be!

Whether Kira was really close to physical death just then or not could simply not be known - and I could not say, even today. But we had sign of great meaning in her mortal fear - in her specific and primal fear of Death.

Long ago, I was given a little pearl of guidance that I always carry close to my heart. And there it whispers to re-mind me, over and over again:

"Wherever is Fear... Meaning is near!"

I simply could not ignore this medicine. I could not ignore the sign and I could not ignore the meaning that awakened in me from the deep terror and that mysterious look of deep *knowing* - the look of knowing something real and terrible - that I saw in my daughter's eyes.

Without a word yet shared between us, we both knew that we were in the very depth of a terrible ordeal. And there was no way out but to find the Way to move ahead! I had no choice but to follow the sign. And without a doubt the most powerfully looming sign - perhaps the only sign there was - was the *Sign of Fear.*

Suddenly, there was a moment of *lightening*... a strange and out-of-place feeling of euphoria. It began with my awakening from whatever trance state I had been in, to suddenly notice that Kira and I were completely alone. Just the two of us... setting out together to face this important milestone, eye-to-eye and heart-to-heart. Suddenly, being there together like that, even through all the fear and dread... felt like a great *privilege.*

We were somehow being honored with a profound medicine ritual which we had not chosen... and a very special moment of deep sharing. A strongly private meaning was growing in us, dancing between us, bonding us in one-ness. It felt as though we were poised at the beginning of yet another profound and amazing Ritual of Initiation... together. And so we were....

Just now, it reminds me of our experience of years later of doing our first Fire Walk together: Kira and I, hand in hand, moving through Fear into Sureness. This spider-dance was like that... but far less obvious. For when we faced the firewalk, our path was clear before us. When we faced the Redback Ritual on that day and all alone, we knew that we were passing through an *Ordeal of Fire*... but we did not know where to walk or what to do!

And then, I felt a chilling realization deep inside: *something* in that look of *inner knowing* that I had seen in Kira's eyes had awakened a feeling of deep, primal grief in me. Yes! And in her as well.... *I could feel it!*

There was already a stream of profound and mutual grief passing between us - somehow touching in to all the pain and grief we had felt when the baby Tiki Sky moved along on his journey around the *'Great Wheel of Birth, Death and Rebirth'*.... We were somehow touching in to the primal archetype of all Grief.

In that single instant, it felt as though we were being *prepared* in that instant for the grief of all the intimate deaths which would come to those we loved.

And were we also being prepared in grief for the death of Kira...? We simply did not know! We both felt it... and talked about it (only later)... but we just could not understand the grief-sign as it flowed through us that day. But as soon as I felt this chill wind blow through my being... I knew that I didn't want to be there and to do that one ever again! If only we had a *choice* in this things....

All we had was this harsh new sign: we had found the meaning of the Sign of Fear in this new presence of grief. But the meaning of the Sign of Grief... had yet to be revealed! So we were still adrift in our experience without sure guidance... and so without any real direction. All we could do... was to *'ride the sign'* as best we could... and to try to be open to whatever may come.

Well, grief is Grief. And as with any primal emotion - be it love, fear, anger or joy - once awakened, *everything* in all our experience that resonates with that primal feeling is reawakened and felt anew... and all at once. So, once primal grief is aroused... *everything is grieved at once!*

And this was power-full medicine indeed! For as primal grief was awakened in our hearts, mourning-song filled our silent sharing, flowing all through us, even as we made commitment and bonded together... even as we took the first brave steps together, to begin to learn the never-before-seen *'Redback Spider Healing Free-Ritual Medicine Dance'* that day!

GUIDED IN - GUIDED THROUGH - GUIDED BEYOND

Up to this point, perhaps only a few minutes of clock-time had elapsed since Kira had been bitten. It takes much longer to describe (and to read), because things were happening on many levels (or dimensions) of experience... and because experience itself is time-less... and infinite. After all of this Word... I do not feel that I have even begun, really, to detail the important content of this experience... or to describe the new medicine process which was unfolding to meet it....

So it is that I don't know how long we were alone, there, together. But I know exactly what we *did*... and what we *shared*... and this is the Medicine Story:

Staying connected, eye-to-eye (even after I closed mine to be more open to what could come from within), I moved to stand over the sitting Kira child. I placed my hand over the bite on Kira's back, and another on her chest. I drew up Breath for both of us - deep and high - to clear us of our private, separating (alienating) Fear and to begin to connect and to bond our future... whatever it was to be and wherever it would take us.

I have seen two of my own children slip into Death before and now, whatever was to come, I knew that I was *not* going to leave this one... *wherever* she might need to go.

I waited a few breaths more, yearning for some mutual reassurance - for her, that I was there and, for me, that I could wholly trust my feeling-link with my little daughter and so find trust that I would be guided through whatever was to come... and from that Sign of Trust... find sureness that I could *act* on whatever was given to me... to do... to feel... to be... for Her.

In Time, we came to be *'of One Mind and One Heart,'* as the Ancient Ones would say. In Time, we were coming to be as *'one'* as we could be... in what time we had.

I drew up with breath, whatever medicine power would come through me and made an *Inner Clearing Ritual Dance* to open to whatever guidance might attend. And all of this happened in a flash: in slow-time, quick-time, no-time, I surrendered all that I could of egoic 'me' to be-come-to-be as *'clear channel'* - as open as I could possibly be - for whatever energy-feeling-guidance-wisdom-healing-Spirit could (or would) come through.

Please remember... at that time, as I have said, I had no objective (medical) perspective on redback spiders. But I *did* trust my medicine. And I knew of the *Power of Surrender*. And so I did... just as wholly as I could... and knew that this would just have to be wholly (and holy) enough!

The still-growing Pain and its twin demon of Confusion seemed likely at first to pose serious threat to Kira's power of focus. But that inner desperation I had seen in her eyes was moving me to a stance of *absolute commitment* and *total determination*... to unravel whatever knot of ignorance or limitation may arise within me... and to find *whatever it would take* to accomplish what I knew to be my absolute need and only path-way: to surrender... to *let go*... and to make whatever medicinc prayer I could to invite Guidance to come through me, there and then... and then to be strong enough to *act* on whatever I was shown to do.

And then we began to dance together....

"Kira! Listen to me! I want you to know that I am here with you. *AND I WILL NOT LEAVE YOU.* I am your Daddy and *I AM HERE FOR YOU!"*

"Listen to me, Little One. Can you hear me?"

"Yes," she replied. Softly. Slightly distant, somehow, perhaps a little disbelieving (but of what I could not tell). I noted her disbelief - or mine, as I could not be sure whose it was - and tried not to let it breed fear in me. And so I went on...

"Kira! We can do this together. *WE CAN DO IT!* Can you feel it...?"

There was a silence. More doubt? My own doubt raised its head once again and was overpowered by Trust. It sounds corny. It happens like that: Fear competes with Trust. Faith competes with Doubt. Shamanic medicine works at this level... but it only works when your Trust is greater than your Fear. And Trust only grows from long and deep experience....

In this realm you must trust that Direct Spiritual Guidance *will* come. If you do... if you can... *It will.* If you do not... then your own fear and doubt - and all other negative expressions of your own ego - will compromise your Openness and cloud your Vision... and you may not see the Way even if it is shown.

"Yes, Daddy... I think I can.... But I'm still afraid, too."

"It's ok, Kira. It's ok to be afraid. Can you feel beyond your fear? Can you feel that *we can do it...* that we can get through this together?"

And then she brightened. She squeezed my arm, pulled it deeper into her chest and said - with a surprising feeling of celebration: *Yes!*"

Not when I had first begun to speak words of reassurance and faith to her... but just as soon as she was finally able to commit herself to our medicine, I felt Kira begin to melt (no other word describes it) into my hands - melting into my yearning for her healing... melting into my open daddy-heart... melting into a deep and wonderful state of absolute Trust.

Finally I felt it: *It was happening!* That was all I knew. *Something* was beginning to move for us, between us, within us. And I felt exalted (even through my fear) at having something to do - anything to do - ecstatic at simply having a way to proceed!

Sometimes this is all you need. Sometimes this is enough: a path to walk and a path clearly shown and a process to help you move. And then the danger and the fear lose their meaning... and so lose their power within you.

My whole being responded to this *Knowing* with a deep feeling of reverent gratitude. I was being blessed: by Spirit, by Life, by Openness... by my daughter's deep Trust and by her profound Surrender.

There is nothing like Trust to awaken Deep Healing and to evoke power-full medicine. At the very instant of Kira's commitment, *I* had become trust-worthy to her... and so was trust-worthy to myself. And I was suddenly empowered to *act* from within this mutual trust.

My hands became stronger... stronger, perhaps, than ever before. I was supporting Kira's entire upper body weight with hands that were doing many things at once: hands that plunged deep into her very center, clearing away obstruction, sweeping away pain and sucking out the vital energy of the poison and (most of all), drawing out the *Fear*.

Even as all this was happening, these empowered hands were gently 'stroking' her breath: lofting breath as a healing force, high and clear and light as a spirit-feather within her chest and back again into total discharge in to the Mother Earth, as we breathed in absolutely bonded unison.

And also at the same time, my hands were communicating my own inner resolution and my inspiration: I was *being* the rock of Father-Power upon which she could lie in trust of my *absolute support*.

To keep this channel open and all this power flowing... I was concentrating *only* upon surrender... surrendering to all the energy, word-flow and guidance that was coming through me. And Kira was surrendering to me... and beyond me... in to *Spirit*.

When I am involved in 'healing' work I know that I only need to keep the channel open. I must only strive to maintain deep openness. And then, *what* 'comes through' me or *how* it occurs does not need to be explained in my all-too-mortal awareness then (or now) for the magic to occur.

The shaman-healer never really heals. The 'healer' can only surrender to become a *living channel* for the greater power and wisdom that comes from without. We may each define this presence as we will: as Spirit, God or Grace... as Ancestor Blessing or Earth-Spirit presence... as Guidance from the Ascended Masters or as the simple Power of Love.

But whatever it *is* and however it comes... when it comes, it is an awesome and deeply humbling experience.

Well... hands... yes. And Breath and Touch and Energy and Light. Yes... all of this and so much more. And however much I might call on experienced Word to share this experience here, there is no way to really encompass the infinity of *'It All.'*

Whatever I can find of Word to share, still more was happening. We were being borne aloft on high winds of clear and pressing urgency - urgency that breathed *process* and *presence* through us both.

We were being swirled in endless vortices of transformation and empowerment. And all the after-questions of 'who?' and 'what?' and 'why?' and 'how?' simply had no relevance in that moment of such desperate glory.

It felt as though every dimension of my awareness (and beyond) was alive and crackling with inrushing empowerment. But my touch... our bonded hearts... our shared breath... and *'The Word'* provided the catalyst, the medium, the energy and the channel for everything else.

Over and over I was moved to speak to my daughter with an unusual and powerfully unyielding commandment:

"I AM HERE! I AM WITH YOU!
I AM YOUR FATHER! AND I WILL NOT LEAVE YOU!
AND WHEREVER THIS JOURNEY TAKES US...
WE WILL GO TOGETHER!"

It shocked me deeply to be saying this. I felt Fear at what this commitment might entail. But I was *not* going to let this child go! (Alone?). And within my Guidance system, I can always ask for a 'screen refresh' - and so update, clarify and check out whatever I receive. And so I did... and so it was still clear: I was not going to 'allow' separation to occur. I was going to ride this trip through in an *absolutely bonded* link with my daughter!

I repeated my reassurance over and over, droning, commanding, inviting, *im-pressing* into her... until, all at once, I knew that it had *'worked!'* And then 'The Word' began to change. Now I found my words inviting Kira to begin to 'take power' for herself and to take control of her *own* healing. I made unnegotiable demands... and so commanded her to act for herself:

"Kira! I want you to *let go* of this poison. *LET GO* of this bite.

Let it go in to my hands. *DO IT NOW!*
Let it go in to my heart. *DO IT NOW!*
Let it *all* go into me, Kira! *DO IT NOW!*
Push it out of your body. *LET ME HAVE IT ALL!"*

I repeated these demanding invitations over and over again, for a long and timeless time. My hands urged and demanded with my voice, working deeply into her body: separating and discharging pockets of fear... smoothing and inviting the streaming energy of her life force to sweep away all the toxins and all the fear... inviting her on a cellular level to *feel* me, to *surrender* to me, to *trust* me... and to *let go of all the pain and all the poison in to me.*

Faster and faster the dance grew. For every inner release yet another wave of insidious poison, pain or fear came up from the bowels of the crisis, crashing in upon our Hope. And yet, with every Fear-fearing withdrawal came a new and more strident invitation.

My hands, my breath, my heart, my will and my words all merged into a unified stream of great power:

"LET ME TAKE IT AWAY!
GIVE IT ALL TO YOUR DADDY!
PLEASE KIRA! AND PLEASE... DO IT NOW!"

Somewhere in the word-touch-breath-mind dance, I also tried to impress upon her that I would not be hurt or harmed by the poison in any way. I assured her and reassured her that, "It is not poison to me and I will be ok if you can just let it all go into me!"

Kira was sitting bolt upright now - physically lifted by my 'lofting' of her breath-chest-heart, but also lifted in a poised stillness of absolute inner concentration. She clutched my arm gently, clinging to Daddy-security and to the Daddy-healing that she had learned to trust, long before, in other dances and other rituals born of other primal needs.

But apart from this primal clutching... she sat with the most elegant poise and balance that I had ever seen... drinking in *The Word*... letting go of all that she could... and constantly *scanning* every inner dimension for any more fear that might be lurking anywhere within range of her conscious effect.

I could tell that she had melted into this healing, to be sure, and at the deepest levels of her receptivity. But on the more usual levels of her (egoic) awareness, she felt reassured (I would say)... but not certain. She was trusting... but not completely sure.

And how could she have been? Nothing was 'certain.' There was no 'surety' built into this situation at all!

As long as we had open-channel to the Guidance... I trusted that we had a chance. But at the level of Little-Me (of ego-me), in many ways I was no more sure than she... no more wise... no more....

And so the Medicine Dance went on. For me, everything was so intense that I was not aware of anything else around me. I did not know anything about anything... except that I was wholly committed and engaged in the 'mission' at hand. Yes... like a 'mission.' A *total commitment*. And *nothing* else existed for me.

As for Kira, I cannot know for sure, of course, the whole of her experience. Perhaps someday she will write this story from her own point of view. But through all of this terror and splendor, Kira achieved and remained in a deep trance.

Once she had discharged her first-fears and had calmed her crying, she became very quiet. It was as though she was *listening* with such total concentration that she did not have energy to spare for anything else!

She listened as she had never listened before. For some time she repeated each word that I said to her, mouthing it silently. Staring into space - completely out of her visual-eyes - she just *listened!*

And then it happened! The moment of our *total mergence* was a feeling that Kira and I will never forget. There was a sudden rise and fall of our breath-link. There was a sudden crashing, imploding union of our one-and-frightened heart. There was a great streaming rush of intensification of all the energies that were pulsing through my hands and through our whole-body connection. There was the ongoing vibration of the sound of word - 'my' word... her word.... all *Medicine Word*. And there was a sheeting and overwhelming stillness of *'The Listening.'* And all at once, we were *ONE* - one breath, one heart, one depth, one mind, one destiny....

Ultimately, 'one what?' is beyond my Word. 'One *with* what?' - I cannot fully say. Then there was a shudder that passed through us - Kira's or mine or ours - or from somewhere far beyond I could not tell - and Kira's eyes (and perhaps mine as well) rolled up and then fluttered a few times as she (or we) let out a great sigh...

It was a sigh of release, as we let go together... and fell down and down and downwards in to and right on through *all* the Fear.... As we fell I had so much time to wonder if we were falling into Death -

hers, mine or ours. It seemed that we had already fallen so far that life must soon run out and so be left behind.

But still we fell further and further into that infinite out-breath-last-breath bottomless void... until *all* the Fear was gone... and we were still... alive!

It had been a great plunge into total Expulsion as all the threat and all the poison was neutralized or cast out....

It had been an endless sigh of Gratitude and Acknowledgement as we both felt the surety of Spirit presence....

It had been a Deep Surrender into Death, Re-Birth and Celebration as Kira opened to a New Life grounded in deeper Trust. And it had been a Free-Ritual Initiation and a Celebration of Kira's destiny of becoming a Wise-Woman-Medicine-Woman of great magic and everlasting power. And so, I can see... she is.

Arising from this State of Grace of *total surrender* into infinite space... we eventually came up to earth-plane awareness once again and looked at each other with New Vision: looked with a long, unblinking, unspeaking, wholly loving gaze into the very depths of each other's souls. For time beyond time we were held there in rapture and in wonder.

And then a smile began to crack on Kira's face. She reached up to encircle my neck with her arms and whispered ever so gently... "Thank you, Daddy."

And then we knew that the Healing was done.

Moving out of the intensely private space of our Medicine Healing Ritual, Kira and I looked around us for the first time in... however long it was. We saw that we were wholly surrounded - untouched, but deeply enfolded by the tear-streaked faces of our family. And as we raised our faces and smiled up at them... one by one they felt the 'news' that we already knew:

Kira was going to be completely healed!

Trying to be Father to the other children as well, I think I muttered something like, "It's all right now. Kira is going to be all right now." Or something equally lame and probably unnecessary anyway. Perhaps it reassured some of us... but mostly, everyone just *knew* that *the Healing had already worked.*

And *now* it was time to go to the hospital!

ALLOPATHIC MEDICINE DECLINES ITS RIGHTFUL PLACE

However strong the medicine magic may be, there is still within me a deep parental responsibility that does not want to make any mistake when child-life or well-being is at risk in any way. And although I 'knew' what had happened between Kira and myself and Spirit (such as I could comprehend it at all), I still felt ignorant as to the long-term bodily effects of redback spider bites.... And I knew that I had to find out.

When conventional western (allopathic) medicine is at hand, I use it as a greatly reassuring resource... and sometimes even for healing... when I can... when it can... when they can... or whatever.

When I have closed a deep head wound and knitted together the loose bits with a butterfly bandage then I call our doctor for feedback and advice. When I undertake an unconventional course in meeting a chronic illness... then I talk it over with a doctor friend and integrate whatever s/he may have to offer.

So to the little country town Aussie hospital we did go. Kira was signed in and bedded down and our diagnosis of the problem tentatively accepted - although they would have liked to see the actual spider to be sure that Leia wasn't doing a paranoid or ignorant parent-number on them. Good medical practice.

Even here, where there are so many separate species of highly poisonous snakes about, hospitals are learning not to administer antivenin unless they are reasonably certain that a bite has even occurred and exactly what did the biting. It's all based upon statistics: how many reported bites turn out to be no bite at all; how many named biters turn out to be something else entirely; how many general malaise complaints turn out to be unnoticed bites... etc. And these statistics prove very strikingly how little people know about what has actually happened to them at the very most important moments of the lives!

There is an antivenin for redback spider poison and I was told much later that this substance is clearly labeled to indicate that it is benign enough that it can be administered even when there is uncertainty if an actual redback bite has occurred... but I guess the nurses just hadn't bothered to read the label.

Kira was given water and we were refused the right to give her the mega-dose of vitamin C that I intuitively wanted to administer. Had to wait for the supposedly on-call doctor to call back before the nurses could allow *anything* to be done, of course. I felt as though I had, once again, signed away all power to go on helping my daughter in this time of need - and had fallen into this (familiar) help-less-ness by the very act of seeking medical help!

An odd irony of the allopathic medical system, is it not? Once you go for help - and whether there is any help to be had or not - you may not be allowed to help yourself!

While we waited for the doctor to respond, a helpful male nurse told me the sequence of what usually happens with redback spider bites. He confirmed that her symptoms were normal for such a bite... and warned me that she was probably due for a long run of increasingly intense pain. He said that an intensely painful lump was likely to form somewhere between the bite site and her heart... and that it might take from twelve to twenty-four hours to go away.

But Kira was not on this predictable track any longer. And as time passed, Kira continued to improve. The lump of painful swelling under her armpit soon began to subside. Her energy was obviously picking up. She was on the mend and everyone could see it.

There were some mildly suspicious inquiries from the other nurses, veiled heavily in that especially saccharin Aussie politeness: "Did we actually *see* the spider? Were we *sure* that it was actually a redback? And what actually happened to the spider after the girl was bitten?" (etc.).

Leia said: "Look... I have lived here all my life. I know what redback spiders look like. After she was bitten I squashed the spider with my sandal and there wasn't anything left to bring here."

The nurses simply could not integrate what they saw and what they felt of Kira's obvious recovery. Where was the textbook pain? And, above all, *where was the fear?* So they tried several different ways to discredit our report that she had indeed been bitten by such a venomous spider:

"Maybe she wasn't actually bitten...?" But then they looked more closely and finally saw the bite marks.

Then they tried another one: "Maybe it was some other kind of spider...?" After all, they reasoned, it really *couldn't* have been a redback, since Kira seemed so peaceful and untroubled.

And when Leia firmly disputed that one they centered on another weak rationale: "Well it must not have been that much of a bite after all..!" And that's what they told the doctor.

In the end, the doctor didn't even come to the hospital. In two hours Kira had been discharged, while the nurses patronizingly affected great patience with us all.

You see, once again, what had been a wonder-full and precious experience of great Medicine Healing to us... was destined to be seen by them as "just another case of mistaken assumption or parental paranoia."

So... as happens in virtually every instance of spontaneous (or miraculous) healing of any morbid condition, Allopathic Medicine once again missed a great chance to grow and learn and to expand its rigid horizons... and Spirit and Healing and Shamanic Ritual Medicine were once again officially recorded as just another case of obvious mis-diagnosis... parental hysteria... and ignorance.

Ah...Sweet Spirit... may we all be filled with such sweet ignorance forever!

THE LESSON OF 'THE KISS OF THE SPIDER-WOMAN'

Kira knows otherwise. And Kira has taken this ordeal very much to heart (no pun): she *uses* her memory of the whole event over and over to help her to make leaps of faith and to find trust in many different situations.

In fact, she has told me that when we first 'walked on Fire'... she used her memory of the redback bite, of its searing pain and of our 'walking through it' so closely together... to gain the courage that she needed to take my hand in hers and to step out with me upon the glowing mass of red hot, fire-breathing coals... to do a *Father-Daughter Fire-Walk Medicine Ritual Dance...* with total confidence and in absolute trust.

So the Redback Spider Healing Ritual goes on, and on, and on... bringing new courage to this rising woman-sprout Medicine Healer.

The medicine story of this event is story enough in itself. But as it happens, I did not write it for several years after that time of our dance through Spider Fear. But now I have learned (and am still learning) how Kira is *using* that medicine... and now I know what is most important to share in this account:

Powerful healing does happen... and there is sometimes dramatic release, discharge and incredible breakthrough in the process. But very often, the real magic of the healing experience occurs *after* the event: after the great release... and long after the Healing Ritual Dance has been danced.

For it is not what 'actually happened'... but what we *learn from...* and what we *do with* the healing experience that becomes the most powerful medicine of all.

We have only begun to see what Kira will do with this deeply power-full Ritual Initiation into Trust... through her meeting with that little redback spider on a long summer afternoon, so many years ago.

And whatever it may be... *that* will be the Healing for us all!

THE ESSENTIAL PROCESS OF FREE-RITUAL SHAMANIC HEALING

For any Free-Ritual Spirit-Guided Shamanic Healing, the *Process* is all-ways the same. It sounds too simple to be true... and it is repetitive to say it over and over again. But this is the all and everything that we can do:

We can just LET GO into Guidance and then follow with *absolute commitment* and *absolute integrity*, whatever is given: whatever impulse, whatever direction, whatever action, whatever inspiration lights up within us.

We can Trust that every impulse *is* Guidance. And trusting ourselves to act from this guidance, we may do many things:

We can Touch into the maelstrom of the dis-ease, pressing deeply on specific energy points or stroking or sweeping energy under our hands. However we feel it is what it is.

We can Breathe with the person who is distress and so learn of their inner experience as it plays through their breath and help them to release all toxins, bondage, dis-ease... and *Fear*.

We can become Living Channels and so be carried into other realms and there confront bizarre energies and entities that play through the moment's trauma or dis-ease. *There is no difference between dream-*

imagination-guidance and Spirit in this process!

We can contact Past (or Future) Incarnations (in ourselves and/or in those we heal) and so help to effect a release of some karmic burden.

We can share a Ritual of Death and Re-Birth - by helping reunite a soul with Mother Earth or Father Spirit and inviting surrender and trust.

We can make Deep Bonding with a lost-child's terror and lead her back in to the Light of Peace.

Or: *We may simply use our Loving Presence* to smooth a tense muscle or awaken a paralyzed limb, to accompany someone on and inner journey of their own... that we may never see or feel.

Over the past several decades, I have seen so many 'miracles' of healing that have happened right under my no-mind touch and before my very eyes in the arms of others, that I know without any doubt whatsoever, that when Healing is evoked from a place of absolute Surrender and absolute Trust:

NOTHING IS IMPOSSIBLE!

And as we place ourselves in the Service of the Healing Process - which seems inevitably to take us far beyond our wide-eyed conceptual understanding - and no matter what we are guided to do, all that is needed from our *Intention* (from our conscious, or egoic selves) is *Deep Surrender* and the *Trust to Act...* in *any* way that we are moved to meet-share-release-discharge-birth the sickness in to wholeness and into health.

Others may beat a 'special drum' in the way of ancient tribes, or do the 'special dance' of some other displaced tribal tradition. But for me there is only one Way: *Deep Surrender and the Trust to Act...* no matter what is required... and no matter where our experience-fantasy-intuition-guidance may take us.

Ultimately, this is the only Free-Ritual Medicine Path. And the work of the Free-Ritual Shamanic Healer is all-ways the same:

We make total commitment to Openness
To find whatever Way we can...
To Surrender as much as we can
To simply let the Guide-Dance flow
Through Body-Mind-Emotion-Spirit.

We make Total Commitment to Follow
Whatever may come
Wherever it may lead!
And then we Trust:

WHATEVER COMES... IS THE GUIDANCE

And in our Trust we know:
It will all-ways BE there
To show us the Way.
And through this Trust and surety
We become living catalysts and Open Channels,
Practitioners of unknown and ancient Healing Arts
Conveyors of endless Magical Processes
That we have never seen before.

From this dedicated Ritual Openness
We Commit to do whatever we are given
To evoke whatever Healing is to come.

HEALING IN THE SAFETY OF THE CIRCLE

There are many times in the life of every individual, when we find ourselves faced with our own or others' needs, for healing, for guidance, for learning. If we feel that we have no way to rise up to meet and fulfill these needs, there are many excuses that will continue to work: "I didn't know what to do." Or, "I thought I'd better wait until someone else showed up." Or, "If only I'd known how to be useful to that person in their time of need."

I use the word 'excuses' because these are the excuses that our culture has taught us - the ways in which we excuse ourselves from having to face the ultimate challenge of meeting 'The Great Unknown' face-to-face, wide open and ready for *anything*.

Even undergoing extensive training in any discipline of healing, therapy or spiritual problem solving does *not* guarantee safety from 'The Great Unknown.' No! Far from it! Virtually every learned practitioner of the validating skills of (western) medicine, psychotherapy or alternative healing has faced these same challenges in the course of her/his work. In fact, it is how we face these challenges that furthers the evolution of these disciplines within our mass-mind consciousness.

For me, the only real benefit that I have ever noticed from having some formal understanding of psychophysical energy systems and processes that operate within the human body-mind is that it gives me enough confidence to open to even stranger guidance. When I first began to do ritual 'healing' work, I found that whenever I felt totally out of touch with my Inner Guidance... I could 'fall back' on specific techniques and processes... and of course, some good would follow.

And even today, if ever it happens that I feel out of touch or when no clear guidance is coming through... I can switch from the innocence of total openness to the surety of the psycho-physical practitioner in a flash. And from this more learned (if less inspired) point of view I can set about to deliberately research such things as restrictions in a person's breathing (or posture or self-awareness) and know pretty well what to do to motivate remedial change in breath-energy-life-flow... and so have confidence that this will begin to break loose associated bits of experience or feeling.

As these new feelings are admitted, 'owned' and finally dis-charged in complete expression... I trust that this release will, in turn, evoke many kinds of other energy release in the body-mind... and that this liberation will *be* a healing of the whole-being system... provided that whatever feeling and content is awakened is *processed-through* and fully self-integrated through that individual's whole-being experience.

But in my earlier years, and just when I began to feel fully competent within these more formal energetic systems, I was shocked to realize that whenever I felt that 'special presence' that comes when we move close to the experience of 'real healing,' it virtually *never* happened through the implementation of these already-known principles and techniques!

On the contrary, I noticed that whenever 'real' healing occurred... it seemed increasingly to happen when *'I'* was almost not there at all. Increasingly, it seemed to happen when my ego-self was drifting around in a trance-state of Deep Surrender (the *'non-doing'* I now knew to do for the Spider Dance with Kira).

As this evolution continued, I began to realize that from deep within that space of uncontrolling *openness*, I might move - touch - breathe - say - sing - dream - demand - celebrate in any way at all. And through that state of openness, whatever 'comes through' is often an extremely powerful *catalyst* of the Healing Process *which all-ways occurs within the individual being healed.*

As we have said: 'we' do not *do* the healing. Whatever healing comes... comes from without and within the one who needs to find Change. The best that any free-ritual shaman-healer can offer is to serve as a *prime energy channel*... as a *messenger*... as a *translator*... as one who speaks Word which has no roots in personal 'knowing'... as one who would trace the steps in an unknown Free-Ritual Shamanic Healing Dance that has never been danced before.

And in so doing, if we are truly surrendered and so wholly open to whatever Guidance may come... we can be privileged to provide the path-way for some spark of connection that unites the injured one with his/her own inner wisdom and cosmic rightness... and so serve to Invite whatever it is that sends actual healing energy and consciousness through us... to come through our Earth-born bodies... and to help us in our endless quest for healing... for wholeness... and for one-ness with *'The All and Everything'* of life... and consciousness... and Spirit.

It is so important to be clear about *who* and *what* we are. And it is always hard to be sure. But when we turn to Openness as the first prerequisite of serving others; when we approach each encounter with 'The Great Unknown' with true humility and true *availability* to be guided... then the *content* of whatever we might 'do' is easily surrendered into the overwhelming experience of what is happening (or being done) *through* us. And then the real healing can begin!

For a broken bone (or a known spider bite), western medicine has many useful solutions. For more subtle, chronic and multi-dimensional ills of the soul, western medicine has painfully little to offer. And sooner or later, these subtle ills prove to be the deepest needs of every living soul.

It is hard to meet them alone. It is always hard to *know* what to do to really care for another individual... and usually impossible to know for ourselves. But whenever we enter a Medicine Circle of like-minded souls - be it a little medicine family of infants on a medicine walk with Daddy, or a powerful gathering of tribal shamanic healers coming together to surrender and serve self and others - we enter a new realm of simple process and deep assurance:

There is wisdom that lives in (and flows through) every Ritual Circle that far exceeds the knowing of any one.

There is Guidance that comes to anyone who opens to the Healing Power of the Circle that may not happen in any other way or place.

And every Healing Circle has a life-rhythm that is all its own:

When the Circle is strong, Release and Revelation is invited and can be evoked from any who surrender to its Power.

When the Circle's clarity wavers - even for an instant - then we can see those who have come to surrender pull back, their inner secrets spontaneously self-concealing from the un-focused circle.

And perhaps the strangest phenomenon of all: whoever seeks to convene or to be served by a Healing Circle also *determines, activates* and *configures* the circle. Perhaps consciously, but often without any awareness at all, we affect and shape the circle's depth, its relative openness, its dynamic potential (its power to elicit change) and its leadership or self-guidance. And then the Circle itself, acting with and through all who are gathered there, will *always* regulate whatever happens to work within the precise parameters of that circle's power and ability.

That is: *nothing* happens in the center of any Circle that has not been accepted and allowed by that Circle's mutual consciousness. And even more powerful is this simple truth of the Circle Process: there is *nothing* that arises in any Circle that cannot be effectively dealt with and processed-through *by* the Circle that elicited/allowed it to come forth! Think about it: this may well be the most miraculous gift of Circle Process that I have ever received!

It is an uncanny and beautiful thing to behold... and I would not expect *anyone* to who has not discovered this from long experience of Circle-Work to even *believe* that this is possible!

So... if we are willing to try it... we will soon learn that the Circle has its own Truth, its own Powers and its own Heart. And *everything which comes up in any committed Circle can be met and dealt with and cleared right there and then.*

Thus we can say that the Healing Circle is self-regulating, self-unfolding and self-limiting. And so *it is safe to 'let go'* into a Circle of committed and surrendered souls.... And *it is safe to Trust* that healing can (and will) occur in direct proportion to the degree of

Surrender that evokes and supports this collective Change.

Underlying these simple miracles... there is another principal of Self which is absolutely essential here: No matter what else may be happening... we all must take responsibility for utilizing *all* of the resources which are available to us.

So while you certainly *can* meet (and heal) the redback spider bites of life while waiting for the ambulance to come... *after* the healing (at least)... be sure to honor your culture's medical-legal traditions as well and: *"Be sure to consult your Doctor!"* Because this is a resource which has also been 'given' for us to use.

Circles which are convened in gentle openness, to offer supportive enfoldment to anyone who needs help of any kind, tend to be *very* safe environments in which to open to compassionate help and nurturing from others.

This special safety lies in what I have come to know as *The Protection of Innocence*: when you are not wholly 'clear' in yourself... you simply will not be a channel for anything (except your own unclarity) and you will receive no impulse or guidance. You can hold someone's hand and wish them wellness and you will not be moved to act beyond this simple companionship and affirmation.

But when we are fully open... *Deep Guidance all-ways comes.* And when we open to shamanic healing within the safety and guidance of the circle... every need can be served, by those who are fully able and fully surrendered to being active channels for the healing energy that is everywhere and all the time... around us, in us and through us... all.

For me... the best circles are those which come together freely, with no specific dogma, no authoritarian leader and with no specific intention except openness and mutual nurturance.

And this heart-centered, *Open Medicine Circle* is the best resource that I have ever seen, to enable people with no formal training or technical expertise, to help each other to explore our inner fears, to find Deep Guidance for all that we need... and to share the Celebration of all that we are.

So... this is the Process... and the Path... of Free-Ritual Shamanic Healing. And *this* is certainly healing enough!

><><

CHAPTER 10

- TALKING STORY - ANCESTORS, ALLIES & ALIENS

INVOCATION MEDICINE SONG

What can we do when God-Light so shines through us
That we fall into tears of amazement
At what is unfolding before us
At what is happening within our Medicine Family

What can we do.... but sing our Medicine Song?
With this Spirit Family around me
My Song comes forth so clear and strong....

Slowly I pick up the sacred pipe.
It feels cold, unused for many moons.

Tonight there is open channel to the stars
And we will offer sacred smoke
To the Four Directions
And to the Earth and to the Sky
And to the Center - within our Hearts and Souls.

Tonight we shall do bhakti *(devotion) to Shiva*
We shall dance with the elements
And bid all elementals to come hither

Enfolding us all in reassurance as they dance
To fill our minds with Spirit Word
And to fill our hearts with Hope.

"Tonight we call you forth,
O Grandmothers and Grandfathers
Of all Life and Consciousness.
Hear our call and come to Us!

Be with us now and bring Lesson to our Circle
As tonight and always do we yearn for your nourishment
And we cry out for your wisdom and your teaching...
Though it be difficult, frightening or painful to feel -
We place our Trust in your compassion
We place our Hearts in your care.
Be with us tonight, O Ancient Ones.

Pass through the veil of Fire in our Circle
Merge with our Hearts and Minds this Night

All beings of Vision who are here in this Light
Come Meet Us and Feel Us and Teach Us to-night!"

THE VANITY OF THE ILLUSION OF KNOWING

There is a way of being aware which seems so hard for us to learn. A way of walking out of the doors of our socially delimited perception and stepping onto the Living Earth with all the pure and simple wonderment of a very young child.

"What is here? What is there? What will I find today...?"

The child does not know what s/he will find. The child does not *pretend* to know.... If not the child, *why do We...?*

The egoic self-security that adults constantly strive for is so dependent upon this feeling of believing that we *know* what's happening: that we know what to do... that we know how to do it... that we know what to expect... and that we know what it all means.

And we easily become so intent upon this quest for the self-stabilizing sophistication of sureness... that we hardly notice what we are missing by strutting around with such affected confidence, in a world that we imagine we so well understand... and which we have hardly yet begun to see.

It is very interesting to note that in its most literal sense, the word 'sophistication' actually means: *'narrowed.'*

This is *Talking-Story* of a learning time of a friend from another world. This is a story that links stone-age consciousness to the world of today... and a takes us on a great leap from total confusion to Deep Knowing... in a flash of time!

STONE-AGE CITY BEACH-SCENE DREAMING

Sitting at the edge of the azure-blue ocean at Bondi Beach in Sydney, Australia, watching the city beach-scene of playfulness and laughter and bravado and joy-full lust. Beside me sat a gentle man from a very different time and place. He was a (real) tribal chieftain from Papua New Guinea and for many years he had been selling vegetables from his garden, day by day, until he had enough money saved to buy a ticket on a magical jetplane to carry him here to visit some of his younger relations.

Together we sat there, watching the sun and the sea and the nearly naked and happy bodies all around. I tried to see things as he was seeing them and to feel anew the amazing glitter and splash of all the color and life and technology of a large western metropolis - as he might be feeling it all on this first day at Australia's most famous (and crowded) tourist beach. And as we sat together, two people from such very different cultures, adrift for a moment together on a newly found island that floated between our contrasting backgrounds, we made a deep, unspoken mergence of feeling and heart.

Time passed. Sun was giving warnings of "Hey! Too much!" for my pallid, white-skin body, while Chada (this is as close as I could come to hearing his name) sat easily erect in the white-hot blaze of blasting UV assault in perfect comfort, pulling absentmindedly at the great gaping hole in his enormously distended earlobe which was accustomed to carrying a massive bone earplug. That and his usual nose-bone and ceremonial bird-of-paradise feathers had all been left behind, in a sweetly humorous attempt to 'fit in' to the culture of this bigger and more modern island of Australia.

As Chada sat with me in silence, and after an hour or more had passed, I noticed that his far-side hand kept fidgeting with something he kept more or less hidden at his side. He said nothing, but his actions grew more and more obvious. Eventually I sneaked a peek to see what he was up to, and saw an ancient brown hand repeatedly clicking its gnarled, long and yellowed nails all around the screw-on top of a small bottle of mineral water which was sitting upright in the sand beside him, shielded by the cloth that he wore around his waist.

I turned away, to allow him privacy for what was obviously meant to be a private action. But try as I could I could not ignore his growing urgency. Inside, this man was full of that genuine stillness and self-peace which tribal people seem to carry so well. But outside, he was becoming increasingly agitated, very intent upon his hand-game with the secret bottle.

After waiting as long as I possibly could, and with all the gentleness I could muster, I finally asked him what he had hidden there and if he needed any help. Throughout the Pacific Islands (and the Orient) as well, maintaining personal dignity - or 'saving face' - is often the most important thing of all! Absolutely essential to maintaining any relationship at all, honor and respect are often more important than life itself!

Chada heard my offer and understood my gesture, and then looked up, instantly embarrassed. I demurred and averted my eyes, so as not to be seen to notice his discomfort. He grew more confident as I looked away. And then we could meet: he flashed a broad shy smile at me and showed me - through a few well-chosen shrugs and some pidgin that I could only barely understand - that he was trying to get the top off so he could have a drink!

Now that seemed a fine idea! So, with a good display of ritual shyness (to match his own) I demurely offered to help. I slowly put out my hand to receive the bottle, and gently unscrewed the cap, making a small show of the force that was needed - and where to apply it. I offered this insight to him as a low-keyed Medicine Gift. And no words here can describe the look of absolute joy and self-accomplishment which lit up Chada's wrinkled face as he took that gift from me: turning the cap the last turn and carefully laying it in the sand, he raised the bottle like a toast - or an offering - and then we shared the best water-spirit-genie that had ever been put in a bottle... and so cleverly capped.

The moment of our mutual success passed in a flash... as Chada discovered the unexpected after-burn of the carbonated water... and then all the tension was dissolved as we shared a good laugh, sitting there together as though we each were intent on watching something far out at sea. Side by side and heart to heart... we laughed. And we were brother-father warriors laughing at the absurdity of the whole world....

Does this all sound obvious to you? Well it wasn't at all obvious to me! I could help this man 'save face' from having to admit his ignorance of modern ways... but even in my role as cultural expert, I could not help myself to save face from my own ignorance of his tribal world. For however ignorant-innocent Chada might be of even the simplest of our modern technology... I knew that he was far better at being in *my* world... than I might be in his. What Chada had to learn from me that day was a very simple mechanical skill. What I stood to learn from him... I am not sure that I can even imagine!

After all... I was sitting next to a genuine stone-age tribal warrior who appeared to be well on the far side of seventy years of age. This man had already succeeded in mastering (by his very survival) a rugged, tribal, earth-centered life that I could only dream of.

Here was a man who had just yesterday removed the nose-bone and bird-of-paradise feathers which had been his people's fashion for untold thousands of years... a man who had been scar-tattooed at puberty with sea shells and charcoal when he became a warrior... a man who had warred with other tribes with stone-crafted weapons and hunted heads and women long before any whiteman ever came to his mountain rainforest home... a man who had likely known tribal ritual cannibalism and had witnessed that first coming of the Whiteman... and the desecration of his tribal life (and untold millennia of traditional medicine lore) by the awesome power and the incredible horrors of World War II in the Pacific.

Papua New Guinea is the home of the 'Cargo Cults' which began during the Second World War. And even today, tribal people in this remote and mountainous country *still* clear mock landing strips in the jungle and build large wooden airplanes and imitation control towers to grace them in the belief that these symbols will actually *attract* the spirit-planes that bring the great wealth of the white man. The head deity of the cargo cults is known (no one knows why) as 'John Frumm.' And the chant or *mantram* (in pidgin) that the cult uses to evoke this deity is: *"John Frumm... he come!"*

And yet, for all of his tribal culture's isolation from the modern world, this man was also a real-time, modern jet-set cross-cultural adventurer who had traveled from the ancient and changeless world of the Upper Sepik River to the relative chaos of Port Moresby by boat and truck for *the very first time* in his life.

Then, in the past few days he had gone through all the high-tech rituals of being photographed to obtain a passport, buying a ticket, checking in his baggage and boarding a living 'John Frumm,' cargo-cult, bird-of-the-Gods.

On board at last, he would have to have been initiated into the rituals of using seat-belts, mastering the complicated aircraft toilets and all the other strangeness of airline food, services and protocols. And after all of this... he arrived in Australia to sit beside me on a busy city beach... *without even understanding how to remove a screw-on bottle cap!*

Live and learn. Live, and learn... if you can! I can remember seeing unspeakably beautiful brown-skinned faces with shining eyes of absolute wonder peering cautiously from behind palm trees and ferns, watching the very first of the great tourist planes come to magical islands in Indonesia and the Philippines. But that was somehow less of a surprise to me than what I saw today. It never awakened the same sort of puzzlement in me as my simple sharing with Chada. For I, too, always stand in wonderment and awe when I watch a big jet go through its metamorphosis from massive earth-bound clumsiness to elegant soaring bird and back again. And all the more when it has landed on a black-paved strip in the middle of nowhere. In fact, anyone who *cannot* feel wonder at such an amazing thing must be... well... very 'sophisticated' indeed!

In other times, I have also had that bizarre experience of being 'The First White Person' ever to be seen by some island people. But this was different: this day in this special space-time I was witness to the closing of a cultural gap in consciousness which might have lasted only five minutes of clock-time... but which spanned many decades of this one man's *experiential time...* and many thousands of years of *Cultural Time*. And it all occurred within the micro-cosmic physical action of unscrewing a simple bottle top... and was celebrated by us both in our joy at mastering this trick of the modern environment... and as a successful meeting of two very different cultural ambassadors.

WE ARE ALL VIRGINS TO OUR EVERY NEXT EXPERIENCE

Ultimately, we all live at the interface of the known and the unknown. We are all balanced on the very edge of *'The Great Unknown'* And we are all primitives to our next meeting with the future:

'We are all virgins to our every next experience.'

All around our planet, a hundred million times a day, truly *primitive* awareness is confronting new concepts, new levels of abstraction, new technology - and the new dimensions of consciousness that these discoveries open within us.

And it happens to all of us, wherever we live. It happens just as it did to Chada on the beach that day - and in big corporation board rooms; in public schools; in ageless, rainforest tribal lands; and in up-market shopping malls everywhere. At any level of sophistication, one step beyond the already known... lies *'The Great Unknown'* in all its splendor... and in all our dread.

I have long felt myself highly privileged to be with Chada on that afternoon, long ago, on that Aussie beach. For ever since that moment of his mechanical *satori* - his *Zen* 'awakening' - I feel that Elder Brother in my own awareness every time I first-touch a new computer system or some new photo-optical hi-tech illusion. I tend to operate closer to the frontier of western techno-cultural evolution than Chada. So the space-time cultural *forum* of my discovery is quite different to his. But the sense of bewilderment, of yearning, of discovery and the celebration of success... well, that is the same for us all. And, yes, the embarrassment, too.

How many 'bottle tops' have we all scratched in just such pitiful helplessness? How many times have you picked at *'The Great Unknown'* without knowing how to get in - waiting for the missing key-bit of information that will awaken deep revelation?

And isn't it all-ways the same? However it comes to you... once you have the vital, transformative *key*... well... once you know... then you *know*!

And from that moment on... through all of your experience to come:

NOTHING WILL EVER BE THE SAME AGAIN!

MEANING AND THE WAY OF FEELING

As things are felt to be
Can be so much more important
Than what they be in material fact.
How we feel *a situation can often be our only Sign*
When the situation itself seems ordinary in all other respects.

But the Magic is no less power-full which comes like this...
With secret Sign... that only you can tell:
The Inner Sign *of your own Feeling*
Which alone can reveal whatever Meaning is to be....

Life is a constant revelation of Meaning
An endless Vision Quest through which we all find Change.
Sometimes we see a Vision that no one else can see
And sometimes we all see the same event
But feel it inside with very different Meaning....

ANCESTOR REMAINS... FOREVER!

Long, long ago, deep in our garden jungle in another land, there was a small English walnut tree. This was Joah's Totem Tree - the *Ally Tree* of his first Earth-initiation with me. And under that special tree, Ami once found a large, shiny lump of jet-black rock. Maybe a kind of basalt - hard and sharp and glassy. Without sharing it with anyone else, she took it to her room and placed it near her bed. There is was carefully covered with one of her special 'ritual cloths.'

A few days later, I noticed it there and asked her why this rock was being honored like this and she said, with no hesitation and with total conviction: "It's my *Ancestor*. I found it in the garden."

Now, some years later, we live in more tropical realms, far to the north of that particular garden faerie-land where she used to play. Last night, as I bent down near her bed to give her a cuddle as she was falling asleep, I bumped into something hard, half hidden by a ritual cloth. It was *'The Ancestor,'* of course, apparently still cherished and still sleeping close beside her on certain, special nights.

Recently, in the blue light of day, I looked at The Ancestor more closely and with new eyes. And when I did, I discovered that The Ancestor seemed more like a very large lump of hard coal than a volcanic basaltic rock! Could it be? Was The Ancestor really an ancient piece of coal? Carbon. Organic matter. The dense life-force of a many-million year old swampland, compressed and contained in this most potentized symbol of organic Life itself.

I don't know where it came from, or how it happened into my family's life. But somehow my daughter has bonded her present-time incarnation with what might be a lump of black coal and she treats it like her ancestor....

What can I say?

It feels funny (and strange) to me, but I trust her *sincerity* (and her mystery) absolutely. What might this child know about this lump of blackness that I cannot even imagine? The answer is obvious: it could be anything... maybe everything.

Sometimes when I think about it I realize that this is no more strange than anything else around here: another sign, new meaning - a thing from some other time and some other incarnation... or... who knows...?

Reality can be the strangest Ally of all!

Anyway, I have placed myself in service to Ami's *Ancestor Vision.* And whatever this thing may be - to the Earth, to my daughter or to me - I guard and tend it with her... as *'The Ancestor'* of my Family.

For who knows how far back our bloodline can be felt and recognized - maybe even into the highly compressed bio-data of Jurassic-land... or even beyond?

BEYOND THE PATRIARCHY OF SCIENCE AND RELIGION

So much of our medicine experience has to do with simple natural phenomena which startle our awareness with unexpected feeling... and so call us back to take a second look. Sign and Meaning. A little leaf, a bent flower, a slowly moving snake: *anything can be Sign. And anything can awaken Meaning and Vision. And Revelation is everywhere.*

We do not choose the resource (the phenomena, the objects, the living beings) as such. We can only choose how to respond. But however they come to us, we know that finding Sign is often the beginning of wondrous medicine adventures in to amazing realms of learning... and always the catalyst of amazing *Change*.

But not all sign comes from such simple things as leaves and rivers and snakes. No indeed! Here we will look at the possibility of meeting life-forms which may not be of this Earth.

The word 'extra-terrestrial' is usually used to describe things which have come here from 'outer space.' But it does not require a great leap of logical reasoning to realize that there may *also* be beings around us which are not *extra*-terrestrial... and yet which are not of our *usual* earth-plane experience.

These mysterious entities may reside in, on or near the earth... without coming into our usual awareness... for many possible reasons:

For example, some living things which have been thought to be extinct for millions of years, may actually be living today and sharing our earth-space with us: unknown... and so, ignored.

Off the coast of Africa lives the ancient *coelacanth* fish. Long believed to have been extinct for millions of years. Within just the past few decades, increasing numbers are being found - alive and well.

As well as wide-ranging reports of sightings of a 'sea monster' which match the characteristics of the ancient *plesiosaur*, a rotting carcass of just such an animal was netted by a Japanese fishing boat just a few years ago. Inconclusively identified... but we know that there was really not much else it could have been.

And there are others: the 'Loch Ness Monster,' the Himalayan *Yeti* and the North American *Sasquatch*, the European *Alma* - and *so many* other life-forms of which we know so very, very little... sometimes knowing so little that every discussion seems to begin with the most basic question of all: "Do these things actually *exist?"*

Another category of 'non-existent' beings - or, we might say, *paranormal entities* - are those which have simply not (yet) been encountered by human beings. There are (still) millions of 'undiscovered' species on this planet. Of course, most of them are obscure variations on this or that basic program - beatle, fly, worm, crustacean, etc. But some of them are bound to be... quite amazing, indeed!

In the past few decades, a great shift in human consciousness has occurred. We have moved on from the Age of Earth Exploration and are immersed in a new quest: to restore and conserve the resources of our planet... and to heal the very Earth herself!

What makes the news today is more likely to be yet another catalog of eco-disasters than news of newly met lifeforms or anyone's explorations of new dimensions of consciousness. And we know that this is a very necessary (if emotionally tedious) thrust: for if we do not solve our ecological problems soon... we will lose our own 'basic question' and humanity may simply cease to exist.

But there is always an up side to evolution as well: as we expand our cultural and technological sensitivities, what we can understand (and admit) as Reality naturally expands as well.

And as our perceptual and intuitive horizons expand, it is quite likely that in the next few decades we will come face to face with new lifeforms (and consciousness) that we have not yet even begun to imagine!

So even though our pressing ecological crises of today demand (and deserve) all the caring we can give them... it is certainly also true that: *The Age of Discovery is not over yet!*

After all, there are still beings - including even tribes of human beings - which our 'organized' society has only recently 'met' for the very first time. In light of this, it is quite reasonable to *assume* that there are still more mysteries - and more new life-forms and more untouched consciousness here on this Earth-base with us... simply here and available to us to meet... whenever we finally open our eyes to notice them!

The next likely category of 'unknown real and conscious beings' is somewhat harder to describe to those who are pre-programmed with denial - i.e., the 'unbelievers' and skeptics who *will not* open to new possibilities... 'on principle.' So, to explore these new perspectives, we might slip the notion in obliquely, as a *"What if...?"* question. And safe within the security of supposed 'fantasy'... we can then begin to delve into even more wondrous realms:

WHAT IF discarnate beings (spirits of once-living humans and other entities) share this earth-plane with us, but (usually) inhabit other dimensions and so are only rarely seen...?

WHAT IF there *are* particular 'spirits' (other tribes have called them *devas* or *elementals*) which live in every plant, every tree, every river, every mountain...?

WHAT IF crystals are alive...?

WHAT IF planetary bodies have consciousness as such... and/or great spiritual presences - actual *living entities* - which live inside-outside the mass of their great bodies...?

WHAT IF beings from other *dimensions* (planes of manifestation) sometimes 'pop through' into our materially isolated, experiential world (consisting of only those three or four dimensions that we can yet comprehend)?

And this one: *WHAT IF* there *are* beings from beyond our earth-plane which have actually come from 'outer space?'

We might first imagine beings that have come here in some form of space craft, of course, because that best matches our own materially-bound experience. But there may also be beings which have come here by some *other* (more practical) means of transportation: teleportation... inter-dimensional 'break-throughs'... or whatever...?

Humans seem naturally to look at the natural world from the biased perspective of being... *human*. We imagine that aliens and their space craft will be more or less on our size-scale. But if we really think about it... this notion is absurd! And once we realize that this assumption is groundless then we quickly see that it is quite likely that these entities may be wholly different from anything that we have even yet imagined!

For example, what about size? If a 'real' and conscious alien lifeform visited our Earth. Just how big do you imagine it might be?

Consciousness seems to require no particular physical size or space in which to live and flourish... and there is ample evidence that it may not require any animate body at all! We do not yet know *how* this can be true... but we can see that it is. And if this is true... then even very highly developed lifeforms may be quite small by our usual physical standards of measurement. Perhaps much smaller than we might ever expect.

A lifeform which could travel through time-space-other dimensions with ease may conceivably be as small as a speck of dust! Or, *just as likely*, be completely non-material: a pure manifestation of *consciousness as energy.*

The actual fact is that on the physical-scientific level... we just don't know to deal with these questions at all. And so we do not. We simply do not entertain such possibilities in any way. For science always sticks to what it is already sure that it knows!

If a 'real' alien lifeform visited our planet... would it come in a space ship? Or would it ride in on a satellite micro-wave bounce-back? Or perhaps it would simply travel on the subtler networking channels of (human) thought... or ride in on a whale song... a meditation... an invocation... or a prayer....

Again, we just don't really 'know' anything with certainty... at least *not* through our organized, linear-scientific way of perceiving and verifying things.

Physical science works with *energy*. If we can detect and measure and manipulate any energy phenomenon... we can then study it and 'get to know it,' scientifically.

But if any phenomenon happens to be out of the range of our current detecting-measuring-manipulating technologies... then, for all practical purposes, according to science... *it is simply does not exist*!

There are reasons why science has to maintain this obviously narrow-minded stance. Some are practical exigencies and some are merely vain expressions of the 'know-it-all' mentality that is the trap of all scientists. And the *'why?'* of this self-restricting policy is not important here.

But it *is* important to realize that when we set out to explore *any* of the possibilities of life that may exist beyond our own three-or-four dimensioned, material-based awareness, the *energies* which may be involved in our adventure (or, more accurately, the particular *energy phenomena* which we may encounter, as all energy is ultimately *one* - a single unified force) are *quite likely* to be too subtle, too powerful, too sophisticated (or whatever) for us to be able to scientifically detect, measure and manipulate them.

So what can we do? Shall we continue to ignore/deny all of our experience which cannot (yet) be scientifically measured or manipulated? Or is there a way to proceed that will take us *beyond* the limitations of our scientifically narrowed, cultural experience...?

Readers of this book - and all followers of the Medicine Path by any name or practice - will be more likely to say "Yes! And let's find it... and just as soon as we can!" And so... we are.

As we follow any growth path-way - of ritual medicine,

psychotherapy, yoga or meditation (or gardening or chess... or whatever) we *all* are invited to look beyond all that we already know - personally, culturally and temporally (in time).

Except for those rigidly 'organized religions' which come to us pre-packaged and with a reigning patriarchal authority... the basic 'practice' of *every* spiritual discipline requires that we continually stretch and exercise our awareness so that it can comprehend ever more subtle (and ever more grand) phenomena... of life... energy... consciousness... and Spirit.

In this realm of endless expansion and growth, the game of 'searching for aliens' is just such an exercise in expanding our horizons and learning new criteria which will help us *notice* the myriad marvels of existence and consciousness which await our dis-covery - beside us and inside us; around us and beyond us; under the Earth and beyond the Stars. And however far we have come, however deep our individual knowing...

We have all only begun our journey of discovery!

For all who walk the medicine path, 'Searching for Aliens' is both *path* and *process*. And whatever our backgrounds... we already know how to voyage in these uncharted realms: we must simply *leave* the synthetic surety of Science. We must go wherever sign and vision lead... to accomplish whatever we can. And somewhere, experiential lightyears from now, we might hope to be able to work our way *back* to scientific plausibility (to recover that physical-plane reassurance that Science does so well).*

Many people today realize that contact with life-forms of 'extra-terrestrial' origin may well have been occurring throughout the whole of the evolution of human consciousness.

---

* That is... we must learn to explore outward and then to return to what our technology can comprehend (and so admit) as being real. This means that we must employ a process of *'retrodiction'* (the literal opposite of *'prediction'*), bringing Home our new discoveries to show Science what we have found. And then, from there... perhaps we can take the Patriarchs of Science - and maybe even the Patriarchs of Religion, who knows? - on a 'Medicine Walk' in to the Living Cosmos that breathes and feels and communicates from far beyond the wildest imaginations of techno-physical science and archaic religion.

These contacts may have occurred through direct visitation, prayer, meditation... or while very sane and 'normal' (and, as often seems to happen, even scientifically trained) people are driving home from work. But whatever the happening, these experiences tend to be systematically 'written off' by our cultural program as hallucinatory or 'distorted' perceptions. We play with them, use them to titillate our fancy in tabloids and TV specials... and then we discard them like yesterday's news... and *never* make sincere effort to integrate them into/with our scientifically and materially dogmatized world-view.

But if we are to *really* 'figure it all out,' then it seems likely that we will have to find ways of *including* these most special, most rare and most exciting of all human experiences in our overall understanding of the nature of Life... and the living cosmos-at-large.

Here are a few common examples which may help to illustrate how many millions of people successfully and regularly utilize energy phenomena which cannot be scientifically substantiated:

* Western Science does not yet understand how the ancient Chinese healing system called *acupuncture* works when we cannot dissect a human body and find material evidence of the existence of the *meridians* (path-ways) of energy which acupuncture treats.

* And another: Science can study telepathy (or ESP) and come up with conflicting results. And yet, very ordinary people have extra-sensory experiences with great frequency... and can often benefit from these unusual openings in awareness *because* they may not need to deny and disbelieve their own experience on grounds that 'it is not scientific.'

* And one last illustration: Science cannot tell us what happens to us when we meditate and experience vast dimensional changes in experience - or when we have the experience of 'leaving our bodies.' And yet these experiences are common enough to all serious students of any discipline of yoga or meditation.

Perhaps it is time at last to begin to include *'The All and Everything'* of human experience (and consciousness) within our working definitions of 'Reality.' (How we have avoided doing so for so long is a total mystery). Just as soon as we begin to expand and refocus our individual 'reality' views... then we are ripe to realize that the best place to begin is right where we are... at home... within *'The All and Everything'* of our own, infinite experience!

And after all... doesn't *everyone* know that old saying:

"Clarity begins at Home?"

WALKING TO REMEMBER AND REMEMBERING TO TELL

Walking down the Darkwood Road which winds between the many bridges which criss-cross the Mother River all along the valley.... It is just after dark. It is spring. The nights are still cool and balmy - our sweltering, tropical summer has not yet come to the valley.

My bus-studio overlooks the river and the steep hill which plunges down to meet its opposite bank. And because of the limited access here, this section of the river is very private... and so my writing, music and private session work is undisturbed. But along the side of the mountain there is a new road... and as I walk along this evening, I can see three, well-spaced pockets of house lights crouched in small gullies and indentations in the steep hillside.

As darkness seeps up from the valley floor, and as I see these homes sparkle with their soft, solar-lighting... I feel the simple peace of this valley: three kilometers to the next bridge... and only three pockets of light along the way. And I know these three homesteads, too: truly magically created dwellings of spirit-conscious people who came here to live close to the Earth.... Yes, in this wild world of change... *this* valley is still a good place to live. And a good place for making medicine.

Without ever realizing it, my walk tonight was setting me up for a deep remembrance. The shape of the hillside, the little pockets of light which adorned it... and the magic in my eyes as I walked free that night and listened to the River Song as the road snaked me through the valley. All of these things were re-awakening Vision Story in me.

Later that same night, after walking-walking had returned me to my bed, I re-lived each detail and all the feeling of a profound ritual initiation that I had experienced in this same valley, many years before.

And since that re-minding, I have swum through this *Dreaming Story* in my dreams of many nights. Now I can *see it all*. And tonight I feel finally ready to *'talk story'* with you. And the story goes like this:

A PILGRIMAGE TO THE FAERIE CAVES OF LIGHT

It is late on a moonless night and I am sitting in a night-fire circle with several others... mostly in silence... just watching the star-show panorama and sometimes poking at the last embers to evoke a few more flames. The soft rain which had been falling most of the day had just begun again. It was sign to me that the end of my day was at hand... and time to leave the forest in peace... for the big-eyed night creatures who were waiting just beyond our fire-light for a chance to come out and play.

I was just preparing myself to move off toward the dry warmth of bed, when suddenly a wild and startling apparition of a darkly bearded man leaped out of the thick lantana bushes near the circle. His eyes were as big as moons and he was obviously very excited about something.

I knew this man from his day-face: his name was Jarrah (named after a beautiful Australian rainforest tree) and I had heard that he had gone out at sunset in search of a sacramental mushroom... or two. And now, here he was... obviously full of mushroom magic and its peculiar medicine power. He calmed himself before he spoke (such as he could) and then told us that we *must* come with him into the bush.

He could not say why. Just, "Please! Come NOW!" And so we did.

We followed Jarrah for several minutes, picking our way through the dense bush which lined the river there, with a few candles to guide our sight as GrandMother Moon would not rise until much later this night. Finally we came to a path which ran along a small, steep hill - a place where some erosion of rain had left the bare, red earth exposed.

In the side of this small hill, just an arm's reach above our heads, were several very small indentations. Not large enough to be seen as 'holes'... more like hand-sized *pockets* which seemed to have been cupped out of the hillside with methodical precision.

Jarrah asked us to extinguish all the candles. So we all stood there for a few moments until our night-sight began to come sluggishly awake.

Soon we could see, a little. And what we saw has come to be one of the most wondrous things I have ever seen. Inside each of these miniature caves was some sort of glowing spider web, shining with that green, un-earthly light of *electro-bio-luminescence* - the light of the fireflies!

We all took turns looking at the magical, glowing webs, shuffling past each other on the narrow (and now quite slippery) path so that everyone could see this beautiful phenomenon. But as beautiful as they were, after a very few minutes, our interest in the luminous webs began to yield to our discomfort in the cold of the night rain.

But just as our little herd of sleepy explorers began to 'baaa' and bleat like restless sheep and moved to shuffle back toward camp, Jarrah said, "No! Wait! You have to look really closely to see *Them!*"

People in the rain, late at night, can be quite petty about creature comforts. So it took some force of determination for me to surrender my attachment to keeping dry clothes - for the sake of this unknown adventure - and to climb on my knees once again up the sodden, muddy hill, to bring my eyes close to one of the webs. But Jarrah's wild eyes were pretty exciting in themselves and I figured that somehow, it would all be worthwhile....

As I approached one of the brightest webs very closely - perhaps four inches, now, from the glowing strands - I literally *fell into* a world of the most amazingly beautiful and intricate... *Magic*! Nothing else could begin to describe this unearthly experience: it was pure Medicine Magic.

What I had supposed was 'merely' a strangely luminescent scatter-web turned out to be a complex and highly organized network of hanging, luminous threads, so delicate that they almost appeared to be unreal: non-material shafts of soft, shining, green light.

Every strand of this magical substance - and there were perhaps twenty or thirty strands in all - was precisely spaced from those around it such that the distance between each of these tiny thread-lamps was no more than a quarter of an inch or so. The strands ranged in length from about half an inch to an inch and a half and each was hanging straight downward, suspended from the ceiling of the mini-cave. But regardless of their individual length, the bottoms of these threads were all on the same plane: exactly even. And the overall effect was of a three-dimensional *curtain* of green-glowing silk.

But there was more: along the length of each of these silken strands were many little jewel-like spheres of different sizes, all glowing with the same eerie green light as the threads. I could soon see that these were actually droplets of some sort of liquid, which seemed to merge right into the vertical filaments, as though they were somehow of the same substance... or as though they had grown out of the hanging threads of silk (or whatever).

But it was strange that instead of looking like (ovoid) bulges or even droplets formed by gravity into the usual tear-drop shape... these little sparkles of faerie-light appeared to be completely spherical.

And then I saw something new: suspended at the very end of each hanging strand, there was a single and larger glob.... all of the same mysterious substance... all of the same size... all equally spaced (as were the light-lines which supported them)... and all of these new globs were perfectly tear-drop shaped.

Each of these little jewels terminated on the same horizontal plane, so that when I looked at these end-bulbs of glowing mucous from a few inches above, they created a visual carpet of soft, green light. And when seen from below, they looked like a suspended platform of softly shining emeralds.

And so the whole event looked like a Faerie Grotto of some sort of barely-materialized, opalescent green, luminous... *energy*. It was a *very* power-full and absolutely fascinating phenomenon!

What *was* this stuff...? What could it possibly be...? I tried to fit some material-plane understanding to the image. Free-Mind sped through all the possibilities it could comprehend:

Were the droplets formed from dew? Or were they raindrops... or what...? And were the web-like strings actually web-silk? Or was there some other source for these strange apparitions?

Then I realized that these were not strands of some sort of silken web-material at all. No, they were individual strands of some sort of *mucous* which were arranged in almost perfect symmetry within each, tiny 'Faerie Light-Cave.'

I well know that these 'picky' details of numbers and measurements can be just as boring to read as they are to write. But since I had never seen such a thing before - and have never seen anything like it since - I feel it is important to at least offer you a picture of the physical presence of this miniature world. And this is as accurately as I can relate the purely material dimensions of the experience... so far!

But beyond the material reality of this 'thing' - whatever it was - this experience was one of great elemental Power: Great Medicine and Deep Magic. And, yes... there was also a powerful feeling of privilege here, the feeling of being in the presence of Spirit... a feeling that I can only describe as the experience of being in the presence of *Grace*.

I have felt this 'presence' often in my life (but never often enough). And whenever this particular feeling comes to me... I know to trust it... and I trust it *absolutely!*

Remember, too, O Reader Dear, that only Jarrah had been 'stalking the wild mushroom' that night. Nothing was unusual about *my* perceptual experience... except the experience I was now having!

Meanwhile, in my eagerness and rapt attention, I scarcely noticed that my hands and toes, which had been clawing into the slippery mud for support, were beginning to slip. All of a sudden I just 'fell off' the hillside and landed in a wet and muddy heap. And just as suddenly, my medicine vision and my feeling of being in the presence of Grace was shocked back into earth-time 'reality.'

And there, looking at me in total wonder, was the most beautiful face and open heart of Jarrah, resplendent in his wildness in this time of majestic, magic mushroom glory.

"What is happening, here.... *What* is here...?" I wondered inside. But I sensed that Jarrah knew (or felt) something more about this amazing discovery than he had yet revealed.

"Jarrah.... Tell me. What do you make of all this...?" I asked aloud, when I my faerie-struck consciousness was finally reconnected with my real-time, human voice.

"Don't know. I just don't know.... It feels like *pure life energy*... like something from another world. Maybe from another planet or even another star. New Life. Something intelligent. *Spirit*.... I don't know exactly.... I just don't know...."

I clambered to my feet, ungainly and clumsy, but lost in wonder. As I looked up at Jarrah, his large, soft eyes looked miles deep... and as deeply inside me. I could feel his total openness to this strange new presence. And I could feel my own. And in this special state of expanded openness I could feel the bond that was forming between us even as we stood apart, each speeding around his inner cosmos, looking for connections, correlations... or anything which might be even remotely familiar from past experiences... on any plane at all... on any dimension whatsoever. And there was... simply nothing there. No precedents. No correspondences. No correlations.

In this amazing micro-cosmos... we were each and all alone... once again, true experiential virgins to this amazing happening.

"All my Ancestors!" echoed in my back-brain, from a thousand fire-circle prayers and as many lifetimes. I breathed out a long and windy sigh... and turned away from Jarrah to climb the hillside yet again. For whatever it was... it was *right up there...* and I wanted *more.*

It was, all in all, a simple visual sight. Unusual, to be sure, but very simple: threads of luminescent mucous hanging from the ceiling of a tiny cave in the soft, wet Mother Earth. But if this was *'the all'* of it... then why oh why did it *affect* us both so strongly?

I felt that I *must* know more. And so I settled into a new commitment to stay there until *some* sense began to emerge from my swirling confusion, my wide-ranging analysis... and from my incredibly charged feelings.

Whatever would come... there was no doubt of this: Sign was here... Meaning was here... Great Medicine was here. And whenever the 'mix' got this rich... I knew that true Revelation could not be far behind!

This time, as I scrambled up the slippery hillside like the gross and clumsy humanoid that I am, I managed to get even closer to the door of the light-cave. As I yet again committed my already wet clothes to the mud and settled in to embrace the hillside once more... I found that I could now very easily and quickly sink into a gentle, meditative trance, every time I looked into the little grotto. And each time I dropped into this trance-state I was instantly admitted in to a new and dramatic world. A place of Deep Vision which was being illuminated by some kind of pure, *Deva* magic... while it prepared for Revelation.

My awareness wafted in and out of this meditative state and I tried my best to give Free-Mind a chance to wander as it would, trying to find trust (and hoping that I could) to be open to whatever it would find.

So... linear clock-time passed and passed in its one-way procession. I don't know how long I was held there, wafting about in timeless space. But all at once, and of course when I least 'expected' it, Sense-Mind suddenly found its focus... and I experienced a great feeling of *"Breakthrough!"* as I suddenly saw through the disguise!

Up until now, my 'worldly' eyes had been transfixed by the vertical shafts and tiny jewels of green light which were framed and hanging in this tiny pocket-cave. But suddenly, something new leaped into my awareness.

Had this new focus just appeared (while I was down the hill and talking with Jarrah) or had I just failed to notice it before, entranced within the splendor of the complex maze of faerie lights and faerie magic that greeted my first visitations? Or could it be that it actually *wasn't* there before... at all? Whichever... whatever... somehow I realized that I would never know.

Anyway, what I now saw somehow and suddenly 'made sense' of this miniature universe which I felt so privileged to fall into. For now I noticed that the individual strands of the hanging light-show and their Christmas ball decorations were *not* evenly spaced. Now I could see that there was a single, linear passageway through the maze of vertical light-lines. And along this passageway was stretched a single line of silk (or mucous... or whatever): a single, glowing line which was perfectly level to the earth and precisely positioned just barely above the jewel-nest of large droplets at the bottom of this whole galaxy of shining, celestial lights.

On this single strand of seemingly heavier, luminous substance, there was a great glistening droplet of... whatever it was... which was also sparkling and beaming out the same un-earthly green light.

This single droplet was much larger than those which hung suspended on the up-down strands around it. It was about the size of the pearl-white egg of a garden snail: about the size of a small match head.

As well as being larger than any of the hanging droplets, this one also seemed to be a brighter light-source as well - clearly the brightest light in the cave! I wondered how I could possibly have missed seeing it on my first excursions into this miniature universe. Just now, it stood out as the obvious center-piece of the whole 'galaxy' of green jewel-stars!

But there was something else about this shining green pearl that was most unusual. To be sure, the smallest droplets in the light-cave - those which hung on each bulging line of light - were unusually round. But I figured that this was because of their very small size.

And all of the larger droplets which hung at the end of each strand of this strange substance of *'materialized light'* were tear-drop shaped, just as one would expect.

It was as though the heavier droplets were viscous enough to respond to gravity's pull... urging toward the Earth... and so everything seemed to be falling in to order on (at least) this one dimension of materiality, after all.

But (alas and hooray!), this new and very large mother-sphere was somehow different. For even though it seemed to be just hanging on this single, horizontal thread of light, the little jewel itself was somehow absolutely round... *a perfect liquid crystal sphere* of extra-powerful, green light. And from this strange and inappropriate roundness I could tell that it was obviously unaffected by its either own surface tension and/or the 'stick' of the mucoid strand it sat on... and perhaps also even unaffected by the tear-shaping pull of gravity herself.

I felt as excited as I had when, as a boy of ten, roaming the (then) wild hills of California all alone, I'd happen to see the mysterious tail of a big snake disappear into a deep rocky crevice or see a mass of frogs' eggs hatching into tadpoles in a slimy, green pond. The feeling was the same: *Look... and look... and look... and surrender in to Deep Wonder!*

No, *I* was the same.... No: *I am* the same: once you are truly Spirit-struck by Earth-Magic... a large part of you *never* grows up! And while many years of wandering had shown me so much about the mysteries of frog-eggs becoming free-swimming tadpoles... Nature had never before shown me *anything* like this!

I felt constantly split into two frames of awareness, throughout this entire experience. On the one hand I was the eager amateur naturalist who wanted to use his fair vocabulary of natural physics, phenomena and processes to under-stand the *'what?'* *'why?'* and *'how?'* questions which were flooding through my emotionally-spurred 'rationality.'

At the same time I was the Shaman-Dreamer of the Rainbow Dreamtime who *knew* that this powerful experience - yea, *any* experience that affected me so deeply - could be a *way in* to the direct experience of Transcendent Magic... of Infinity... of Medicine... and Spirit. And *this* level of my awareness also knew that there was absolutely nothing to 'find out,' nothing that needed to be asked... and nothing that could be 'known.' But also... that now there was something new to *be*.

Where these two *yin-yang* streams of awareness and intention overlapped, I felt that I was experiencing a 'meeting' - some sort of special introduction or initiation into a wholly new perspective - perhaps about to discover what would be (for me) an entirely new *dimension of consciousness*, which had been waiting for me here, in this most unlikely of places.

True to this sense of magical meeting... I reached out in reverent softness to *make touch* with the light. I reached out to 'shake hands' with my new acquaintance. My finger moved carefully because everything here (except me) was rendered in such a miniature scale. So I very carefully moved my gross fingertip up to a few of the delicate strands of barely materialized, glowing substance and ever so gently and with great feelings of tenderness and trust... I allowed my skin to touch a single strand.

The effect was almost instantaneous: the steady light which emanated from the whole complex of whatever-it-was suddenly fell sharply away from my touch - a wave of rapid dimming of the light which moved exactly from my point of touch to affect the entire 'community' of light-lines and jewel-stars within that micro-cosmic Cave of Light.

In just a second or two, the single strand which I had touched had now lost all of its light and showed no tinge of its usual green color whatsoever. Those strands closest to the site of my penetration - my touch now felt like a 'rape' of the integrity and sanctity of this subtle and tiny organism - were barely glowing, while those farthest from my crude intrusion were now shining at only a small fraction of their original intensity.

"Stop! croaked Jarrah, moving toward me rapidly from where he had been standing in the shadows behind me. "Stop! DON'T TOUCH THEM! It doesn't *feel right* to touch them...!"

"I know.... I'm sorry, Jarrah.... I'm sorry...."

The light returned to this little apparition-friend - slowly, as though cautiously. But in time it finally came back, strong and clear once again (to my great relief)!

Then I just watched - star-struck - for an endless time... meditating on the crowded 'nothing-ness' of everything within and everything that was around me at that moment. In its own time... time itself returned. And with time's rebirth within my awareness, my eager-to-know *quasi*-rationality was fired up once again and *yang*-linear Logic-Mind was once again speeding along its desperate and hungry course of cause-and-effect plotting and internal dialoguing-with-itself:

"What *was* this thing (on the comfortable physical plane of biology, for example)? How was it formed...? How could it suddenly fade like it had when I disturbed it...? What did that mean...? And why does my entire experience of this... thing... feel so eerie and mysterious...?"

True, Brother Jarrah was under the influence (and guidance) of a consciousness-changing sacramental medicine. But I was not. I had come to this meeting from a very 'usual' space in my own consciousness: pretty well earthed, fairly reasonable and clear-headed I was, for me (at least...for me). And, too, several others had experienced this same phenomenon. So whatever was happening to/through/within Jarrah... I knew that I, at least, was not lost or 'spaced out' in some wholly private world of wish or fantasy. And because it was share-able, I knew that I was not 'spacing out' into some kind of purely personal cosmic 'discovery.'

No. Not at all alone: many of us had come to this place together. And, as so often happens, we apparently all needed Jarrah to be in his special state of mushroom-consciousness to *find* this medicine and to guide us all to it with all of his great caring - and the insistent intensity which so effectively called us all away from the easy space of our Night-Fire Story sharing... and the inviting warmth of our nearby beds.

So, still *in-time* connected, Concept-Mind eventually drifted back to trying to comprehend this 'thing.' (I left it un-named and undefined... because it was still a total mystery to my mind-sense). *What WAS this thing?*

However I labeled it or referred to it in my internal self-self dialogue - as special, as incredible, as amazing, as magical... or as holy - *'IT'* still avoided being processed into a peacefully self-assured state of intellectual *understanding*, emotional *clarity* and/or spiritual *knowing*.

"But wait...! It wasn't *a* 'thing'.... No! It was a whole *hillside* of 'things!' For there were dozens of these little microcosmic galaxies inset in this stark brown mud-slide.

I had been so lost in but one of them that I had forgotten.... We were in the midst of a whole *city* of these 'things' - what*ever* they might be!

Cave after cave, each mini-universe seemed to include the same elements of strands and spheres and lights. And also... all of these *Light Beings* were ensconced in caves which were almost exactly the same size and appeared to have been scooped out of the hillside with mechanical precision. So even the tiny *caves* in the hillside were un-earthly, and beyond any explanation that I could generate.

A community of any kind of living being will form wherever the ecology is right. But this was a very *temporary* setting. At the very next hard rain, it was more than likely that this fragile community of faerie grottoes and magic lights... would simply be washed away!

"So why would they even 'set up house' here in the first place...?

"...And who (or what) had scooped out the tiny caves that housed these mini-galaxies? What parent(s) had seeded (or spored) the whole system...?"

I was once amazed to find in this special valley, a small mushroom, shining brightly in the night with the same, green bio-luminescence. And I have also seen other types of fungi and mildew here which emanate this same soft, cold-green light.

But if what I was seeing now was 'just' some sort of exotic fungus or mold culture... then how did they form these complex galleries of light...? In fact, how did they form at all...? And most puzzling of all: why had none of the others who saw these lights ever seen anything like this before - including Jarrah himself, a long-time resident of this Valley...?

"Ah well..." Smoothing-Mind tried to content me... "too many questions with no answers to be found in this City of Light-Caves so late on a rainy night! Perhaps if I return to this place tomorrow, the more 'rational' light of day will show me some answers...?"

Once again, I was about to move on... to return to earth-plane, to find our camp... and then my bed... and to use what was left of the rain-softened night... for sleep.

While I was running all of these mind-trips and trying - in vain, alas, in vain - to place and fix this etheric experience solidly and matter-of-factly within the dimensions of the knowable material plane... I had been looking away from the center-stage of the grotto that was just above my eye-level.

I had been looking at the mud... somctimes briefly glancing upward at the *'City of Faerie Lights'* that was sparkling before me... and sometimes just moving *out* of my visual-eyes for awhile, as I meditated openly (and then pondered mentally) on all of the riddles and mysteries of this amazing experience.

Feeling finally to move on, I turned to say good-bye to the little green light-globs and slippery stuff once again. But as I re-focused on the micro-cosmic world before me... I was shocked to see that the little round ball of matter which had been so prominent but a moment before... was nowhere to be seen!

I checked the dirt at the bottom of the little cave... but it had not fallen. I looked at the thickness of the horizontal strand... but it had not been 'absorbed.' And as I looked all around with my out-reaching and analytical eyes... I suddenly saw the little crystal sphere slide outwards, ever so slowly, from a place of seclusion at the rear of the light-cave. It came from a hidden place at the far end of the horizontal strand - a strand that had suddenly become a monorail track upon which the living sphere could move!

As I watched - with, truly, an open mouth hanging unconsciously slack and agape - the glowing crystal sphere began to move very gently towards me. And then it stopped. After a moment, it began to slide toward me once again, but slower now... then it stopped once again... then moved a bit closer... stopped... and then moved back the other way, away from me, faster than before... stopped.... And then it began to... well... how can I describe it? It began to *quiver* or shimmer or *pulse* ever so slightly on its threadlike highway.

It was such a subtle expression that I could not tell exactly what it was doing! Was it the wind? No, no wind moved in this protected grotto. Was it a vibration? No, the Earth was still. We were still. In fact, stillness was everywhere... except in my pounding heart!

A person-noise sounded behind me and as I 'popped out' of my trance-state, I slightly turned toward the sound, off-balanced and ended up sliding unceremoniously and backwards down the mud bank yet again.

Once on my own two feet and back in the real-time world once again, I found that I had been so engrossed in the magic that I had not even noticed the soft comings of yet a few more pilgrims who were *Walking the Path of Jarrah's Medicine* on that rainy night.

The others came, looked, loved, ooo'd and ahh'd... and then went on to warmer places. In no time I was all alone once again - except for one tall brother-totem-friend who was standing in silence, smiling all over and in total peace with everything and every one.

It was Jarrah (of course), standing well back from the hillside in perfect patience, giving me the gift of all the time and space I might need to experience what he already had seen and felt so well....

As I raised my eyes to meet his, I saw tears of love and tears of joy shining back at me... through my own tears of wonder...and through my instant and unaccountable tears of deep *thankfulness*....

As we looked into at each other so deeply... through an opening in Forever... I remembered what he had said earlier when I asked him what *he* made of the phenomenon:

"Something from another world: Intelligence... Spirit!"

And now I knew exactly what he had meant!

Suddenly, it was all so overwhelmingly obvious! The 'phenomenon' of faerie-lights and magical grottoes was amazing in itself. And the single droplet of moving, volitional ooze was incredible, of course.

But beyond all of that, there was the *feeling* of a 'presence' - the feeling that some *being* or *entity* was there with us... unfamiliar and yet deeply familiar as well. It was a feeling of some precious, deep and delicate *intimacy*. It was a feeling of being so *privileged* to witness this wondrous event... or being... or Spirit. And feeling so blessed to attend this amazing *Visitation*... of a consciousness I know I may never really understand....

The powerful and moving time of this profound discovery seemed to be over... for now. I was beginning to feel signs of emotional overload. I had been so deeply touched by this meeting with... whatever it was... out there, in there, in 'The Great Unknown.'

Yes... touched, moved, turned inside-out and flipped back again. And I knew that I would need time and a great deal of unhurried, gentle reflection to process this experience and to 'sort out' even its most basic implications for me, for my life... and perhaps (who knows?) for *all* life! For who could say how *far* the implications of such an encounter might go...?

Indeed... *Who could say...?*

This night I knew only that I *knew* that I had experienced some sort of 'audience' with a decidedly conscious entity. It felt as though the depth if this sharing had already changed me on many levels of psycho-physical, mental-emotional and spiritual reality.

And buoyed by Jarrah's loving support... I found the strength to summon whatever objective detachment I could claim... and whatever and spiritual openness I could *be*... to go back again for one last look... just to re-discover... and to reconfirm... that 'they' were actually there at all! Just to be sure that I had not just floated along on some magic-wish of my own... or perhaps empathetically tuned in to Jarrah's *Mushroom-Dreaming Vision*.

So I turned for a third time to face the plain, brown mud of the ever more slippery hillside with whatever clarity I could muster... but also with a strong and prickly chill running up my spine. As I clambered to the top of the little hill, I held my breath for a moment - perhaps to hold away any more overwhelming experience - and paused before I even dared to look again.

And then... Yes! I saw the entire City of Light, just as it had been before. And yes - they were still and really *there*. All of them: glowing, pulsing and radiating their cool, green light. Some were back in the recesses of their little star-worlds, while others were 'out front' and very easy to see.

In a voice so soft and tremulous that it was scarcely there... I said, "Goodbye... for now.... Goodbye... and *namaste*!" [*'Namaste'* is a sanskrit word which is used in India as a ritual greeting and a ritual farewell. It means: *"I honor the God within you."*]

And then I sank back onto the Earth, sliding down the hill: it was finally time to move away from this magical encounter....

We walked together in silence, Jarrah and I, back to the last curl of smoke from the Night-Fire Circle. For some time our only spoken words were warnings of branches at eye-height, or talk of the best way to move through the forest in the darkness, helped along ever so little by the late-rising part-moon light.

Just as we were to part to seek our own bed-places... Jarrah took my hand for a moment and said, simply, "I really wanted *you* to come. I needed to know if you'd see what I saw...."

"Ahh! Yes, Jarrah.... Yes! And thank you *so* much, Brother.... *Thank You!"*

And that was all that I could say from between my own tears - tears of gratitude and tears of pure wonder.

IN THE LIGHT OF THE VERY NEXT DAY

The next day I was occupied with other things for most of the daylight hours. When I was finally free, I picked up my camera and a good close-up lens... and set off to try to find the hillside-of-magic-grottoes once again. It was not all that easy, because I had been led in and out of the forest - and the Darkness - by Jarrah.

But in time I succeeded. There before me was the hillside, for sure - my own body-sliding streak-marks in the mud marked it beyond a doubt. And there were the little pocket caves dotted into the damp earth. Everything looked smaller in the raw day-light, but otherwise, it was all exactly the same as when I had left it.

I climbed up the mud-bank once again. Now I was *so* close... Breath caught and gasped in my chest and Heart thumped in excitement...! I felt as though I was somehow 'Coming Home' once again!

Quizi-Mind was racing with my heart: "*Why* is this experience so immediately power-full? *What* is here for me? *How* might I open even further to this Teaching, to this Revelation - *whatever it might be...?"*

My experienced arm reached automatically for the topmost handhold I had used the night before and as I raised myself to eye-level with the tiny home of the Liquid Crystal Light-Being... I was completely startled and taken aback when I looked inside... for *there was simply nothing there at all*!

A small depression in the mud-hill, strewn with a few tiny bits of leaf and twig, a pebble or two... and nothing else whatsoever! I quickly checked all the *other* holes... and found the same thing: no-thing there at all.

I clambered-fell back down to ground-level and there, half stomped into the earth, was the stub of the candle that I had brought here last night. So this *was* The Place...

And then I realized that, yes, this was the *place*... but this was clearly *not* the time! My pilgrimage to the Faerie Light-Cave - and my meeting with whatever life-form was there - had already happened. Real and/or un-real, for better and worse: it was over. And there was nothing I could do to re-create that medicine again.

When I left this place last night... I left an altered state of experience and had re-turned to human-being. And whatever I had met there in the dark of night past, seemed to have returned to its own place, as well (wherever that place may be). The 'City of Lights' was no more. And in the light of day, there was nothing whatsoever remaining of intricate *living structures*.

So... the *Ritual of Visitation* was over. But I knew that the profoundly deep *communion* that I had experienced on that rainy rainforest night... would go on changing me and expanding my Vision... forever.

And the lessons that were to come from it have continued to

unravel within my mind and go on awakening my Spirit in new ways... even today.

AND A LITTLE TIME TO BREATHE IT IN...?

Now I know this is an unusual request, but ask you to pause for a moment, here... please. Let yourself *feel through* this story. I know that this tale was not your own experience... at least at first. But now, it is *Medicine Story* that lives between us. For I have *gifted* this Medicine Story to you in *Spirit*... and it *is* in your experience, now. And so it will remain!

This story is sign. Mine at first and, just maybe, now, yours as well. Discount it, love it, whatever: make of it what you will... but do take a moment to *let it in* just now while its energy is fresh so that whatever meaning it may bring... can come alive within you....

THE LESSON OF THE LESSONS

I have kept and nurtured this experience inside myself, now, for about twelve years. I have told very few people about it... not often as medicine story (for the medicine was still too private). No, when I have spoken of this it has been more as an edge-of-science event - as an encounter with a paranormal phenomenon.

Taken simply as a bizarre phenomenon, this experience is still important because it evokes some realizations about what we can actually *know* about consciousness *per se* and about conscious *beings* - be they of terrestrial or other origins - and how consciousness can sometimes manifest in very unexpected ways.

This is an endless study for we of human consciousness (and mortal, human form). This is one area of exploration in which we can bring together every dimension of knowledge-belief-inquiry-process-awareness. It is here that Science meets Medicine. It is here that mythology meets materialism. And for the philosophers among us, it is here that epistemology (the study of that which is knowable) meets infinity ('the all and everything').

And it is here that we might come to be still more intimate with that larger *pool of consciousness* which opens to us when we very least expect it... which expresses itself in forms we cannot easily recognize and often find difficult to believe... and which moves *through* us in ways which we can never fully understand.

Somewhere - perhaps everywhere - there is consciousness: alive and flowing through an infinity of forms and formlessness, through countless dimensions and endless ages. And whenever and *however* this larger and more primal consciousness may manifest in our experience... all who feel it seem immediately to *know* that, somehow, this is *The Source of all Awareness*... it is the bringer of *'The Word'*... it is the *Mother-Father Spirit* that surrounds and nourishes us all... and it is the messenger of all the lessons that we have come here to learn.

We separate and so-human beings too easily fall prey to the illusion that our own limited awareness is all we have to tap and use... for whatever we are here to do. But as soon as we can open to *The Living Revelation of 'The All and Everything'* in any of its aspects or dimensions... we instantly discover what yogis and meditators have known for thousands of years:

All Consciousness is a Living Being
And this Living Consciousness is Whole and Unified
Throughout the Living Cosmos.

Consciousness is *ONE* unto itself: one being, one force, one entity, one shared experience. And we are all participants in this glistening pool of omnipresence... this wellspring of pure *Infinity.*

As I walk the medicine path... I carry my small part of the ultimate Ritual Celebration that attends the gathering of this universal consciousness with amazement. And in pride. And, I would hope, in humility. And my hope is that I can remain trusting enough - of myself, others and Spirit - to continue to open and share my most intimate shamanic experience to any who might find it of use.

Today, I am excited to share this story. There is deep and power-full *lesson* in this story of 'The Faerie Caves of Light' - lesson for me, of course... and perhaps also lesson for any who can really *feel* these words.

Meetings of this higher order are so very, very rare. And so few of these special moments survive the harsh examination of the defensively 'objective' mind which so delights in being the tyrant of the clear light of day....

But sometimes there are chance meetings. Or are they ever by 'chance?' Chance, destiny or synchronicity, such meetings are so powerful and so *real* and so absolutely life-changing that we would be as fools who would throw them care-lessly away!

So I invite you to come with me... in to the *feeling* of the *'Faerie Caves of Light'*... and I will show you such a sacred place and such a sacred meeting, clean and clear... that you, too, might find the Sign and the Meaning and the Vision that was there for all to see... one night, so long ago, for Jarrah... and for me.

THE SHAMANIC PATH OF OPENNESS

As my awareness moves back into that long-ago rainy night in the Mother-Valley Rainforest, I realize that I still do not know 'what' I saw in the mud-slide hill that night. It could have been a mold culture, a fungus, a cosmic joke, God Herself... or the brief visitation of a life-form from some other dimension, planet or star-system. Whatever it was, I cannot say with any 'scientific objectivity' that I really know much about it at all....

Beyond science (and the religion of *Scientism*), the great blessing - and perhaps the hardest task - of the Medicine Path is that we struggle to leave *all* possibilities wide open and somehow maintain a position which recognizes that there is some essential (i.e., necessary) Truth in all that is said... in all that is felt... in all that is imagined... and in all that is experienced.

Ultimately, *everything that we experience is real*... if only in our feelings... in our thoughts... in our consciousness. And all that I (or you) *must* do to stay clear and flowing on this medicine path, is to be wholly true to the *'All and Everything'* of our own experience, *whatever it may be*. Known, unknown, not yet known, seemingly unknowable... or whatever: *all* experience is absolutely real... within your own reality.

To 'Walk this path in a sacred manner' is to make commitment to whole-being Openness... to make commitment to remain just as surrendered and as open as we can to everything which we can possibly imagine... and to remain open to all that lies beyond even our wildest fantasies.

From within this special state of Openness... who are we to judge or dismiss *any* feeling? Or to judge any image or any impulse (our own or others') as 'un-real?' As soon as we are closed to anything/everything (*'The All'*) that lies beyond that which we already know... then we are no longer open to the enlightenment of pure *Revelation!*

'Beyond our wildest dreams?' We cannot even imagine what we will discover. If we cannot foresee the destination... then we can only pay attention to the *Process*. If we cannot see through the clouds or over the hill that lies ahead... then there is nothing else to do but to focus on the *Path*.

The spiritual path of the free-ritual shaman is the *Path of Openness*: that openness which alone allows whatever bits of ultimate 'truth' that might penetrate our ego-protective masks, to simply *pass through* our awareness, unimpeded. To *pass through* our experience in any way (or shape or form or feeling or image) whatsoever... without judgment, without denial and, if we are but clear enough, without Fear. And as this *experiential infinity* passes through us... *Change is our endless reward!*

This same (and only) state of openness also allows all that has meaning to enter our awareness. We surrender in to Deep Openness so that *we can feel the truth within the feeling*... so that we can know the moment... read the Sign... be *one* with all the meanings... outcomes... realities... of every morsel of experience.

This is the Medicine Vision that I follow... and this is the Medicine Path that I walk. It is my *yoga*. I know that not *all* of Nature and the living cosmos-at-large will be knowable from within this all-too-frail human vehicle. Not all will likely be revealed to me. And yet, there is no blame for any personal limitation... as long as I am wholly committed, and walk this path with the clearest integrity that I can muster.

And so I make commitment to accept and honor *'The All'* of my experience... to open to the guidance of every dream... every medicine vision... every idle fantasy... every medicine sign.

And through and beyond all of this (which feels already to be path enough for many lifetimes yet to come)... I make continual re-commitment to my primal surrender... that I may be as open as I possibly can... to *'The All and Everything'* which lies beyond my wildest imaginations.

For all that lies beyond 'The All' that any mortal being can even imagine, there are two Medicine Words: We can call it, simply... *'Spirit.'* Or we can call it, simply... *'GOD'*

And however 'it' is called - once we open to the direct experience of this presence... *then* (and only then) can we know that

Spirit is all ways One with-in us, all and each....

THE ULTIMATE REALITY OF EXPERIENCE

What did I see and feel so strongly late one night in the ancient, Australian Rainforest... in that magical valley of the Mother River? Well, perhaps you can tell me...?

I have shared with you (almost) all that I know about this experience. I 'have' the experience (as we say, as though we possess or own it), to share... but about this experience I have no clear 'answers' for you... or for myself.

The whole phenomenon might simply have been just some bio-luminescent mold, easily named and cataloged by any competent biologist. But maybe that was only what 'it' was 'wearing' when we met!

No, I experienced something more than an esoteric biological event. Whether the magic resided in the light-cave itself, or in my own *Dreamtime Vision* experience, is something that I cannot know. But does it even matter?

For my medicine path is the *Path of Surrender*: I do not *have* to 'know' anything at all! I merely have to be able to *bear* the incredible power of *'The All and Everything'* of my own experience and somehow learn to channel through me the (often frightening) intensity of all the beauty, Grace and absolute wonder which this path brings through this one human being. This is 'The All' of my Medicine Wheel Free-Ritual Shamanic work. And this is surely enough for me!

When we follow *the Path of Innocence...* there is nowhere we cannot walk. And that traditional spiritual tyranny which demands that we judge all experience as 'real' or 'unreal' - and the vanity that imagines that we even can - is one of the outworn superstitions of our old cultural God of Scientism.

But remember: science can only relate to those things (events) which it can study over time. By contrast, most people realize that the very most meaning-full experiences of life - those which change our consciousness most profoundly - seem to have only one thing in common: they are unique and unsolicited experiences which occur instantaneously and without warning.

And as they are truly 'phenomenal' - these experiences simply cannot be repeated by any act of egoic will alone. So with its intrinsic bias that denies the reality of everything which it cannot control, alas, poor Science is left out of the many wonders that full-fill the life of all who walk the path of Spirit.

For me, for us, for better or worse, all that can be 'known' of the very *most* important experiences in our lives... is ultimately nothing more and nothing less than whatever Meaning it evokes... in our experience. Or, we might say: whatever meaning comes to us through our direct experience... is all the truth that we can know. So here is yet another perfect circle: *the Circle of the Living Medicine Wheel.*

And what was the ultimate Meaning (the personal meaning) of my vision quest in to the realm of the light-cave Devas...? Well, this is all I know:

Through that one, long night of high medicine and Earth Magic - during this one night's pilgrimage to the 'Faerie Light Caves' - I was profoundly *changed!* Changed inside and out, on many levels of awareness... and changed, I trust, on planes and dimensions of consciousness far beyond whatever I can yet comprehend.

I *know* that I was so changed... because *I feel so changed.* And no science or any other 'objective' process can override this simple truth of my own experience. For in the realm of the shaman...

'Change is the Sign of all Experience.
Change Reflects all Meaning.
And Experience is the Revelation of all Reality.'

To be true to my medicine vision and the meaning it evoked in me, I must reveal *all* that I know of this experience... or say nothing of it at all. And the most that I can tell you, even so, is that on that incredible night... while clinging to a mud-slide hill... I reached through 'human being' and was met by a consciousness from beyond the far horizons of my experience and imagination.

And somehow, within me, I know it was *a visitation of Spirit.*

For on that magical night...

SPIRIT WAS THERE... FOR ME!

><><

CHAPTER 11

ECO-MEDICINE

THE EMERGENCE OF EARTH-AWARENESS

Change is all-ways with us through our ever-evolving cultural consciousness. Until very recently, the world of Nature was introduced to children as a wide-open, free-range realm of mystery and wonder. Before the age of scientific conservation, the world-at-large was seen as a place where unknown lifeforms still roamed in uncharted lands... and virtually anything could (still) happen.

From within this naive (and, yes, imperialist) mindset, every animal was believed to exist in inexhaustible supply - 'placed' here solely to satisfy our carnal pleasures of the hunt. This exploitation mythology was not only a *belief* set... it was the *religion* of western culture! And from within this grand self-delusion, we met Nature eagerly and bravely... and with a voracious greed. With loaded guns, big tree saws and competitive self-centeredness, we stalked and killed and vanquished all that had ever tempted us... or threatened us... and (why not?)... all that did not pose any threat at all.

In those days, children were told stories of the terrors of the ocean deep; programmed to believe that every lion and tiger wanted to eat every tasty child; and convinced that if any snake held poison in its bite... that it would bite us all if it could! Nature was ripe for our projections of 'Beware!'... and Nature was ripe for consumerism and abuse.

In time (perhaps just in time), we began to realize that Nature was also ripe for the seeding of our newly emerging religion of *'Scientism:'* we were determined to become the masters of all Nature.

Tired of always being *'at effect'* in a world we feared and plundered, humankind set a course toward *total objectivity* and the industrial revolution... and Scientism became the only path to God.

As we began to lose our spiritual innocence and deep sense of myth and mystery, Nature, too, was defrocked and denatured in our laboratories, zoos and schools. In time we finally succeeded in putting everything that was small enough/large enough under the microscope; shuffled everything larger into cages and zoos; and consciously and unconsciously pushed whatever was left to the very brink of extinction (or beyond) in ever-shrinking natural habitats.

Then and now, the newly scientific 'natural world' was made up of all that we had so far noticed: all those species that had received our 'seal of official existence' and the award of a Latin name; all those phenomena which we could 'explain' scientifically (and no others); and all that our technology could possibly help us to exploit-kill-master-control.

And while we roamed the planet on our missions of scientific mastery, we preached the dogmas of the new cultural religion of Scientism to every one. We told every child that 'Nature is nothing more or less than an expression of immutable scientific laws and principals.' And somehow... we all believed it!

And so we were still further reinforced in our historic and vain mythology that *homo sapiens* was the ultimate lifeform and that it was 'natural' for humanity to be a destructive parasite on the Earth, squandering all natural beauty and resources and subjugating everything to the rise of technological culture and insatiable (and in-sane) economic greed. We believed that we were the God-gifted receivers of all the bounties of the Earth... so long as we could continue to find more and more ways of manipulating the Natural Laws of Science to our (commercial and political) benefit.

What chance might any child have, amidst this naive thrust of cultural egotism, to grow up with a natural sense of Magic and Mystery intact?

Sure... the wholly uneducated could retain their wonder in the face of whatever Natural splendor they could still find. True, the most enlightened scientists could still marvel at the infinite intricacy of the Living Cosmos (the word *cosmos* means 'ordered'). But for the vast new middle classes... Nature was nothing more than a weekend's drive, a tired slave, a captive who had grown old and less interesting over time. And how we thought about the natural world; how we felt all natural phenomena; and how we held ourselves away from any experience which was feared to be *unscientific* (and so invalid)... was all controlled by the prevailing cultural dogma of *Scientism.*

In the ever-shrinking wilderness, big animals were ritually hunted, filmed, zoo'd and stuffed. Whenever a photograph of a mighty bear or whale or python was seen, the first comments you would hear were, "How'd you like to meet *that* in a dark forest someday!" Or, "Boy, I bet that fella would put up quite a fight!"

And through these times - from the 'fifties to well into the 'seventies - virtually *no one* ever imagined what was to come as our consciousness ever so slowly began to recover from a million years of predation and fear... and to lead us into the new dimensions of awareness that exploded within us when the concept of *'Ecology'* entered the mainstream of the human mind!

THE LIGHT OF HOPE!

Somehow, through all of this exploitation - and for the first time since white, European imperialism set out to conquer the rest of the world - these same last few decades have seen a parallel rise in our awareness of the mystery and the magic of the Natural world... and the living universe beyond.

Somehow, through all of our materialism and in some vestigial corner of our awareness, it seems that our western culture retained the 'cute' notion of the Earth as a kind of 'mother' - although we hadn't dared to imagine the great depth of truth of this image ever since the middle ages, when the Grand Inquisition of the Patriarchal Catholic Church tried to kill off *all* expressions of the sacred feminine (the Goddess), earth-wisdom and mother-magic. And then the industrial revolution tried to squelch and suppress whatever was left.

Well, however it happened, we are now in the midst of a new development: for some three decades now, *the birth of eco-awareness* has been reawakening our understanding of our *place* in the medicine wheel of all creation. Finally we are beginning to dis-cover that:

We are all Children of the Earth!

Every tribal culture sings out this wisdom. Every open-minded observation confirms it. And as western culture opens once again to this awareness, it is beginning to help us to feel (once again), the ultimate *security* of knowing our rightful place and the experience of living within the enfolding nurturance of *'The Great Mother.'*

No, alas, not all of us... the leading edge of our evolution is never shared by everyone at once. But there is a movement among the billions of individualized person-cells that channel our human, mass-mind awareness - a stirring that may be our 'wake-up' call - to re-enter the sacred space that our ancestors knew.... so that we can once again celebrate and consecrate each new child's *rightness-of-being* and each child's inherent *rightness-of-place.*

And the *new and ancient awareness* that shines from the eyes of our newborn babes today is living proof that when our children grow with-in loving affirmation and encouragement, they *can* retain their natural sense of wonder... and their innate connection to the deeper realms of magic... and consciousness... and Spirit.

BUT STILL THERE IS DESPAIR

But alas, there is a downside to this picture. We have so squandered and violenced the natural world that it has become necessary to include the ecological-survival perspective in (almost) every aspect of our relationship with Nature.

So when children today see creative and life-affirming documentaries on TV; when children today go on nature walks and treks; when children today are introduced to the wonders of the Earth... there is always the accompanying message of how few of any species remain, how devastated are its habitats, how destructive humankind has been... and how grim the overall picture is becoming.

Today, every beautiful revelation of the magical consciousness of the great whales always seems to begin or end with shots of the slaughter (past and present), which has led to the endangerment of these great beings.

Every guided walk in the forest teaches children to be aware of the unnatural overgrowth of understory foliage; of the damage from feral (introduced) species; of the permanent devastation of erosion... etc. And once we open to this level of awareness... well... we easily see that our Mother Earth is in a tragically sorry state indeed!

True, a very few children may be able to integrate this incessant revelation of despair with a positive appreciation of the beauties that still remain. But probably far fewer than our well meaning eco-educators would imagine. And even for these fortunate few, to become aware of the hopelessness of the overall perspective *and* still find positive joy in Nature (in spite of it all) simply cannot happen if the only messages they hear are the endless and repetitive expressions of our great *Cultural Guilt*.

As the 'caring minority' today, we are coming to be so ashamed of our atrocious past in relation to trees, land, wildlife of all kind… and the Earth herself… that virtually *every* glimpse that our children get into the otherwise inaccessible realms of ocean, rainforest, desert or mountaintop comes complete with a massive download of this stridently urgent, accumulated guilt.

And *this* is the severe limitation of the 'green' consciousness today: that we have overthrown the tyranny of *exploitative, materialistic Scientism…* and replaced it with the despair of the new, *scientific Eco-materialism*! And if we are to feel and love Nature today… we must all live within this oppressive paradox: in order to have any 'nature' left to enjoy (in hope-fully innocent wonder), we must *all* become sensitive to the damage that has occurred and we must *all* become 'masters' of the material plane so that we can actively and effectively participate in the Healing of the Earth.

But in order to feel *empowered* to accomplish this urgent work… and if we are ever again to be free to feel the Deep Magic, wonder, and sacredness of all Life… then somehow and sometimes we must find ways to be *freed* from this terrible guilt… so that we can surrender into whole-being openness like the Children that we all are… so that we can find ways to surrender into the belly and breasts of our earthly archetype of *'The Mother'* - in-to our birth-mothers and in-to our Earth-Mother as well.

We need moments (at least) of freedom from the guilt and ravages of our historic desecration so that we can find new ways into the experience of *trusting* mother-love, of *trusting* her nourishment and her sufficiency, of *trusting* her great powers… and so coming to trust the ultimate *rightness* of our individual (and collective) lives. These are the *Blessings of the Mother* that can only come through woman… and the Earth. To the extent that we have denied and desecrated either or both… we are forlorn and desolate and so our children cannot be whole… and free… and in-touch with their natural wisdom, their natural magic and their birth-right of spiritual inspiration.

It is a choice. And it is a choice that has been made badly - by tradition and by arrogance - for far too many generations of humankind. How we meet (and hopefully redress) this *crisis in our collective consciousness*... is a more urgent and pressing problem than the *material* conservation of any forest or any species on this planet. For in this *New Medicine Ritual Dance of Earth-Healing* and the *Free-Ritual Re-Initiation* of our collective childhood within the loving embrace of father-mother Spirit... lies perhaps the only chance for the future of our kind... and of the Earth Herself.

If we constantly blame each other and tell everyone that *we are 'the problem,'* then we are back to square one in the 'original sin' arena - merely substituting *eco-guilt* for spiritual unworthiness. And when we hear this message, we tend to respond in a binary (polarized) way: either we try to *ignore* the 'bad news' and so form an even thicker shell of insulation to protect our cultural traditions of selfish denial and greedy consumerism... or we assume the burden of collective eco-guilt in good faith (and despair) and set about to do penance for our whole race... and for our collective sins of global overpopulation and cultural greed. And as we assume this burden... we naturally become dis-empowered... and so ineffective as shamans... as *Medicine Healers of the Mother Earth.*

If we are convinced that Tiger is all but lost... we will (and must) seal off our active caring for the non-viable lifeform called 'Tiger' and turn our attention to whatever still has any chance of success - like those aid workers in every famine who must choose who shall and who shall not receive food, the food that is Life itself.

Ironically, so much of our deep-seated feeling of collective disempowerment, helplessness, apathy, depression and striking-out violence comes from the endless messages of despair which are beamed outward from the very medicine heart of our *most* caring ecological awareness!

Nevertheless, the messages of shock and horror at how we have mistreated the Earth are absolutely essential today. We cannot ignore the reality of our desperate situation.

But still... even where tidal waves destroy an idyllic island beach scene... even as the waters withdraw, the magic of earth-life-healing-change goes on and on... and on. And somehow we have to learn to balance the messages of doom and despair that so assault all hope and trust today.

True, human overpopulation, human greed, strange ideals of land 'improvement' - and all the rest of our ecological sins and innocence - are also 'natural' forces. But if we concentrate too much on the horror... we will not be attuned to the *rebirth* that is happening all around us. And so we will too easily pull our children's hearts and hope down into an abyss of despair, as they are forced to assume far too early, the stifling burden of all the past generations' blindness.

RETURNING TO GAIA... AND GOING BEYOND

Far removed from eco-destruction for many thousands of years... and still far removed from most of our 'civilized' ecological concerns... The Medicine Way, the Path of the Shaman, has evolved through untold millennia of tribal experience - through ages of people living harmoniously *with* the Earth. Today, more and more people are struggling to reawaken this primal earth-consciousness and give it new life in the very heart of our highly industrialized culture. In growing numbers we are beginning to recognize that the very survival of our eco-desecrated planet may depend upon the power of this feeling that we might call, *'The Returning'* - this wave of what is often now called *'Gaia Consciousness'* that urges us all to celebrate and heal our Living Mother planet Earth.

As the magic and the beauty of the Living Earth begins to flow again through our every experience, so we come naturally to look for all our 'medicine' in the splendor and magic of Nature, in the realm of the Ancient Ones, within this state of natural wonder.

We honor the gifts of Gaia by learning once again how to live simply on the Earth and try to live in harmony with all other living things. We try to de-fuse our dependence on material things and seek release from our addiction to the false wealth of the consumer culture.

Many of us study natural nutrition and so learn of the perils of consumer-food: the dangers to ourselves, to our children... and to the Earth herself. Minimalism. Simplicity. Renunciation. Sounds good. Feels good, mostly, too. But if we are not careful... all of this accelerated caring and self-responsibility can so easily turn into a morbid and guilt-ridden state of deep depression. That is, it is so easy to become so overwhelmed by ecological issues that we begin to deny all of our natural appetites and so to stifle all our natural exuberance for Life itself. [It is interesting that we only need attend the meetings of virtually any ecological group and feel its mood to see the dangers of acknowledging the guilt... without liberating the celebration!]

By now we know the grim truth of human-earth ecology: *nothing* is wholly 'safe' for the planet. Even normal human bodily functions become gross ecological problems when there are so many of us here. In fact, everything that humans do takes its toll on the environment. And the very most conscientious among us often feel so dis-empowered that we are able to do little else but to curb our personal excesses and indulgences on a very individual level.. and agonize over the whole situation.

To preserve our zest for life even *through* our awareness of the global ecological crisis, we need to find some balance between the forces of Conscience and those of Pleasure.

We need to find some *up*-energy to help us retain that eager-child hunger for experience, understanding and integration which is the driving spirit of our evolution.

And so... along come the Children!

Children are not born with pre-implanted eco-guilt (anymore than they are born into 'original sin'). They are born with a *natural wholeness* that (naturally) celebrates every aspect of Life: all its feelings, every new sensation, every adventure and every learning.

And we - the newly self-appointed, *'Eco-Guardians of Gaia'* who are trying to wrest public enchantment away from consumerism and redirect public pleasure away from the jet skis and back to seeking the natural inspiration of quiet oceans, of the *Tao* of Mother Earth and Father Sky - are now living in the vortex of the next generation's eager outreach... for *everything*... for everything that is so naturally wondrous, fulfilling and exciting.

How will we re-act to our children's natural desires as they blossom forth in ways that we might not choose and could not even imagine ?

Will we deny their natural explorations and try to program them with our generation's 'politically correct' minimalist guilt? As the 'revolutionary' zeal of the 'sixties fades into a limp eco-apology to our children in the 'nineties... will all our supposed spirituality and eco-awareness come to nothing more than a feeble trade-in of the tired, patriarchal notion of 'Original Sin' for a more noble and Earth-centered, *'Original Guilt?'*

We cannot remain detached from the current situation that we have created. We all resonate with our collective-historical failure at profoundly deep levels... and yet we know we must *find the beauty* afresh and anew for every new child... however we can. And the pressures that this dilemma is placing upon the psyche of every (conscious) individual today is perhaps our single greatest crisis-of-heart.

If we are determined to redress this imbalance of feeling... where will we begin? How can we help ourselves and our children move from dis-empowered eco-despair and doom-consciousness... into the empowering light of natural beauty and wonder... and magic?

Somehow we must discover a new emotional-spiritual stance that can remain closely attuned to the urgent needs and the devastation of the earth as it progresses day by day... while also remaining attuned to the *natural wonder* that is the birth-right heritage of every medicine child. In the academic and intellectual community, the new discipline of *eco-psychology* is beginning to address this issue on both philosophical and pragmatic (therapeutic) grounds. And in the realm of pure feeling and experiential flowering... we offer the enduring inspiration of the Medicine Wheel... and all the adventures of Life that come with the Earth-reverent understanding of the Medicine Path.

If these new-old path-ways are to be effective in leading us out of the eco-social downhill slide that is happening all around us now... then we will all need to discover (and consecrate) a *New Rightness-of-Place*... so that we can find new security and new sense of belonging on the Earth and so that we may 'live long and prosper' within the context of our long run of cultural and spiritual evolution.

For our family, this new security - and our *New Medicine Celebration* - begins when we take Spirit to Heart... and when we find ways to honor the old and new wisdoms that abound *everywhere* in Nature... as we 'walk in a sacred manner' between the Earth and the Sky.

><><

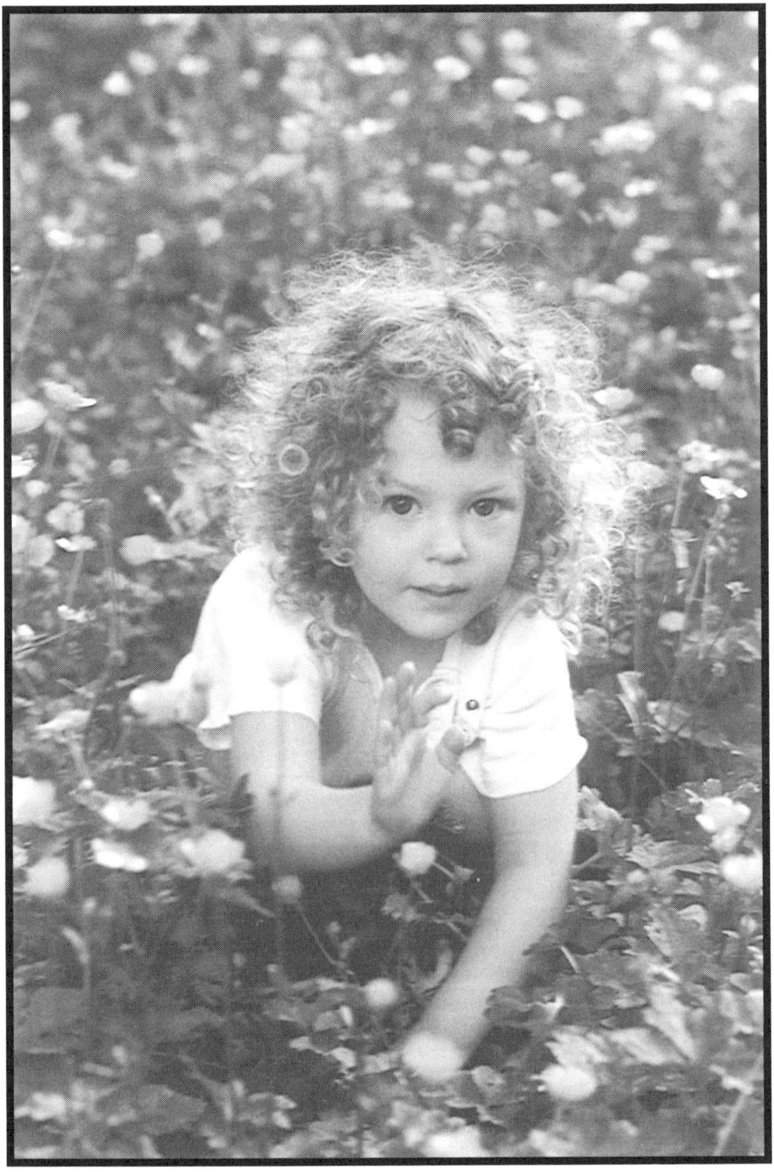

CHAPTER 12

REAL WORLD MEDICINE

- IN THE REALM OF MAYA -
THE SACRED THRUST OF DESIRE

Children are bubbling with desire and hunger and eagerness from even before their first breath. Children naturally reach out to taste and try *everything* that comes into their awareness.

Desire is the 'strange attractor' of all growth. Ultimately, all yogis will admit that even the urge to become a renunciate saint... is just a different (and more evolved) form of any little child's desire for a bright new toy... or a piece of brightly colored cake. The very same Desire. The one and only Desire. And we all know from when we were children ourselves... that perhaps the surest way to intensify desire... is to forbid its fulfillment!

Even if some adults might want to seclude themselves away in a wholly natural environment, far from all the trappings (and traps) of the techno-consumer-world, to meditate on Vision and Spirit for the rest of their lives... one thing is absolutely predictable: *their children certainly will not!*

DESIRE: The desire to evolve. The desire to change. Children are naturally inquisitive and naturally worldly. They urge to explore everything - to find out about anything that feels new or bizarre or exciting. And so they should! To hold any child back in their eager search for excitement and meaning is to oppress them, to stifle their vitality and to subvert their amazing auto-firing, high intensity self-integrating, self-evolving learning systems.

But even beyond what harm can come to individual children if their creative desire is thwarted, there is another level of urgency here: we *need* all of our children to experience this world; to know how everything works, inside out; to feel all of its glory and all of its horror... just as we have passed it on to them. For only through such in-depth experience will they become competent to deal with whatever is to come, with whatever the world will become. And, whatever it may be, we all know that it is going to be very intense... and very demanding... and very carefully balanced between careful living... and extinction!

After all (and after us), it will be up to them to steer and shepherd the Earth through its next generation. And the choices that they will have to make are *so* important to the ecological-economic-political future of this planet... that I, for one, want them to have all the experience that they can possibly glean from the world-at-large (of *whatever* is 'out there') to guide them in their healing and custodianship of this precious, living planet Earth.

Sure, we old-timers can hold stubbornly true to our idealized 'medicine visions' of waterfalls and sacred pools. We can live as we need to, such as we can. But there is always the danger of being too narrow in what we are willing to include as worthy and real in life. These rigidities (these defenses) may be hiding anywhere at all: within our well-spoken spiritual ways; within our over-zealous organic food dogmas; within our acceptance/denial of computers, information technology and real-time, whole-planet, internet communications; or within our fixed attitudes (pro or con) about drugs - from sacramental medicine plants to mind expanding chemicals to alcohol and tobacco... and whatever is yet to come.

Wherever our limitations lurk, our children are pre-programmed to find our every closed door and pre-energized to break them down. They will buy into some of our games, of course. And they will be prone to other silliness that they buy into from the mass-marketing of the culture-at-large. But somewhere deep inside, we *know* that they will sense every flaw in our total openness... and that they have come here to do so!

They will try to invite us to 'come out to play' in the simpler, black and white world that they see around them. And if we do... then we will make medicine together. If we can... and to the extent that we can just 'let it be'... we can be 'medicine families' together, still.

But if we refuse to be moved - if we wholly refuse to accept any aspect of their precious, now-time experience as *real and necessary* - whether such denial comes from our own limitations of vision, or from some rigid dogma of eco-moralism that we dare not admit and release - one thing is absolutely certain: if we cannot accept *The Invitation of the Children*, we Old Ones will soon find ourselves sitting in our Sacred Circles and staring at our Sacred Fires... alone!

And even while we sit there, meditating on our precious 'natural lifestyles' (and wondering what happened to our medicine families), our medicine children will be racing toward the city lights by the fastest possible means... eating and trying and consuming and testing and *celebrating everything* as they go... as they go away!

It is a strange paradox, is it not? But even 'though we can never know what the future will bring... still, we can choose our Path....

We may not be able to choose the ending... but we can choose how to *begin*, anew, each and every moment.

Every next step is a first step to the future. And...

The very first step on the path of Free-Ritual Shamanism
And the deep sharing of all Medicine Family Dreaming
Begins with the discovery that: EVERYTHING that flows
Through our every feeling-breath-experience-dream...
Is Medicine... is Consciousness... is Spirit... is REAL!

So it is. And thus it must be true: if we want to continue to 'make medicine' together, to sit in High Council together, to walk together in a sacred manner with those we love, we simply must be willing to include *'the all'* of our children's experience... and be willing to walk with them... *wherever* they may lead... us all.

In time, for a time, we may have to be wholeheartedly willing to leave the pristine, natural settings of our idyllic medicine circles. We may have to say farewell to the simplicity of medicine journeys through far-away and still unspoiled rainforests, seashores and mountains. We may have to accept that those precious, formative times of first-look wonder are now passed... and hope that the lessons and the openness and the magic of those times will carry us (all) into an unknown and very different future.

To make this transition, cvcn though wc will be carrying our babes and shepherding our older children into their meeting with the world-at-large, we need to recognize that we are also *following them.* We are responding to *The Invitation of the Children* - that flows through their eagerness and their ultimate need - to 'come out' and to find the way to relate our medicine to the world-at-large.

We must be willing to explore with the fresh heart and open eyes of youth, to discover anew that which many of us left, long ago: that strange place which is strangely known as the *'Real World'*.

The 'real world' - the world of commerce and employment; the world of fast cars, wild music and exciting new technology; the world of sense-glut and boundless 'gimmie.' And it is also the dark world of global madness that plunges into war after war, caring not who lives or dies... the world that endlessly rapes and plunders the Earth... the world that commits unspeakable atrocities on sister-brother human beings, caring not for suffering... and all in the name of some in-sane *'God-of-Fear-and-Greed'* (or another).

To keep our family and our selves and our 'eco-mission' intact and happening, then, we will all learn to go out into the world together, as much as we can, for as long as we can.... Or we simply prepare to say, "Goodbye!" The choice is largely ours to make. And however we choose, for every one and every family, every departure from the safety of the home-temple-nest is the start of a journey into *'The Great Unknown.'*

In many ways it will be frightening, for we will inevitably have to confront things that we have never before been able to endure-change-tolerate-accept... or *integrate* in to our more secluded spiritual life. But wherever it takes us, it will be the greatest Medicine Walk of all! For as we literally follow our children out of the magical forests and special ritual places, we will be moving in a wholly new direction.

Instead of Earth-centered rituals to evoke the special *knowing* of the Ancient Ones... we will now be seeking *Vision of the Future...* and we will learn to 'walk in a sacred manner'... in strange, new lands... walking toward *the Tomorrow of the Earth.*

THE POWER OF ACCEPTANCE

As we move beyond our usual medicine walk and 'new age' environments, we soon come to a whole new universe of stimulation, guidance and experience. For our children, this new magic is the real-time world of the peers. And to any kid it is immediately attractive, immediately challenging and *absolutely essential.*

The World of the Peers is a whole new *dimension of effect.* And within its endless variety, it has great power to affect any child's attitude and behavior - Medicine Power that will, in time, inevitably surpass even the most glorious and gifted powers of parenthood.

As we parent, so may we be remembered. And if we 'succeed' in our relationships with our children, then we may have ongoing connection that will be rich for us all... and for several generations to come. But if we try to pretend - even for the barest moment - that we can dictate or control or demand certain feelings, behavior or attitudes from our children as they grow into the separate persons that they need to become... then we have already lost the game... then we have already given up the chance to serve them in that most basic and essential way of helping them to connect their parent-child and inner family experiences with the amazing onrush of possibilities that await them in the world beyond.

There are many ways to help, of course, and many strongly held and differing perspectives as to what is enough and what is too much. But perhaps the most important way to help... is to be trust-worthy enough that you even *get* to hear what is happening to your child in his/her real-world adventures... and response-able enough to find a way to *include* their new ways of feeling within your family sharing.

As our children grow in years and power and come to individuate themselves, first within and then from the Family Circle, *acceptance* may become the most powerful tool and the greatest ally we could have in preserving the family union.

In its full-blown magic, acceptance is the task of finding the *rightness* (for them) in whatever your children may become... in whatever they may do... and in whatever they may feel.

We have all seen instances of parents who have used this vehicle (this medicine tool) of acceptance to completely transcend their own values and judgments. These parents succeed at being friends for life when they are able to celebrate the 'rightness' and the worthiness of their children's life-paths - even when those paths take them far away from parental values.

To allow our children full access to all of their birth-right freedom-of-becoming, we need to accept them even when we cannot comprehend their choices... even when we cannot hear the distant drummer that they follow.

Now if we were all-ways wholly accepting of each other, then of course there would be no need for healing within our relationships. Somehow... we can never quite be as open as we would like. But in this dimension of family sharing - as in every other - there is a simple *Ritual Circle Process* that can help us to move-through times of conflict and denial. And it goes like this:

ACCEPTANCE - FORGIVENESS - TRUST -
RELEASE - HOPE... and ACCEPTANCE

It is a *Circle of Commitment.* It is, once again, the Medicine Wheel. It is a path-way to maintaining closeness. And through all of the (little and big) crises that parent-child sharing brings (and however we may change the wording of the process to suit our family's specific needs)... ultimately some form of this *Ritual of Acceptance* may be the *only* way, the only medicine that will really work to keep our families intact and pulsing and alive!

Most parents who feel that they have succeeded in becoming *friends* with their children as they grow up, will say that they have come to a similar realization: that *acceptance is the only path-way to Deep Intimacy...* with anyone.

So... if medicine families we would be... then sooner or later, we will find ourselves listening to a new bird call that drifts to our ears on winds that come from somewhere far away. It is the song of the City Lights. It is the real-time beckoning of the inevitable future. And once we begin to hear its call... then there is no point in denying it as *Sign* - for it is surely sign for us all.

And there is no point in mis-reading its *Meaning...* for it has come to in-form our future awareness. No... once the Song is heard, then we have no other honorable choice: we must do whatever we need to do to find ways to carry our medicine out of the special valleys and away from our traditional sacred circle sites. And we must prepare to take our Medicine Show to town!

DEEP MEDICINE IN THE CITY CENTER

In the very center of the city there is much medicine to meet. When you can 'walk in a sacred manner' amidst all the confusing and imposing energies that always threaten to overwhelm everyone there... then you will meet some truly amazing wonders.

One warm night, our family was walking around in the city of Brisbane (Australia). It was a medicine walk: we had consecrated it carefully by each sharing our intentions... and our hopes... and our excitement. We had agreed to 'make medicine'... and then moved out into the city night to *find* it... whatever it was to be!

Almost immediately we found ourselves moving toward the sounds of a church carillon as it sent out its muffled metal song across the noisy and empty airways of the canyons of the night-city streets. But as we moved toward this sound... we were suddenly attracted by the feeling of cleaner, fresher air. Never actually finding our way to the bells, still the bells led us instead to another churchyard. And suddenly, there we were, sitting beside the most beautiful stone pond, filled with many-colored fish and the splendor of tropical water-flowers: lotus and hyacinths. The electric lighting that would have felt so harsh and discordant in our peaceful forest homeland was quite natural here... changing colors constantly, as different underwater lights sequenced through unseen electronics. And it was *all* Sign.

Later, when we talked about the trip and shared our different Meanings... the one that was most important to me was the unspoken joy I could feel in my children's wholehearted affirmation of *all* the people in the world-at-large who *cared* enough to make such beautiful things as church bells and colored-water flower pools... such wonderful mandalas as the graceful arcs of bridges reflected in still waters... or the circle-magic of Victorian wrought iron street lights... such wonders of materiality as sweeping freeway ramps and many-tiered, sparkling, parking ramps... such marvels as shining store windows and used car dealers' flags... and those nice places for pigeons to live in the park. And I felt proud, too, that for all of the woes of the *Realm of Maya*... that there was such caring and love still to be found there... and even more, that my newly city-dazzled children could notice and affirm it for us all.

Hello there, brave Humanity!
We see your Spirit is still alight
In all the Cities of the Night.
Let the cynics cry and moan
As they deplore cement and steel
Some of us who had already fled
Are coming back to see it in new ways
With Children to reawaken Wonder in us all.

There is so much magic in the city. There is so much to process and so much to learn. One of the greatest lessons is the phenomenon of the city itself: that so many people have come together to live in such strangely non-intimate intimacy. They share looking at each other night and day, hardly able to be truly alone. They share such intimate touch - jostling each other as they pass, rubbing thighs and shoulders and bellies and breasts so tenderly in the trains. They share their smoke and breath and sweat and fumes and the stained and intimate wrappings of their most private foods and personal needs. They share their voices and the sounds of their anger and their pain, their weddings and their funerals. They share their skills and their breakdowns, their genius and their madness... and they share all their love and all their hatred... with whoever just happens to be around!

It takes a very impressive and specialized skill to even survive in the city, with your sensitivity intact. And seeing us sharing such deep intimacy with those we too often try to regard as 'total strangers' - as nameless and irrelevant others - is deeply re-affirming to our family... and feels hopeful in its own, strangely alienated way....

Well... that's what we learned on *our* Medicine Walk today.

AND HOW WAS YOURS...?

LIVING WITH OUR FAMILY'S DIFFERENCE

So... this is the Way of our Medicine Family Vision. And it is working well for us, for now. If it continues to be meaning-full in the lives of every one as the months and years flow by... it will be because we are not afraid of Change... or difference.

If we can allow our process full freedom to be constantly adapting and evolving - the always fluid state of *becoming* - then perhaps we will 'walk in a sacred manner' together for many more decades to come.

Yes, for now, this works for us. And I can only offer other families what has come from our direct experience. But I also know that my family lives differently than most. And so it is important to try to relate our medicine family process to the world-at-large.

What we are doing as a family is different than any other family that my children know. This says a lot! And so it is important for me to try to share this difference with my children, to try to help us all evolve a perspective that includes our way... and also the ways of the culture that we live in:

"None of my friends go on Medicine Walks with their families.... And they don't make any wishes to the Father Sky or sing to the Mother River when *they* go swimming...!"

"Why *don't* other families do these things, Daddy?"

And after all these years... the best (and only) answer that I can give them is: "I don't know.... I simply cannot imagine why...!"

And yet... *I* have to find answers that help my children to integrate our lifestyle with the way others live. And I know that if I were to speak judgmentally of others' lack of interest in their own consciousness, spirituality, wholeness and family one-ness... then I may come to be a patterning force of alienation in my children's lives.

In some ways, this is almost inevitable. Because to the exact extent that my children hold respect for my opinion, they will be very sensitively attuned to my every reaction (pro or con) to any human behavior. If I judge... then they will also (for now) carry judgment within them. If I accept others' choices without reaction... then they will see me 'not caring' about things I tell them are very important. And which ever way it goes, there will always be some confusion. And there will all-ways be some contradiction.

The up side of this is, of course, that we can guide our children to internalize at least some of our best values. The down side is that they will also naturally hear and internalize even the barest hint of any message that even implicitly says: "We're different... and therefore... we're special!"

Every conscientious parent who moves into non-traditional realms with their families knows this one. And, like all parents, I struggle with the paradox that says: yes, I *do* want to draw clear hierarchies of social behavior. I want them to feel that it is *better* to be one who picks up trash than one who throws it on the Earth. It is *better* to look for ways to clear through our personal dramas than to always impose our own unclarity on others.

And yet... it is also important to convey that those who do things differently may *act* in less responsible ways... but *must* still be worthy as people. Worthy of our love, our respect, our openness (etc.). Because no matter what or who or how we are... all of humankind is still *'All One Family'* in our essence and in our Spirit. And *that* is a very wonderful thing, indeed!

So... I know that if my children's effort to understand their apparent 'difference' became too difficult… it would be too easy for them to fall into some kind of smug (and alienating) sense of superiority. After all, self-alienation is one obvious way of coping with contradiction. And if this occurred… then my children may not feel open to find the magic of intimate sharing with others who simply do not live as we do… or care about the same kinds of things.

And if ever this happened, then they would miss out on sharing their hearts and their lives with others - finding new friends, other teachers, lovers (in time), etc. And this is *not* what our process is about… of course.

This is a common paradox that all families must face.

But what can you do…?

> *[We are all such innocently pure reflections of our culture's contradictions! So perhaps it is understandable that most of our 'tribal' friends tend to be dogmatically suspicious of all technology and media; and our high-tech friends equally suspicious of anything that smacks of Earth Ritual and/or Spiritual Guidance.*
>
> *Our yogic friends tend to fear anything that is based in the physical-emotional world (how they dread and fear that ol' 'Realm of Desire!')… while our new age friends are innately suspicious of empowered maleness ('The Patriarchy,' you know).*
>
> *And so it goes, on and on: our academic friends still believe that 'shamanism' is something that you can (only) learn by reading a book, doing a 'certifying' weekend workshop and learning to imitate the practices of other cultures, philosophies and times.*
>
> *And of course, our eco-political friends are suspicious of… well, almost everything…. And our dear old hippie friends, well they are still more pure and more globally essential than they ever suspect… and more 'retro' (and more emotionally regressive) than they will ever imagine. All in all, this culture is a very weird mix!]*

So what about us? What about the 'Medicine Family?' Well, we are not 'above it all' by any means. In fact, we tend to embody *all* of these same weird energetics and social genetics (of course) in some way or another. And yet… and still… our goal is to try to accept it all: *'the all'* of human experience (and as much of human behavior as we can as well). And so we try to ride the waves of cultural change as best we can, somewhat self-isolated within our own *Medicine-Magic-Nature-Bubble* just for now, perhaps… but still hopefully open to every meeting with kindred and semi-kindred souls alike… whenever and wherever we find each other....

Ultimately, we all tend to understand 'reality' in terms of what we experience on a day to day level. And once we feel that we 'know' what life is - i.e., what is 'real' and what is not - we naturally (and unconsciously) tend to overlay our personal beliefs upon everyone else's experience.

And once we have set up our walls of explanation... they tend to inadvertently become self-isolating walls of denial and defense. There is all-ways that risk... but even so...

My task here seems simple enough: I seek a way to invite families everywhere to open to the 'medicine' that is all around us... to the deep streams of Earth-magic that flow through every new conception and up through every child's outstretched arms.

But if it is to work... for *you*... then this Medicine Way must be able to live and flourish within your *own* family process, within your own family's rituals of sharing and within the unique ways of being that have evolved for you.

And after all these years... and after seeing so many families find new hope through this process... I really trust that it can!

I know that the spiritual path we are following is unfamiliar to most other families (in this culture, at least). I also know that most families live in a state of constant and conscious *compromise* - 'making do' with brushing past each other many times each day and yet rarely (if ever) experiencing the deep sort of communion that is built into the family situation as a natural, birth-right potential.

Real intimacy is hard to realize... and harder still to share... until we come to realize that *there is simply nothing else to do* than to share *everything* that we experience with and toward each other: everything that we sense and feel and wonder... everything that we love... and everything that we dislike and resent... and especially: *everything that we fear.*

And through that sharing... comes the only effective path-way to emotional clarity... that I have ever seen:

Whatever flows through our experience is Real.
Whatever is felt can be Shared.
And whatever is shared... brings Change.
And where change and growth are Celebrated...

ANYTHING IS POSSIBLE!

I invite you to think of this next time you feel tempted to take the 'easy way out' and allow your precious moments to pass by... resigning yourself to living with unshared love... or unshared inner pain... resigned to failure... and ultimately... resigned to deadly *compromise*!

It is 'different,' to be sure. And it will make your family 'different' as well. At least for now. But if enough of us medicine monkeys learn to wash our selves clearer in this way... then maybe we can hold tightly together, now and then, in celebrations and gatherings of all kinds... until the hundredth monkey takes the plunge... and we all learn to celebrate wholeness together!

In the end, there is no need to worry too much about being 'different'... because if you have children... pretty soon *they* will find you (and make you) 'different' anyway! All it takes is a little Desire... and a few squirts of those ol' hormones of sweet budding adolescence....

And lookout! Here they come already!

PEERS AND FEARS

Ami is having her eleventh birthday party this week. She has a new school and new friends and they are very important to these first hormonal explosions of adolescence. For now we are suddenly in the time of the *Peer-God* when the opinions and judgments of 'The Pack' are suddenly more important than everything else in life.

This is an important developmental phase in the *Ritual of Finding Place*... and a key moment in the conditioning-programing process of the Living Culture. It is a time of wild emotionality and although our parent-efforts may only rarely bring any real comfort to the child, this moment needs to be handled with great compassion and delicacy.

In our family, we are *all* becoming highly sensitized by this rush of constant judgment which now sweeps through our ranks like a moralistic S.W.A.T. team scanning for any little sign of whatever is 'uncool' that day.

We, the pitifully ponderous and hopelessly habituated, parental adults, have been told how to behave in the company of *The Party:* we are informed that it is 'fully uncool' to have Ami's birthday guests sitting around in a circle on the floor to eat. Totally uncool to have *any* actually healthy food in sight. Horrifically uncool to make any fuss over the birthday cake... and maybe even uncool to sing 'Happy Birthday' (in English *or* Chinese - we usually do both). Likewise, it is uncool for Daddy to expect any public notice of the ritual of profound change which turning eleven is bringing into our entire family circle. It is uncool to mark or celebrate this new direction in any way at the Grand Sleepover Party. And above all else... whatever else may happen or does not... "*Please* let's not make any medicine prayers at the party!"

It was a ponderous moment. "What?" I said in a very subdued voice... but which probably had all the overtones and effect of a great howl of outrage and indignation in the ears of our hyper-sensitized child-woman. "*No* holy-sweet gushy-syrupy medicine prayers...???"

She danced around me, cajoling and secretly testing just how much of whatever she imagined I was feeling was mine... and how much was her own projection. But this was really just an empty ritual observance because in fact she couldn't care less about anything that went beyond her own ever-tightening circle-of-self.

I played along with her charade of responsibility for awhile, played mock hurt, defeated sadness, rejection. Then I noticed that my play-acting was actually nothing more than a brave front which was holding me secure against the revelation of my real (and unfelt) inner feelings of dread and sadness and disorientation: "How am I supposed to *be* with all of this? What am I to do now with all of our traditions of medicine processes and medicine ways...?"

Feeling inside my only half-conscious game, I discovered a much deeper reaction: after all this parenting, guidance, teaching, sharing and celebration of the Medicine Way... after all these years of fairly unswerving (and only lightly tested) faith that *my* family would no doubt glide through life fully empowered and filled with joy and self-worth, through their long experience of whole-being earthing and conscious liberation in and through the spiritual path they would know so well from countless circles, rituals and medicine walks, etc., etc., etc.... after all of that... now *THIS?*

Forget about the drugs-and-smoking peer taunts of teen-time yet to come temptations... here-and-now, at this very first hint of a real-life trial - facing our first terrible ordeal of *'Trial by Peer Group Judgment'* - we were immediately informed that everything that even hinted of 'medicine' had to be immediately thrown out, denied, pretended away and buried as deeply as it could be!

Every medicine ritual object was potentially offensive. Even the slightest glimpse of a ritual blanket or medicine wheel mandala was believed likely to ruin all of Ami's social chances in this small-valley, small-time community of newly born-again almost-teenaged consumer-materialists. And this was more ironic still since Ami's new friends were the very daughters and sons of the very heart of the eco-spiritual, self-sufficient, bio-diverse, sustainable lifestyle, low-impact, permacultural, 'new age' stream of consciousness in this land.

Of course the denial I could feel was not so absolute within the reality of Ami's feeling. And so I came to see. It was just that in this secluded valley which is filled with one-time hippies living out their ultimate, let's-go-back-to-the-land-organic-garden-owner-built-home stuff... all of their (our?) children seem to know only one thing for sure about 'real life' and it is this: *"HIPPIES ARE TOTALLY UNCOOL!"* And anything that smacks of hippiedom in any way... may mean the social ruin of any eager, up and coming, peer-pack conformist clone.

"HIPPIES...? *US...???"*

I licked my wounds with exagerated gesture (actually healed pretty quickly), then returned to genuine mirth and merriment as we prepared for the Great Eleventh Party - and soon recovered my own inner celebration of this amazing world of almost-teen which was descending like a turbulent cloud into the very heart of my family circle. Beautiful. Passional. Rich and so eager for the next scene... eager, that is, as long as everything was 'passed' as acceptable by The Peers... and so long as every move, gesture, action or choice could be governed by the Laws of the Pack!

From this happy recovery, I carefully assumed a well stylized waiting stance and just... well... waited. And I watched the neo-fascism of teenage coercion run its (quite predictable and more than a little boring) course through our lives. And then it came to pass one day that Ami came sniffing around for a little hit of the ol' medicine magic. But alas... it was out to lunch. No one there.

I made out not to notice and not to care. After all, she was only hinting around. Nothing specific had yet been said. Wholesale rebuffed as I (and my path) had been... I certainly needed more overt invitation than that! Maybe a little begging, even.... And so we danced around for awhile in a precarious balance.

Then one evening I found a rare chance to settle in with my little boy-babies (then of three and six years) and to have a good old

Boy-Circle with them - an event which came to little more than a quick cuddle-heap as they passed out on my lap in a pile of steamy, warm-puppy curls.

Ami was being excluded. Hey! This was simply "*not* excellent!" It was all right for her to exclude us... but to be shut out of even a partial-family cuddle was a pretty big blow to her. I explained it in terms of needing to make time for the little ones to get *their* fair share of those old Faeries and Elves and all that kind of 'old fashioned' kid-sort of medicine stuff... just as Ami had when she was that age. She agreed, in principle at least. And she accepted the momentary separation. With a brave affirmation of their right to have that kind of time with me also... and with more than a twinge of mutual regret, we let go of the night.

I kept this dynamic current dancing between us for several days, alluding to it now and then in silly jokes and subtle jibes, interspersed with sincere sharing and processing-through of whatever each of us were feeling. Inside, I was always waiting for her to take responsibility for making a specific outreach - for declaring her need and her desire to re-consecrate our medicine space. And through all of this I could see Ami growing inside like a banana plant... changing at a deep cellular level, but changing so fast that I could see her expansion pushing and stretching her whole being from the inside out.

AND SPIRIT STILL RUNS DEEP

A PAGAN GRACE:

Arise ye budding soft green Life
Move thru the mire of Earth and Wet
And Grace our table... and our Hearts
With all Goodness of your Earthly delights.

The Great Feast and Deep Family Circle for Ami's 'Real Birthday' came at last... several days before the Grand Sleepover Mega-Drama. As she nestled in the curve of my reclining self and blew out her candles all-in-one-breath, she made a wish. A *real* Wish. I playfully asked her to tell, but of course we agreed that she really didn't have to share her wish if she didn't want to....

She thought it through, felt it through, and then said "I'd like to tell you, Daddy. I wished that the Mother Earth and Father Spirit would help to guide me on my Medicine Path in this next year... and forever in my life."

And so our Medicine Way was chosen and re-created once again. And with a wee tear welling in the father eye, I could feel that our medicine family was still on track and steamin' along. I shared this little joy with Ami - very carefully of course, lest the bubble be shattered by some care-less off-hand denial - and she said, only...

"Yes. Fully!"

THE BIG DAZE PARTY-TIME

The Big-Time Sleepover came and went with a thousand shared secrets, all too secret to be told, giggled and shouted and clucked over all through the long night. And throughout the entire free-ritual chaos, Leia and I were easy: we tried not to impose our process or style on them in any way. Mostly.

We did not make them sit on the floor - instead they kneeled against a makeshift long table and ate like a double line of piglets at a trough.

We did not enforce a whole-food regimen at The Party and did not care that Leia had to sing 'Happy Birthday' almost all alone as she brought out the cake. The decorations were tasteful - not strictly black and white only, as requested, but tastefully monochromatic nevertheless.

And were we 'cool?' Hey! 'Cool' doesn't begin to describe it. We were beyond cool. We were totally chilled! No one even looked in the direction of a feather or a drum. No one let loose so much as a single word about rituals or the Earth or any of that.

All of our local elves and faeries and devas and nymphs were shut out stone cold and no one cared at all if they pressed puzzled and lonely faces against the windows all night long. We (well, some of us) watched really cool rock videos and we were very grown up, indeed!

And above all, and in absolute obeisance to the terrible peer-fear which all-ways runs this archly conservative denial, no one blessed the meal, blessed the daughter or made even the barest hint of a spirit-prayer of thanksgiving for a magical eleven years. And when all the after-gossip was in, we heard that it had been decreed by one and all: the Party-Eleven was a smashing success!

And the very next night, as our family all lounged around together on our biggest bed and went through our party 'debriefing' stuff... we opened a new lesson, a new frontier of exploration which I know will need many months to process-through... and as many children to meet it in their time.

For now we have begun a new journey together: we are setting out to consciously explore how we can interface the Medicine Way with the world-at-large. So... *Watch out World... here they come!*

MOTOR MADNESS MEDICINE SPIRIT DANCING!

There is medicine in everything. It simply must be so! But as our children grow and change and hurl surprises at us one after another, we are often stretched to find it. But still we can know that it *must* be in there, somewhere, awaiting our discovery, in everything that our evermore free-ranging children can find to explore... to do... to learn... to share... to become.

It must be there... or there's no medicine anywhere! And so the earnest parents commit to learn new medicine ways.

Just now, our family is moving deep into the medicine of the mini-motorcycle. We are making a new kind of 'Sacred Circle' in the pasture, enfolding everything in two-cycle sputter.

"Wait! How could you do this?" some readers might say. Well... *'how?'* is the essential question, all right... but 'how *could* you' simply ignores Reality!

My big-little Joah is now nine and moving up fast on twelve. His friends all have mini-bikes (50-80-125cc trail bikes). And I began to get the eager requests, hints of the Medicine Dance to come: "Can I go to Eric's and ride his trail bike? He has a new 125!"

A lame visage of my former self arises from somewhere deep within my inner eye: I see that younger medicine man of ages past who nodded with silent, affirming power when his children said... "some people eat chocolate cake...but we don't *like* chocolate, do we, Daddy?"

Nodding sagely, he was, in honor of his children being given the chance to pattern their desire-bodies with several loving years of very devoted natural nutrition and sugar-free wholeness. And silent he was to maintain some integrity in the face of his own tendencies and ancient historic addictions.

"There will be time enough for them to learn of everything worldly. Everything in its time," he intoned, inwardly, as if to remind himself. It felt right to the Medicine Father and so he was at peace. Except... except... now... and already ...

it is suddenly time... for EVERYTHING!

Now I don't personally feel that nine year old body-minds have any intrinsic need for hands-on motorcycle experience. There is nothing in their internal essence that needs to be gasoline powered just yet. I could relate this to something about relative coordination, judgment, etc. But the *Power of the Peers* has spoken and it says otherwise.

The peers are *The Future*... of everything. And here and now, the peers have gotten a foot in the door of motorized excitement... and they are not going to let go!

Some parents around the valley have approved it. Others will reluctantly, begrudgingly acquiesce to the unrelenting pressures. Still other parents will try to deny 'The Force' and will try to hold back the river with their bare hands. But the Living Culture has spoken. And however anyone feels... no one can deny that this is what's happening all around us now. No one can wholly deny the *Power of the Peers* (and only a fool would try)!

My choice has been simple and stolid, my path no braver than that of any other parent: I stalled for awhile (got no time to come to grips with the issue). Then I came around somewhat and began to 'talk motorcycle' with other boys and other dads for awhile. Then money stalled us even longer. And then, the time to have it all my way was plain and simply up!

We had come down to the line: either my son was to be included in what was real for his age, in his world, in his time... or he would have to stand lamely aside while everyone else buzzed off into the bold frontier of gas-headed boy-bliss... and he would not be able to learn and grow with them. I knew that this would mean that they would (quite literally) leave him behind! Read the Sign. *Remember the Sign?* I can remember the sight and smell of dust myself....

If we have the Power of Denial running strongly within our blood... then I would hope to bring it to bear on the truly dangerous temptations of The Peers: drugs, alcohol and tobacco; theft and vandalism; unsafe sex and teen pregnancy.

Thus it came to be that we knew we had to expand some of the outer limits of our ideals and we had to expand our medicine vision to take on a new Free-Ritual Medicine Object: an ancient and ragged 80cc Yamaha 'DT-80' trail bike, half again older than its newest owner - our own Starship Enterprise which would take us to explore new worlds where no Joah had ever gone before....

[N.B.: For those of you who are by now worried that my daughters might somehow be suffering sexist exclusion (and come on now, you know who you are who run this program every time boys get-do-feel-need anything boyish at all)... *please* let go of your programmed fears: the bike is there for everyone!]

Biggest daughter thinks it's "Hell!" (which of course means 'Heaven' this week). The other can take it or leave it, but mostly leaves it. Leia hasn't tried it. Beny Sky is too little to reach the Earth. And I don't care about it at all, of course, being far too dignified for such things as this (much too little) mini-bike. But I do take it for a few whirls around the pasture now and then (and then and then)... 'testing its settings' and 'checking it out' for the kids - you know, just 'making sure it's all right,' like dads do....

"Uhh... Dad! Uhh... Dad...? Hey Dad! Come back! It's *my* turn!"

So, anyway, the bike has different levels of meaning to each of us. Some more, some less. But to Joah... it is a New Revelation: it is pure Testosterone God!

When the tired old machine first arrived, we made a little medicine ritual to inform all the nature spirits, elves, fairies and devas of this land of our truly peaceful (?) intentions. The bike will be staying in a large and well-fenced pasture. A neighbor who lives across the creek lets a few cows roam in and out of that field. He says they are well-accustomed to motor bikes from the sons of the last family who lived there. So the cows were cool. And sure enough, they never even looked up.

Next we walked around and around in the paddock together and sort of 'asked' everything to be at peace with the bedlam that was soon to come. We reassured every living thing that, "We will always drive the bike as gently and with as little disruption as possible. Probably we won't ever go fast or even rev the motor or anything."

We asked the daisies, the grass, the prickers, the snakes, the creek, the platypus and the trees... and once again, just to be polite, those soft 'house cows' who seem to hang out in this pasture, when it suits their mood. Whatever these various entities thought of it all, I cannot say. For they said nothing at all. But anyway, we knew that we were cool... 'cause at least we *asked*!

Soon it became obvious (to some of us, at least) that to some of us, at least, this ritual was a walk-through. Mere lip service. A simple courtesy-gesture from a newly empowered broker (and breaker) of all peace: *the Mini-Shaman of Noise and Speed.*

And oh was he ever reverent that day! Joah was hotly keen to do *whatever* medicine I might decree... and as quickly as possible, if you please! "Let's get on with it!" panted every well-controlled and pious breath. "Let's do it... and let's do it NOW!" blared forth from Joah's strained toning of every medicine word. And so all beings knew peace - or such 'peace' as was to be their fate - and then the *Ritual Initiation of the Motorhead* began!

A couple of suns later... and now he can ride and ride and ride! In just an eyeblink of time I have seen my son take many giant steps toward the competence and poise that he will need as a man... and, I must say, as a shaman as well.

He is learning fast. Not just how to ride a bike, for no learning is ever about just one thing at a time. No, he is working far beyond mere mechanics: he is working to master the disciplines of many spiritual path-ways all at once.

On the most obvious levels, this is a mechanical thing. And Joah is meeting his first big hurdles of that mechanics-time-money-energy equation that so taxes us all, as he strives to get on top of this new *Maya Machine*.

But he is also learning to feel the limits of his own ability, learning how to listen to that little inner voice that sets the day's limits of daring and tells him when to push himself and when to honor his fatigue... and when to honor the *Guide-Dance of Fear.*

He is also learning how to dance with the Power of Gravity as he floats and grinds across the Earth in this outrageous new way. There is so much boyish excitement to contain and release... and so much resistance and fear to meet. And there is no end in-sight. For the motorcycle has transported Joah into a vast new realm of truly magical learning:

Riding a trail bike is a pure *Zen* discipline of movement meditation and endless awakenings (in Zen Buddhism, *satori*)... if only we let it be so. Bouncing around our simple *Medicine Wheel*

Motorbike Circle-Track traced in bending grass brings such wonderful lessons: lessons of balance - grace - focus - control - power - gravity - flight - falling - surrender - protection - safety - pain - healing - recovery - ecology - sharing - ego strengthening - humility - fear - pride - and so many *Revelations of pure Joy!*

And so our medicine family is exploring *'Motorcycle Dreaming'*... and we are working together so that Joah Jai can take his place in a larger medicine circle... and be full-filled with the *Power of the Peers*.

And I...? Well, I am privileged to be the channel (one more time) for this new learning... and the father-shaman who is privileged to initiate him (one more time) into the next level of his empowerment and competence, in steady preparation for his manhood to come.

On the physical, worldly plane, getting the bike was a great choice. For I have the great security of knowing that he will be home taught, slowly taught (and well-taught) in the craft and the yoga of *Mini-Motorcycle Dreaming*.

He will learn what to do... what not to do... and above all else, what to watch out for. In this way I can best guarantee his safety. And someday, whenever he is finally ready to pass through the gates to other pastures and ready to seek higher trails with his peer pack, *I will know it*. We will share it. And I will certify him to proceed, level by level. And through my direct involvement in this process, I (hope that I) will have strengthened his trust in my judgment... and that he will shine with-in my *acceptance*.

And as a dad, I will be reassured in knowing that he has learned to ride with all the subtlety and sensitivity, with all the power and the sureness, that our medicine - and yes, our ever-growing feeling of Spirit - can bring to this most egoic and worldly adventure.

Through it all, I can laugh and make fun of his full-bore enthusiasm. But in all fairness to my little motor-head, I must add this: Joah loves the bike. But riding a trail bike has in no way alienated him from all the other things he loves.

We still make medicine near the creek at sunset; we still spend quiet time in sacred circles together. What has changed is that he has expanded his experience and his prowess into some new realms and has opened up several new dimensions of experience... and potential.

The new dimensions he now inhabits are those very realms of learning that we named above. So his new love and all the learning that goes with it... represents true growth for this already sensitive boy... and so a new fulfillment for all of us.

There is a way in which a pocket knife, a vehicle, a computer, electricity and fire are all the same. Ultimately, it's not so much what it is... but *how we use it* that develops and reveals (and facilitates) our consciousness. Up until now, my children have handled all of these things well: all signs have been good. I trust what Joah will do with this new power (or the bike would simply not be living with us). And I trust what Joah will become....

And I know that this is just the first of many times to come... when I and we will be forced to grow *with* our children... committed to find our family's medicine 'Way In' - to wholly new dimensions of experience.

EVERYWHERE IS ALL AROUND US

The medicine of the trail bike is a good example of extending subtle energy-medicine-consciousness into the world-at-large. Because if we can find the medicine in the motorcycle... we can probably find it anywhere! So let us look again at the world of *Maya* (in yoga, *maya* is the material world, the *world of illusion*), and see what medicine may await our revelation.

If there be medicine at all... it is everywhere around us, in us... for us. If there is vision at all, then vision may come to us anywhere.

Hidden away in a secret cave, *we* are less distracted and so *we* can tune-in better to feel the very subtle nuances of softly channeled awareness. But Vision needs no cave... Spirit needs no church... and meditation needs no ashram!

You have already heard it well. But we meet it everywhere... so here it is again: Sign, Meaning, Vision, Revelation and Guidance are *everywhere*. And as soon as we can fine-tune our perception and still our minds enough so that we can open our awareness to these subtle energies wherever we happen to be... then medicine will be with us wherever we are.

MEDITATING IN THE MARKETPLACE

We have all known people who react with a strange and defensive kind of annoyance whenever a friend expresses a need for a peaceful surround in order to work on their meditation, yoga or medicine. And these folks often say, "Well, if you were *really* able to meditate... then you could do it anywhere... even on a busy street corner!" And this is true, in a way - or at least partially true - but only up to a point....

Most people who use meditation to relax, to focus our awareness and to deliberately tune-out background distractions, could well use some practice on a busy public street. But where this misses the point is when meditation progresses to such rarefied levels of total stillness and subtle breath and consciousness that even the slightest pollution (of sound, vibration, airborne smog, etc.) *de-tunes* the receptivity of the meditator... and so sets an artificial (material plane) limit upon his/her sensitivity and balance... thus delimiting consciousness and inner growth.

The same is true for any discipline which requires great balance and sensitivity - be it tight rope walking, music, meditation or mastering the game of chess. But meditation and medicine (in any form) are different than these other acts of *will*. Because meditation and medicine involve our opening to subtle energy and consciousness which must come from (somewhere) *beyond* our ego-selves - to connect us with something beyond our individual self-self limitations.

So, sure... you can meditate on any street corner. And if you can remain wholly detached and unruffled by all that swirls around you, you can 'connect'... you can receive some kinds of guidance. But even so, the most dedicated yogis (like the most dedicated shamans) *always* seek the tranquility of a peaceful privacy on the natural Earth as the beginning point of their most subtle interface... with consciousness... and with Spirit.

PROTECTING THE PEACE

In the beginning, when the process is new and fresh, medicine walks *always* work best in the most tranquil, natural settings. By the very nature of the process itself, medicine walks and vision quests require a very special receptivity: the more we can open to very subtle energies and feelings, the more 'medicine' we will discover.

This sensitivity is an *'altered state of consciousness'* - one that is wholly new to many who might like to try this new way of relating... to everything.

Opening to medicine involves an awakening of the power of *Deep Sensing* - a process of profoundly *sensitizing* ourselves to increasingly subtle nuances of feeling, meaning, energy and Spirit.

But care is needed here! For as we become more open, more sensitive, more aware... we also, inevitably, become more *vulnerable*. Even in the midst of our highest experiences of magic and spiritual empowerment, the same 'altered state' of expanded sensitivity which has permitted such magic also renders us very fragile and *very* susceptible to distractions and intrusions.

This little truth simply cannot be overstated:

> *We are ALL vulnerable and fragile! So it is all-ways important to provide care-full nourishment and support for ourselves (and each other) whenever we would enter sacred space.*

Whenever we set out to 'make medicine,' we can honor this special state of awareness and its special needs by beginning any free-ritual medicine process in an environment that best supports and nourishes it... and us.

It is also important to be aware (at every instant) that every medicine quest involves walking-running-leaping-exploding into *'The Great Unknown'* with eyes and hearts just as open as we can possibly be.

With-in this openness we have a new chance to learn about our own limits - a renewable chance to see some of the ways in which our ego-eagerness intrudes into our clarity and clouds our inner vision.

With this new vision we can then begin to unravel our complex knots of defense: we can come to see how we (all) *stop* the medicine (usually before we ever even know that it has come), with silly noise, by falling over in the dark, by bumping into each other and laughing, or simply by coughing loudly just as the hidden deva-flower-spirit calls to us! It is a process of learning to know ourselves very, very well. And for every one of us... there is so much learning to do!

If medicine is, as we say here, a wholly natural occurrence for *everyone* who will come open to listen with a fresh ear and see with virgin eyes... then our greatest task in learning the *Dance of Vision* is just to work on this level of unfolding self-revelation: watching and learning how we block our own awareness... of the deeper levels of awareness (and Spirit) that are all-ways nearby.

Consider... if we take the subtle-energy workshop of the medicine walk into a busy city street, there are so many outside distractions that we have no hope of really seeing the workings of our inner games of self-limiting denial... and we may never see how we are holding Meaning and Vision and Spirit away... always imagining that we 'just had to cough' or that there was nothing else to do but trip in the gutter and fall in the mud right at that moment, with a great shout of genuine surprise.

But there is *always* something else to do! And in the end, there may be *nothing* else to do... but to find out what *IT* is... and how to *let it be!*

In the early days, we enter our apprenticeship into the world of subtle energy medicine magic through carefully prepared free-rituals, medicine walks and vision quests - in the most undisturbed and natural environments that we can possibly find.

As time goes by and we become more sure of ourselves and more secure in our own medicine processes... then we can begin to stretch out and explore new possibilities, relating our medicine to everything we meet, wherever we may be. And then, one day, we realize that we are becoming very 'good at it' - that we really know how to Dance with Spirit - and we are finally ready to take our Traveling Medicine Show to town.

The very first time we enter the 'outside world' with-in the deep openness of Medicine Spirit, is a big step indeed! The little medicine-birds with untried wings are making their first flight away from the temple-nest of Mother Earth's wooded glens, open deserts and high alpine meadows. It is a big leap to take. More than a little scary... and very exciting. But whenever it is time... then it is time... to go for it!

When our family opened to include the motorbike in our medicine... we did it *very* carefully. The best tool for us then, was that we placed the motorbike within the very environment of our medicine walks - within the rolling pasture land on the river flat below our house. So we did not have to go 'to town' to find the bike. No... this time, 'the mountain came to Mohammed.' When time was right, the motor-medicine came to the medicine family.

We did not go out looking for it, only to drag it home like one of those 'shopping buffaloes' that I might capture in the marketplace-at-large and then bring home to feed and clothe and excite my family. No, this bike actually came to us. And though it seemed strange to some of us at first (and to all of us at one time or another as the days unfolded) we knew that we had actually *invited* the trail bike to come to us through a more or less conscious *Ritual of Evocation*.

The bike was brought into our Family Circle from high in the mountain rainforest valley by a medicine messenger of *Motorcycle Dreaming* - the Last Dad in the long chain of this machine's long medicine history of Ritual Initiation in families scattered all over the mountain. And from the moment it arrived we could *all* see that *it was Sign*... and one look into Joah-eye revealed that it brought Deep Meaning... for sure!

If we had first met our motorbike differently - perhaps by going into a big city and tasting every motorcycle that we saw with our newly awakened Desire - then I know that the little lesson that was begging us to hear it... the one that said, "Hey, this is Medicine, too!" would have been harder for us to notice.

But to see that ragged little bike suddenly putting away gently in our Sacred Circle... was to immediately *know* its message... and its lessons: about things... and experience... and growing up... and about becoming sure and strong and able in the world-at-large.

><><

CHAPTER 13

THE ELECTRONIC MEDICINE WHEEL

MEDICINE FAMILY MEDIA

In a time when it is becoming so urgent for us all to appreciate our home-planet, Earth as a living being of very finite resources and great vulnerability... we need an expanded and unifying global perspective more than ever before. And yet, as population and the complexity of life increases faster than ever before... we can so easily become effectively disempowered.

We try to believe that if we follow the paradigm that says: *'think globally, act locally,'* we can somehow hope to solve the looming ecological and demographic crises that are so close at hand. But in devoting ourselves to practicing this (now) dogmatic wisdom we also isolate ourselves from the one force that has even the barest chance of succeeding at this critical moment: the great power of the force of *us*, the Great Medicine that comes when the Whole Circle of *US* comes together as One Heart and One Mind... to meet whatever is at hand.

To bring about this global empowerment just as we need it most, humankind has a new Medicine Ally: we have the Gift of Media. And with this gift we can begin to work from a new paradigm, which would be well expressed in a *New Medicine* 'bumper sticker' which says:

'THINK UNIVERSALLY... ACT GLOBALLY!'

The earth has been... the Earth... for billions of years. And yet, most of us could never see its simple reality, its fragility and its aloneness... until humankind gained the expanded perspective that came when we first viewed the earth as we orbited in space.

Once we began to see the *Whole Earth* all at once, then a mass cultural leap in awareness occurred: we could finally see our planet for what it was! And no one outside NASA would have had this revelation... if we had not seen it in our homes, on the good ol' TV.

In our medicine family, we *use* this gift of media - TV, video, recording, computers, modems, etc. We use it *all* as consciously as we possibly can, to expand our world-view and to learn about the inner workings of nature, ecology and human society, far beyond our local experience. We use media to extend our awareness far beyond our limited visual horizons.

We use media to in-spire (i.e., to 'bring Spirit to') our creative work and to help us to understand how we can (and must) learn to relate to the world-at-large as one great organism... and in time, perhaps, how to move into the living cosmos, beyond this nursery planet of our birth.

To illustrate this great resource, here is a little medicine story which shows the great worth and the great power of consciousness-expanding media experience:

'WHAT ABOUT THE CHILDREN?'

When Ami was in the last months of her ninth year, we happened to see a rich and moving documentary: a deep look into the tragic plight of the rainforests of the Amazon.

Ami was very moved by what she had seen. We lived in rainforest too (or at least what is left of it), but far from the Amazon Basin. She was too young to even imagine what had happened here, how the great rainforest mahogany, red cedar and teak trees were cut from the Earth, rolled down long 'shoots' to be loaded on sailing vessels bound for England. And without the benefit of the local historical perspective, how could she imagine the whole-forest reality?

Well, as it happened, a few days later I was teaching Ami simple three-chord progressions on the keyboard in my bus-studio. I left her to practice on her own, reminding her of the simple sequence that was required to start the recording gear, in case she wanted to save anything she played.

Ami met me later and as she brushed past she said: "I turned the recorder on when I was playing and I think I liked some of it.... And by the way, there is some silly stuff at the very end... words and singing. I don't know where it came from but you can erase it if you want to...."

Next day - I let the tape run as I worked at the computer. The keyboard music was uncertain but quite sweet. And then came the vocals, that 'stuff at the end' that Ami had told me about. What I heard was a sort of roughly hewn 'protest song' about the rainforests in Brazil.

This barely sketched song said so much of what so many of us have been saying for so long. Nothing really new in content... and yet it was somehow all new... in its *perspective*.

There was a theme that ran through the short piece that asked again and again, *"What about the Children...?"* But the most moving thing about this song... was that it was such a clear and powerful message, coming directly from the heart of such a very young child... who was awakening to feel what was coming to the Earth.

I had no idea that Ami could sing like this... let alone create such beautiful Song. Her voice is like a bell, like her mother's. It is clean and clear, with harmonics and phrasing that awaken powerful response in everyone who hears it. Very magical!

The melody of the song was complex and far beyond the three-chord stuff I had been showing her. I was, once again (as so often in the presence of my children's beauty and magic), absolutely amazed.

I committed there and then to doing whatever was needed to help her develop this song. It was powerful medicine. I felt that it had the potential to deeply move people... to awaken more caring about the devastation of all the rainforests of the world.

And so we went to work. I asked her to spend whatever time she needed to just *be* with that song, alone. I suggested that could "let it find its own form... its melody... and its own natural progression." I also tried to help her feel that she could just slip into a gentle meditative trance-state whenever she wanted to, so that she could "let all the words come out." And so she did.

I don't know exactly when she found the time to do it, but the very next evening she came to me to announce that the song was all finished! She sang it through for me, many verses of a slow waltz in the key of A major, joined by a very etheric minor bridge in 4/4 time. Somehow, without accessing the original PCM digital tape (that was tied to the complexities of the studio setting), she had managed to keep in touch with the heart of the song and completely develop it into... a truly finished piece. And a very beautiful song it was!

On the next day, we went into the studio after school and set the magical machinery running and... off she went, like she'd been recording all her life. The song was now greatly expanded. Some chorus lines and verses were to be repeated and there was a well modulated change from the major verses to the minor bridge... with a repeated chorus ending that could perhaps be sung for a long time by a live audience someday.

I was more than impressed. Beyond my endless father pride, I could see that she had done something that I simply could not have done. I find it exciting being around anyone who does things that I cannot... and especially so when it's one of my children.

It took us two long afternoons to record a good 'demo' version of the song - which was now firmly titled: *"WHAT ABOUT THE CHILDREN?"* Ami's mother honored the process with her presence and support during our producing-recording sessions... and finally we had a finished tape. For those who understand the recording process, it may be of interest to mention that although we were equipped to record digitally, we were limited to two tracks only. This meant that we could not multi-track and we could not edit our recordings in any way. So what we needed to make up a working end result, was straight-through perfect takes. Any slight mistake and we just had to begin again... and again... and again... and again.

Ami stayed with it, hour after hour, until we got it right - well, as right as we felt that we could. I coached her on every inflection, many pronunciations, her phrasing, her breathing, her emphasis, her volume and had to teach her first-time microphone technique as well (as well as engineering and playing a too-crude keyboard backing). And somehow we did it!

The next morning (pure synchronicity?) I received a rare call from the head of the distribution company that packages and markets my own music in Australia and Europe. I was still so excited by Ami's song that I played it to him over the phone. He was so immediately moved - to tears, he said - that he asked me to rush him the master. He then ordered a few hundred copies of the tape and sent some off to London to the 'Gaia Foundation' - front-line workers in the rainforest movement - for free distribution in aid of their work. Then he ordered another dupe run and told us he wanted to send copies to every public school in Australia... and all at his own expense, saying that it was important to return energy to worthwhile projects in the community. His action was a kind of tithe - a deliberate *returning* of energy to the community at large.

Soon, people began calling us - radio people, media people, ecology people, healing people - asking if they could use the song on air, in classes, in a teaching video (etc.). So many of those I spoke to said that when they first heard that song... it brought an immediate rush of tears. It was power-full medicine indeed!

As this all was unfolding, I became very impressed by what adults could do when they brought all of their professional adult-type skills to focus upon the work of a little child. I have, of course, experienced what it is like to be alone in the great and confusing maze of the music industry. But in this first-time project, everything was different: there were no egos, no competitive, super-cool brush-offs. No un-returned calls. Just whole-hearted and immediate commitment that "I want to do whatever we can to get this heart-message out to people everywhere!"

I recalled all the wonderful things that I'd seen children produce: artwork, poetry, dance, free-ritual sharing... and heart-songs. The rush of such sincere response to Ami's song seemed prophetic in some way. Perhaps I could encourage adult pros in the broad range of media/PR/production (etc.) to rise up like they were for this song... for some of the other wonderful things that children do all the time... which too rarely ever get noticed.

So Ami and I sketched out a project which we called *'Young Earth Action' (Y.E.A.!)*. It was to be a Children's Ecological Action Network which could hopefully discover powerful Earth-saving messages from children in any medium of expression... and then use adult skills and connections to coach, invite, arrange, edit, reproduce, package and distribute whatever magic might come forth.

Like so many powerful visions and good intentions, the Young Earth Action Network has never (yet) taken off. We collected a few members, some letters were shared, and the lifestream went off in other directions. But the song, however, went on and on....

We changed the name of our studio to *'YoungEarth Media'* (wholly unmindful at the time of the direct tie-in of this name with the Christian Creationist movement) and we wrote a statement (an insert) to accompany the first tape as it wended its way around the planet. And I would like to share this vision-statement with you:

"WHAT ABOUT THE CHILDREN?"

Original words and music by AMI DAEMION
[written when she was 9 years old]

This demo cassette was made from a digital PCM original
Recorded 1989 by YoungEarth Media, Byron Bay, Australia.

PLEASE SHARE THIS SONG!

Any action group or event which is wholly non-profit and aimed at helping to save the rainforests and the planet can use this song and recording in any way including direct reproduction for free distribution and for broadcast on commercial radio or TV for environmental purposes. Commercial rights reserved. Please ask!

This tape is the first project of the YOUNG EARTH ACTION NETWORK (Y.E.A.!) - an Earth-Saver Network of Kids (and adults) who want to help young voices and eco-action get out to the world. Any proceeds from this song will go directly toward the work of Y.E.A.

"HELLO WORLD! WE BELIEVE THAT ALL OUR NEEDS AND HOPES AND INSPIRATION FOR THE HEALING OF THIS PLANET AND THE PRESERVATION OF HER FORESTS, WATERS, SOIL AND AIR - AND THE ULTIMATE MEANS TO ACCOMPLISH THIS - ARE ALREADY ALIVE WITHIN THE HEARTS OF ALL THE WORLD'S CHILDREN.
AND WE HOPE THIS SONG CAN FIND ITS PLACE IN THE GLOBAL MOVEMENT TO HELP SAVE THE RAINFORESTS... AND ALL THE CHILDREN OF THE EARTH!"

- YoungEarth Action Network [Y.E.A.!]

~ ~ ~

Ami is now fourteen. Over the years since *'What About the Children?'* came through her, many things have happened. The song has been spread around the planet and has affected so many lives. People still cry when they hear it... and yes, even I sometimes still let out a tear or two when I share it with them.

We have performed together on many stages at various New Age Festivals. I sing, do shamanic chanting and play through the MIDI electronic universe of sound in my keyboards... and I accompany Ami. Most of all, it feels, I accompany Ami. I have gotten used to people sweeping toward us with open arms to praise our music... then passing me by completely to wrap Ami in hugs and strokes and celebration... while I stand around awkwardly, looking down and drawing in the dirt with my toes.

Her little song inspired a Hollywood producer to invite Ami to sing it at the opening of a Children's Environmental Theater in Beverly Hills... and to perform with Olivia Newton John, but Ami felt that she was "already committed" to a play a major role in her sixth grade play in Melbourne... and so could not make the trip from Oz. In the end Ami's song was shortened and sung at the event by Olivia 's very young daughter.

So the song goes on and on. Wherever she goes, she is still pressed into singing it... and everyone still loves it.

Here, we were talking about media and how it can be used. How the expanded perspective of the media world-view has become essential - to expand our perspectives, to bring understanding and direction, and the guidance that we so urgently need if we are ever to begin to reverse our planetary slide into ecological disaster. And this innocent little song-story is a powerful example of media used in this way:

Now, about that TV: if Ami had not been with me on that night long ago, to share that deeply impassioned TV-revelation of the bizarre and tragic cycle of destruction that is happening *right now* in the rainforests of the Amazon Basin (and all around the planet)... then she would never have discovered her sorrow for the trees when she did.

She would not have been able to understand, in those tender years, whatever feelings of vague sadness might loom inside her whenever she walked on tree-cleared land. And she would not (just then) have opened her heart to be such a clear and evocative *channel* for the creation-channeling of that beautiful Rainforest Medicine Song which has since touched so many lives... and awakened so much caring for the trees in so many loving hearts.

If our medicine family had a policy of rejecting television completely (as so many supposedly spiritual families do), and closed ourselves off to all that it can bring to our hearts and all that it can awaken in our awareness... then many thousands of people would never have shared the tears that fall for the rainforests... and for all the Children of the Earth... whenever they hear Ami sing, *"What About the Children...?"*

We have already shared enough medicine in this song-story for it to be a valuable tool in revealing the medicine process we are trying to share with you here. But there is still more to relate. There are two very mysterious things about this little song, which provide Sign that points to its source... and clues to its universal Meaning:

After we had completed a second recording of *'What About the Children'* (when Ami had just turned twelve), I came across the original recording of her 'practice session' which had brought this song to life. I listened all through her keyboard stuff and it was still sweet. When Ami's bell-like voice first sounded... asking that ancient question once again: 'What about the children...?' I settled back to re-experience that original magical moment of discovery. And what I heard sent shivers through my whole body (and still does so now in this retelling). For what I heard on that birth-tape was... nothing at all!

On the original tape there was none of the haunting melody, none of the subtle changes, no verses, no chorus, no bridge. There was none of the poetic subtlety. In fact, there was no sense of a song at all! Just a few words of the eventual song, that called out:

> *"What about the Children?*
> *What will they be living in....?*
> *The rainforests in Brazil*
> *Are being burnt to ash."*

I cannot say how these few word-sketches ignited such passion within me that I immediately 'took over' the task of getting this 'song' completed. I know that if I had never felt so compelled, I never would have encouraged (and guided) Ami to finish it. I know that if I had not at once abandoned all my own work and focused my total energies on shaping, producing, coaching, recording and *networking* this song for awhile... that it would never have appeared. But for all of that, I cannot hear anything in that original recording that would inspire such absolute devotion and commitment. Nor can I hear the seed of the obvious deep inspiration that led Ami to create - entirely on her own and without reference to the original - the finished version of this beautiful song.

And because of this I knew that I was acting through Guidance - that I was needed as a catalyst if this message were ever to come to light... and that I was needed to serve the long and involved *Ritual of Initiation* which followed: this 'coming out' party into the world of music and recording and performing for my eldest daughter.

And more... through *'the all'* of this happening, I know that Ami experienced direct *in-spirit-ation* (inspiration) that lifted her so cleanly from her groping, first-touch experience of composing on a keyboard into the ecstatic high of a truly magical sound experience... and the lasting experience of being able to *affect* something important in the world - something so very many people long for... without ever finding out *how* they can do it.... And at the age of nine... Ami has found her Way!

So you see, this story illustrates and reveals medicine process on many different levels.

For me, all the time and energy I have put into this project has been repaid a thousandfold in seeing all those glowing, tear-streaked faces, looking up so intently at Ami... whenever she stands alone in front of the entire adult world and demands response to that most primal question - a question that fills the hearts of every parent... and every child... when she cries out: *"And What About the Children...?"**

I said there were *two* mysterious things about that song. Here is the second: it has been four and a half years since that song came through Ami. Since then we have written some medicine words for Brahms' *'Lullaby,'*. We have chanted together (but only very rarely) and Ami sometimes sings along with her CD's. But Ami has never really written another song of that depth.

I have offered invitation, encouragement, time, a few 'shoulds'

---

* A cassette recording containing two versions of Ami's 'demo' tape is available from AJNA MEDIA - [see order form inside back cover]

and 'oughts' and the hopeful incentive of connecting her to the L.A. people, some professional studios, etc. But it has not felt right, in the end... and she has never written another song. And part (but not all) of her self-resistance, I suspect, is that she cannot imagine what could possibly follow that creation.

Do not despair (I am sure I have already done enough of that for all of us). Ami is now into acting and her first (Australian) feature film is just now coming out... and even though she is still living in this beach scene rainforest medicine family paradise... she now regularly leaps into the skies whenever her agent rings, off to follow the casting call to auditions of many kinds. And though she may not be writing songs... she writes good Medicine Word poetry endlessly and so keeps her Spirit (and her open channel) fresh and alive.

[See Ami's update 'Letter...' in AFTERWORD - pages 391-392].

And what of the *Young Earth Action Network?* Well, years later, now, I realize that I was so inspired by everyone's reaction to Ami's song - by that rush of wonderfully competent and eager energy from so many well-positioned adults - that I completely missed something:

'What About the Children?' was not received with such enthusiasm *just* because it was a moving voice of a child pleading to adults to care about all the Children of the Earth... and all the children yet to come. No, so much of what people were responding to was Ami herself - *her* incredible voice, *her* heart... *her Medicine.*

All of us grown-up types who have danced together with this song and with Ami... feel privileged to have had such profound opportunity. For her vision is so clear... and her shaman-spirit is powerfully magical... indeed!

And we all know that with children such as this... coming through us everywhere today... the Earth still has a chance!

THE LIVING ARCHETYPES OF LEARNING

Human consciousness is largely based in our experience of what I have come to call *'Living Archetypes.'* Archetypes are the very essence of a particular stream of consciousness. Father, Mother, Heart, Love, etc., can all be archetypes. And archetypes are actually *alive* - they live in concept, feeling and experience. An archetype can be a new possibility, an essence, an entity, a process, a skill, a state of being (etc.). In our medicine terms, every archetype awakens a new *dimension* or possibility of Meaning.

Children grow and learn by integrating the new possibilities that each new archetype brings, into their whole-being experience. And there is time... and a clear time for everything.

There is a time for learning the living archetypes of *'The Mother'* and *'The Father'* - what each can offer, what each is there for, what each can awaken within the child's potential. The process of learning about these two primal archetypes begins sometime before birth (some would say even before conception) and lasts throughout our entire lifetimes... and even beyond.

There is a time to learn of the archetype of anger, another time to learn the archetype of pain and another time to learn the archetype of sharing. And so it goes... *archetypal awareness* grows with every new feeling that we encounter, every new experience, every new *dimension of consciousness* that we visit... or *let through* our awareness.

In the natural unfoldment of human awareness, children (and adults) will assimilate each new archetype as we are able to understand them. Newborns who do not see much beyond mother-face and mother-breast do not need to understand the archetype of writing. It is obvious. And since very young children do not have responsibility for managing family economics... they do not need to comprehend the function of a bank... or a credit card.

As we need them - as we develop the mind to understand things - new archetypes come *naturally* into our awareness. When we are ready... we notice a dead bird and imagine being dead ourselves. Until we are ready to deal with this implication of dead-bird medicine, we believe that 'only birds die young.'

We could say that this is the underlying wisdom of learning as a natural flow: *Life is the Teacher... and everything is here that we need to learn... all that we need to learn.* What each individual supplies in this process is a self-sequencing procession of discovery... and the feeling to react to whatever experience comes along... and the feeling to motivate the whole-being self-integration of whatever lessons are met.

Today we live in a constant in-rush of media input: magazines, billboards, radio, numbers, signs... and television. It is startling to realize, but I have come to realize the truth of what one of my art history professors once said to me, long ago: "Every individual who lives in any modern city of today sees more graphic imagery in any single day than Rembrandt would have seen in his entire lifetime!" Something to think about... and something we cannot easily ignore....

MAGICAL CONSCIOUSNESS THAT LIVES IN A BOX

In this ocean of endless media stimulation, one channel clearly dominates all the rest: more than any other medium, television has changed the flow of our childhood awakening... has changed how we process new archetypes... has changed the natural rhythm of our learning experience. For whenever we switch it on... it will immediately *try* to show you something you have never seen before.

All of a sudden, little babies do not need to see very far or travel to dangerous places in order to receive visions of every kind of wildlife... every environment... and every imaginable human experience. So now we are all regularly exposed to a vast range of 'living archetypes'... which are no longer naturally paced to our needs or our development. Now we see *everything and all at once.* And far too often, children come upon these new archetypes alone, without parental empathy, accompaniment, interpretation or guidance.

If we are walking with a loving parent-guide and we come upon a dying animal, there is father-mother consciousness to help us *under-stand* what this sign means... to us. But if we see a beautiful antelope shot in living color and bleeding before our eyes on TV... sadly, there is usually no one there at all to help us process this encounter, this awakening of yet another new *archetype of violence.*

So our children 'watch TV' as we call it. Yes... they *watch* and they listen and they imagine and they strive to understand. But to them, it is no easier to see an elephant slaughtered on TV than it is to see it actually dying before them. Adults too easily say, "Well, it's only TV. It's not *real* so it can't really hurt them." And we say many other foolish things as well. But every new parent meets the child's universal TV reality sooner or later: every child believes that whatever is 'on TV' is actually real-ly happening *inside* the box.

No... TV is not a passive fantasy of unreality. It is just as real as Real can be. And it demands just as much care as any other dimension of real-time experience... and much more, when we consider what is actually shown in the name of 'entertainment'... or 'news!'

So... the next time the mini-shamans of your own family are

lying around vegetating in front of the TV... *PLEASE BE THERE! Please control the TV... or it will control them!*

Uncontrolled, unregulated and, especially, *unexplained*, it will all too easily dominate your children's emotional growth - amazing them, delighting them, scaring them, confusing them, overwhelming them... and be-numbing them. And it will do all of this simultaneously: *TV does 'It All'... all at once.*

As members of this mega-culture, it is so important to come to grips with this ever present force which channels so much information (and dis-information), feeling and meaning. As individuals we owe it to ourselves to understand when and how (and if) we can use this medium to enhance our perspective, stimulate our creativity and expand our horizons of what is... and to help us to explore what is possible. But as parents... it is *absolutely essential* that we find a way to understand what this technology is - in essence, in potential and in reality - for the sake of every open child-spirit.

Is it a demon or a tool? Is it an essential part of our evolution... or (just) a mind-numbing diversion that is robbing us of our individuality and motivation?

In fact it can be either... and both. And *it is up to us to choose* which it will be for our children.

And if we (ever) get that one together... then perhaps we can begin to try to choose for all the other children of the planet as well.

As I give this piece its final edit... there are *supposedly* sincere debates going on at the highest levels of our (American) government that are *supposedly* trying to understand this simple question:

"If a child sees people endlessly raped, tortured, dismembered, killed and incinerated... at the hands of every kind of warpo, sadistic, murderous villain that our media producers can imagine (at the far reaches of un-sanity)... then will this have any effect on the developing consciousness of our children...?"

Uh... what can we possibly say except: "*Of course* it will! How could it possibly be otherwise?" And... *"Why do you even need to ask?"*

Well, we can reel and stagger around in shock and disbelief at this hypocrisy as long as we need to and we can even try to detach ourselves from this pedantic and pitiful process. But 'they' who are debating this - and even as ridiculous as they look in their mock sincerity - well, they are *'us!'* And even while our bureaucrats fumble the ball and obfuscate the issue (and its solution) I believe that it is high time that we all figure out this simple answer for ourselves... and for all the children of the world:

'Of course! Everything affects everything.
Everything that our children hear-see-feel-know
Will affect everything that they feel-see-think-grow-are!'
And all that they will come to BE.

EVERYTHING IN ITS TIME...

Protecting the natural unfoldment of every child's awareness is such a profound responsibility of parenting. In the natural way of life, archetypes come when we are (more or less) ready to feel them, ready to understand them (and whether we believe this or not). It is exciting for me to have found that we *can* still approximate this natural rhythm, even amidst the incredible overstimulation that our modern lifestyles - and our television sets - force upon us.

For example... I am at peace with my feeling that very young children do not need to know about such archetypes as guns or the potential for humans to commit murder, rape or any other gross violence. Sure, these things are all around us, in our culture, all the time. But nowhere are they celebrated in such distorted ways... in such exaggerated concentration and in such hideous variety... as they are on the family TV every night.

So even while our family *uses* television as a channel to expand experience... we are determined not to let the medium use us! We simply do not watch the gore and violence that our culture loves to celebrate there, in every gruesome detail. Our children have learned that they sleep better when they *voluntarily* turn away from gross violence and all of the sudden intensities of the shooting orgies which pop up unannounced during otherwise good family programing as 'promos' for later thrills-to-come.

As they grow older, I invite my children (and often with solemn ritual formality) to bite off more... and more... and more... of the cultural apple... and so to begin to learn to deal with all the cultural worms (and insecticide pollutants) that they will inevitably encounter! These invitations are significant *Rituals of Initiation* - not all that different from a tribal father presenting his child with a first bow and arrow and saying: "Now you are ready to learn about this...." Not different... just enormously more complicated!

In time, of course, they will find their own time to watch whatever they want to, anyway, at home or away. Knowing this... we find that the subtle art of creating effective Rituals of Initiation into these new (and more violent) dimensions of our cultural experience lies in their timing: they must occur while you still have something new to offer... and, hopefully, just before the new offering (the new object-power-feeling-tool) is needed.

It is a dance of finesse... like finding the right moment to talk to your children about AIDS, birth-control, drugs (etc.), so that they experience you giving them needed information, reassurance (etc.) rather than clouding their still childlike feelings with ominous and confusing issues of unimagined futures.

Whatever I have to offer my children - whether it is a ritual tool for ecological awareness or access to some new reality of bizarre human behavior - I know that they will (have to) find their own perspective in the end. But by consciously *initiating* my children into worldly things, I know that they are moving out to meet the world with awareness of my position (my values, beliefs, opinions)... and all the *perspective* and support that I can possibly offer them.

They know that they have my confidence and trust. And they have my *Father-Blessing*. And I would urge parents everywhere to *never* underestimate the guiding and stabilizing effect that these precious affirmations can have in your children's lives.

When Joah Jai was six years old, he came to ask me with some formality, "Daddy, what is *'war?'*" Now he is almost ten and he knows a little more. He knows, I hope, what ten needs to know. But he still cannot imagine the horror that humans continue to inflict upon each other... and I am not yet ready to show him.

But we have begun to talk about the overall craziness of trying to settle disputes by armed combat when we see (on our television, of course) live coverage of the supposedly dignified New Russian Government blasting away with tanks at its own House of Parliament. And we are sad... and amazed... together. But still we have not yet met the real Horrors of War.

When it is time... then we will have an even deeper sadness to share: when we find out how far this military madness can be carried... and still more when we come to realize (together) that this global madness never ends!

We will react to it all together... feel it through... and find, I trust, some way to trust humanity even so. And I will no doubt share some different form of this ongoing ritual stream with every other child as well, each in his or her own time. But then... living in this time and this specific cultural consciousness there is nothing else to do.

Sometime... *it must be met and shared and processed.* Sometime and somehow... every individual has to integrate our cultural reality of ritualized violence into his/her life-view. But in our every child's journey from whole-being innocence to their first-meeting with the archetype of *War*, it is so important for parents to realize that in its effect on our children, a murder on TV is *no* different than one in the street. At least, if feeling is still alive... it certainly shouldn't be!

Yes... there is so much violence on TV and more each minute as American media plunges ever deeper into its orgy of desecration. But there is no need to blame the messenger that brings our inner cravings such sweet fulfillment, is there?

No... parents who equate TV with violence have simply missed the point. For within that very same box, there is also incredible wonder and beauty and magic. And even in the very center of the fire-storm of TV horrors... and even though what it reveals of human nature is often very frightening (at any age)... I maintain my respect for the medium. And I remind myself again and again that the humble TV is just a passive channel for the mindset and desires of our culture. Nothing more and nothing less.

Television is a cultural window like no other, that allows us direct access to our collective consciousness... or *un*consciousness... or whatever. And in this way, television may be the most democratic institution in the world: it shows the masses what the masses want to see. It reflects for us all the leading edge of our desires - and our sickness.

And if the programing tries to pull the audience in any direction that they do not want to go... then the masses revolt at once: they stop buying the products that pay for all commercial programing. The 'TV' reacts instantly to this rebellion and returns to feeding the people what they want... *whatever* they may want to see!

So *whatever we see on the TV... is an exact mirror of our cultural mind-set.* And for better or worse, in sickness or in health, our cultural experience is the home turf of our incarnation. This is the mass-mind that my children will live *in* for the rest of their lives. So I hope they learn it's essence well....

In the hyper-intense world of television, I see two streams of meaning: we owe it to our children to allow them access to the world-at-large and the TV is undoubtedly one of our most powerful tools of understanding... *and* we owe it to our children to guide them gently into meeting the archetypes of *all* of human consciousness and all kinds of human behavior, including all the varieties of *our* violence: from the violence of outright rape, murder and warfare... to the irresponsible violence of mass starvation... to the subtle violence of celebrating mindless commercial greed and wholesale consumerism... to the self-destructive violence of our gross ecological care-less-ness.

It is how we balance these two streams of response-ability - these two obligations which are also profound privileges, if we can see them as such - that will determine whether our children are enlightened or afflicted by all that they see around them ... and whether they will be able to preserve their natural innocence and their trust in human nature as they mature... and whether they will learn all they will need to know to be positive forces, in their time, for the healing of our planet and (we may well hope) for the urgent healing of our *Cultural Mind.*

AT THE DAWNING OF THE INFORMATION AGE

Many people who would walk the path of tribal wisdom are consciously trying to simplify their lives. And for many, this involves moving away from dependence upon technology of any kind. These are the *minimalists* among us who show the world that it is possible to live and love and celebrate life and honor the Earth without need for the fast lane - without hungering for the glitz of the consumer culture.

It is true, of course, that much of the technology that we have produced is, by its very nature, exploitative of the Earth's resources and dehumanizing to her people... limiting their experience (and thus their consciousness)... and so delimiting their personal (and spiritual) freedom.

But there are also technologies which are uniquely empowered to effect changes in our cultural drift: to begin to changc what we are doing to the Earth... to actually *heal* the Earth... to feed and educate the world's burgeoning population... and to provide us with clear channels and real-time networking of our most important communications, consciousness and inspiration.

The technology which offers all of this (and just in the very nick of time) is the humble *integrated circuit* - the much maligned computer chip and its virtually infinite applications.

We've all heard it and it is true: this is *The Age of Information*. This is the very moment in our evolution when the entire planet (and beyond) is at last becoming linked in a *Global Circle*, a planetary Medicine Wheel... of instantaneous, real-time mutuality... of immediate connection and communication which has the ultimate capacity to transcend all space-time barriers, all sensory limitations, all political boundaries and all patriarchal competitive nationalism.

Let's face it: many people still do not like computers. And those that do not... rarely even understand why. For all that it promises, the computer is still only loved by those who have already found it love-able! Ironically, virtually everyone who preaches against information and media technology has never experienced what it can do.

It is an understandable reaction: deep inside, those of us who believe that they dislike computers (or TV, for that matter) are usually holding unresolved *fears* of what technology will 'do' to us.

We associate information technology with what we see as a cultural trend toward depersonalization. We have been *conditioned* to fear that the technology itself will somehow oppress our human spirit and 'turn us into mere numbers.'

We can say that these frightened ones are simply stuck in nineteen sixties Hollywood scenarios of computers 'taking over the world.' It's all true enough... but how can we invite them to come out of their shells and take a look around?

Those who are already at peace with high technology, please bear with us here: it is *so* important to share this medicine with those who have not yet discovered what is so clearly *the most important new dimension of human experience and the greatest resource for evolution... since we learned to use Fire!*

Are *you* afraid that computers will take over your mind, your feelings or your freedom? Are *you* afraid that they will one day 'run the entire planet?'

Hey there, good people: *it has already happened!* All around the planet, *everything* that is produced or grown... everything that moves across the Earth by any means at all... and all the fuel and coordination that it takes to move it... and everything that relates to economics or energy or resources or time or human effort... is *already* being fully coordinated and regulated by computers. And it simply cannot be otherwise!

It is a simple fact: our world is becoming more and more complex. And it will continue to do so whether we eat vegetarian or not, whether we use plastic bags or not... and whether we travel or stay isolated on our organic subsistence farms. The world is growing up. And we will either grow up with her... or we will become the dinosaurs of future myths and movies.

That's just the way it is. Without computers to process and regulate and coordinate our efforts and resources... without computers to expand our perceptions and our perspectives... without computers to communicate via telephones, satellites, television, the internet (etc.)... virtually all large-scale and state-of-the art human activities - such as food supply, transport, communications, economics, science, medicine (etc.) - would be wholly impossible or so grossly inefficient that we could not *afford* to do anything at all! The cost in money, time, resources - i.e., the cost to the Earth and to her people - would be completely prohibitive.

Yet again we meet the irony that those who already know this... already know... and those who have not yet met the future of global communications and this new invitation to planetary bonding... are so often afraid to find out.

Let's put it this way: computer technology is opening up vast new dimensions and untold new realms of consciousness. But until we are *initiated* into this amazing world... until we see it and touch it for ourselves... until we hear it speak to us directly and personally... it is completely impossible to even imagine what this *'new-consciousness channel'* can do for humanity... and what it can do for Mother Earth!

SHAMAN-CHILDREN OF THE NEW ELECTRONIC NEXUS

Everywhere our children turn in the world-at-large, they will be interacting with computers. Computers will soon be wholly integrated with-in our experience - controlling an infrastructure that we may never see and facilitating experience that we cannot yet even imagine. And wherever they appear, they will be serving to simplify our lives.

They will extend our natural sensitivity and powers beyond

anything that we can now predict. They will (have to) regulate and economize on all public energy use. They will track and preserve virtually whatever can remain of the natural environment and lifeforms on this planet - as the only way to save it from human greed and human *need*. They will enable us to communicate with each other when time-space-distance does not permit us to make contact in any other way. And for all our fears of 'Big Brother,' this is the link that will (finally) enable us to unite all humanity into one stream of consciousness, as the political and nationalistic boundaries of the old patriarchal order give way to truly global awareness... and then invite us to move far beyond.

So I am a 'believer.' And as for our little medicine family, well... we would rather live in a lovely rainforest valley, close to a thousand miles of unspoiled white-sand tropical beach. And so we do! Just as far from archetypal City as we can get. But one of the marvels of our present time and our evolving high technology that makes this lifestyle even possible... is that we can communicate and be *in touch* with the world-at-large from the very center of our idyllic temple-nest... *and the World can communicate with us!*

IN THE MAGICAL REALM OF NINTENDO-SEGA

You already know our family's love of Nature. And you will be able to feel where I stand - in deep appreciation and awe - in relation to technology in its highest forms. But this book is not the place for lengthy praises of high tech state-of-the-art. This is the place for *Medicine*. What we need to do here is to see if and how technology can be included in the notion of *'Real-World Medicine.'* If it can be... if it *must* be... then we need to explore how to expand our simple nature-based medicine family process to include the *Magical Realms of Nintendo-Sega*... and we need to discover the driving importance of finding the Way....

Every child of today will meet up with this new world of computer games sooner or later. For they are everywhere... and breeding fast! And this new realm is no different than any other arena of human activity: how we approach it, how we use it and how we integrate it in the rest of our lives... will determine how it affects us.

It can be a new frontier of discovery, a conscious expanding inspiration... or it can be a mindless (and mind-numbing) addiction.

The choice is (all-ways) ours. But there is one choice we cannot make: this new technology is here to stay... Nintendo-Sega will *never* go away!

When our children first enter this new world, they are opening up many new *dimensions* of possibility. Unfortunately, perhaps, like TV - exactly like TV, in fact - the content of computer games is a *pure reflection* of our culture's values: there is violence, there is noise, there is conflict.

Yes, like it or not, we cannot cringe away from this simple truth: computer games reflect our culture, plain and simple, horrific and grotesque... and beautiful and exciting. It is up to us to find the way through the ugly part so that we can help to reveal what is worthy and inspiring and positive to our children.

The mass-marketing rule applies in this new arena of consumerism, just as it does in all media: the first wave of programs was aimed at the very lowest common denominator of our mass-mind cultural consciousness: shoot-em-up, kill them all, shoot them down, blow them up. The Popeye and G.I. Joe characters of our children's grandparents' days are still alive and... well... tortured. Although now they all take Ninja training and are more lethal than ever before!

The first-wave of computer games could do nothing but animate our cultural traditions of violence and good-vs-evil. But today, things are beginning to change. Now there are also computer games which are beautiful, artistic, creative and most definitely *consciousness-expanding*. And still there are many that are not, of course. But if we choose the time and 'choose the channel' then there is absolutely nothing to fear in entering the New World of Nintendo-Sega... and an amazing wealth of personal skills and integrated learning to be gained.

The next time your child picks up a control pad (or wants to)... have a look at what is actually happening. If you can manage to look at the game through 'medicine eyes,' you may find that there are many dimensions of growth and consciousness which are being stimulated, clarified and sharpened as the game unfolds. Let us look at just a few of the dynamic meditations and the special learning that occur spontaneously in the *video-game-Zen* of this new realm:

COORDINATING HANDS - EYES - TIMING - STRATEGIES: When asked what computer games have to offer, most of us don't see much beyond the obvious benefits of increasing hand-eye coordination. And, sure, this is part of it. But there is much, much more! In the video game world, timing is everything. And a player's overall sense of inner-outer time and how to move through and with in Time's dimensions develops in direct relationship to how much hands-on experience s/he accrues.

DANCING AHEAD OF TIME - Even while any player is moving through very complex and precisely timed hand-signal patterns, s/he is always counting down to precisely match a control movement with an upcoming, screen-timed event. S/he is also continually looking ahead at what will come from any here-and-now choice and working out complex strategies to deal with that future - by integrating *all* previous experience of what has worked and what has not... with new tips and rumors from friends... and allowing for the real-time feeling of how the machine is working today (where it feels very responsive, where it might be sluggish, etc.). And all of this must be coordinated with the split second timing of the multi-dimensional rush of color-light-sound-movement that floods into us from the Program.

SAVING LIVES AND LOSING LIVES - Whenever a player makes a mistake, s/he (usually) 'loses a life.' Each game gives so many 'lives' - often three or four. 'Extra lives' can be earned by playing very well. And then you make mistakes: there are time-wasting mistakes that cause loss of lives if the clock runs out before you get where you need to be. There are also *'fatal errors'* - which cause immediate loss of life.

Losing lives is like getting 'outs' in a baseball game. The more you have in reserve... the farther you will be able to progress through the different levels (or *dimensions*) of the game. However it happens... lose a few lives and it's *'GAME OVER'* for you! And 'game over' usually means passing Control over to your friend.

GAINS, LOSSES AND CONSERVATION - Losing a life or a game represents an important waste of much time and effort: when all lives are lost the player has to begin again at the very beginning and work through all the easy levels, up to the point which represents the actual *frontier* of the player's discovery - the dynamic frontier of the player's ability, understanding, accomplishment... and integration. And then, whatever lives are left can be used to chip away at the leading edge of discovery - trying different approaches, techniques, sequences, timing, etc. - until a breakthrough occurs... or... *'GAME OVER!'*

PATH-FINDING: LEVELS AND META-LEVELS - The latest video games have over one hundred different *levels*, usually progressing from fairly easy to extremely difficult. Different levels have different graphics, different tasks, different dangers and different goals. Often there are no instructions to guide you... and you can only get through the hardest levels by finding a *hidden pattern* of timings, movements, etc., that allows you to pass. Some games even have 'blind' levels - where you cannot see anything on the screen at all except your own little icon (figure)... until you either lose your life... or get through the unseen maze... and on to the next level... and a wholly new set of challenges!

PATIENCE AND THE PERFECT STILLNESS OF MIND AND BODY - All of this requires enormous levels of patience. It is the same kind of patience that an adult might use to practice meditational stillness: you have to still the mind and try to rise above its distracting chatter as it talks to you, about you, with you, for you... senses everything they possibly can... and then reacts to everything it senses with a full spectrum of desires, judgments and plans. *And it all happens at once.* To succeed, you have to still your body and try to invite it, coax it, threaten it to "Be still!" and to please let you get on with your game without the interference of eager muscles or any distracting feelings of any kind. And hey, parents: how long can *you* sit in such focused stillness...?

The stillness required to concentrate on a video game is different than that dullness which comes over us like a drug whenever we sink into passive (uncreative) TV watching. Television induces a state of true lethargy which easily leads to a more general state of apathy... which, over the hours-days-months of abuse can easily lead to a dangerous state of general (psycho-physiological) depression.

TOTAL FOCUS AND ONE-POINTEDNESS - *Videogame Zen* is different than couch potato TV: the stillness that is needed here comes amidst a continual rush of sensations, excitement, despair, elation, frustration (etc.). During the course of any game, every player experiences *many* different emotions rushing through every cell of their body-minds.

ACTION AND NON-ACTION - Video games are about *action.* These games involve players *totally*... and then demand that they stay light on the controls no matter how excited they may become. You can thrill, scream, need-until-you-burst, celebrate, despair and rage... but you must always *stay light* on the controls and you must remain precisely focused and yet detached: highly attuned to the *process* and the *timing* and the *sequence* and the *strategy* and the unrelenting unfoldment of the game at a real-time pace which is literally mind-boggling and overwhelming to most adults!

SHARING - There are also many new lesson of how to share that come to us when we first pick up a video game controller. Usually whenever a player loses a game, the controller is passed to the next person. For beginners, this means that each turn is very short. But if a player is very good, a game can last for a long, long time. And for however long it lasts, everyone else just sits - riding along, advising on strategy, celebrating their friend's successes and enjoying the risk-taking that leads to dramatic failures.

MUTUAL AFFIRMATION - What is especially striking when you watch a few kids playing these games is that instead of wanting everyone else to fail - so that they can get the controller for themselves - in this game-culture, *everyone seems to want each other to succeed*!

Those who wait while others play show more genuine patience than I have ever seen in any other children's games. I believe that this is because everyone is sharing each other's experience so closely. They are 'living through' each other's actions, choices and results with a *total presence* that most adults (playing golf, for example) simply can not achieve. Together they are, in the adventure and in the learning process, no matter who holds the *Ritual Power* of the *Magic Controller.* Together they work out strategies, remind each other of everything that needs planning and care... and together they celebrate it all.

THE MEDITATION OF PLAYING ALONE - Videogame Zen can be also practiced alone. When there is no one there to share our most spectacular successes - or failures - we have only ourselves to meet... only our own learning curve to discover... only our own self-control to perfect. When friends are elsewhere and Little Brother is not following our every move... we can easily slip into a deep meditational trance-state as we fly through obstacles and move through level after level after level. We learn how to retain perfect focus and we learn to move as little as possible... with a minimal pulsing to signal the controller... and allowing *nothing* to distract our attention.

When playing alone, it is easier to break into new territories of experience: visual-eyes widen to include the entire screen (or even multiple screens) at once. Mind speaks only to fingers, telling them what to do without awakening any other bodily desires. Learning accelerates until we transcend all expectation... until we *know* that we have entered a wholly new dimension of consciousness. And then - as every serious player knows - we know the meaning of *Zen.*

As with any meditation, if we notice too much, then we will suddenly 'pop out' of the trance state and be left in a bewildering daze, sitting in an all-too familiar and wholly unfamiliar world. And as with any meditation... if we can find the way to move through new levels of awareness without letting big-ego distract us... then new vistas will open before us... through us... within us... without 'reason'... and without end.

THE TOOLS OF MEDITATION - From the ancient *yogas* (and their equivalent in many cultures) we learn of many *para-sensory* aids to achieving the state of meditational *no-mind.* And all of these practices can be seen to be operative in the spiritual discipline of *Videogame Zen:*

> There is *MANTRA*: the use of repetitive syllables and chanting to defocus the ego-mind.
>
> There is *YANTRA*: the use of graphic images and designs to hold the mind still until Spirit can be heard.
>
> There is *REPETITION*: prayer wheels, beads and many other devices can be used to lull awareness into new openness, helping us to be more receptive to whatever comes from beyond the Mind.
>
> There is also *TRANSFIXION*: using the flame of a candle or any other moving object as an aid in the induction of trance

states of all kinds.

There are yoga postures or *ASANAS*: used to open subtle energy channels in the body-mind and as an aid in achieving the perfect stillness which alone will allow Spirit to come through.

There are hand positions or *MUDRA*: which symbolize (and so evoke) certain spiritual energies.

There are *NUMBER SEQUENCES* and the 'million and one names of God' which can be recited to evoke Spirit and induce receptive openness.

There is also *REFLECTION*: the use of mirrors (in the discipline of *tratak*) to reflect Self back upon us until we can see the Divinity within... and the consciousness beyond.

The *INTERACTIVE TOOL*: and today there is yet another tool - a medicine tool that encompasses all of the above. It is the world of the computer and the information technology which is expanding to meet and inspire human consciousness at its highest potentials - technology which is evolving faster than any technology ever known by humankind... and growing faster than any other body of knowledge which has *ever* been wholly accessible to every one.

One of my yoga teachers once said: "Everything that you use in your spiritual practice (your *sadhana*) - all the asanas, mantra, yantra, music, chanting, breathing, mudras, repetition - *all* of these things exist only to help still the Mind! There is no other purpose and there is no other use for any of these things: they are all nothing more than tools that can be used to help us to *still the mind!*"

Of course, all of these medicine tools for meditation were 'invented' many thousands of years before the advent of the electronic age. And now we have some new tools. If we look closely we can see that they are not all that different than the meditational tools of ages past. What has changed is that now we have a new *medium* - a new playground in which to explore... whatever we want to know... or feel... or master... or evoke.

There is a catch phrase that is being applied to the electronic information technology more and more these days: "Garbage in... garbage out." And what it means is that whatever we will get out of our new yoga-machine is directly related to what we put in: when we finally begin to use our collective awareness to program computers for *consciousness... then* we will begin to activate and realize the Medicine in the Machine... and *then* we will come to meet the ultimate interface between electronics and consciousness.

Until then... some of us can taste the future just enough to know that there is amazing Revelation just ahead...!

For now, our little mini-shamans burn though the intensity of 'levels' games... learning and reveling in the crassness and insensitivity of the culture-at-large. And as they do they are also learning the skills and the focus and the commitment that they will need to someday put this technology to a higher use - to evoke the catalyst for their own growth and flowering... when tomorrow comes.

For now, *they* may think that they are just 'playing the game.' But I have watched and *breathed with them* as they play... and I know that they are actually doing far more than they possibly (yet) imagine.

Personally, I must confess that I have no personal interest and no time for computer games. Never have. And no, I don't mean 'no interest' like I don't like motorcycles. I mean real non-interest. Like zero charge... like nothing at all. Thus I am not a good one for enthusing when I hear kid reports of great mastery in this or that maze or level... or whatever.

I don't really even like to hear about it... anymore than I like to hear a third-person account of the plot of any film or book. But I can still celebrate the rush of mastery and revelation and accomplishment that my children are trying to share with me. And this brings such a beautiful richness that through it, I have come to know and trust the deep medicine of *'The Electronic Medicine Wheel.'*

In many ways, Videogame-Zen is like Motorcycle Medicine, but even more so. For while riding a motorbike is still - regardless of what my son thinks - actually an *optional* activity... today, Video-Zen (or its near successor) is not.

The Electronic Information Age IS the Present:
It is the Primal Reality of our rapidly evolving world.
And as such it is absolutely undeniable...
And increasingly indispensable to every child's education!

And so I know that I must meet it, breathe it in, offer my children a taste of this latest *cultural medicine...* and hopefully, guide them into a sane use and celebration of whatever it may have to offer.

Ultimately, I have come to trust this entry-level initiation experience into the joys of the electronic world as much as I trust any other mass-media cultural expression: despite all the obvious violence, habituation pitfalls and other limitations of video games as we know them today:

Our Living Culture is US - it's all of us - and like every cultural expression, somehow it must be right for our times (and consciousness)!

And yes, it is painfully true that it is getting harder and harder to believe in this foundation of all spiritual evolution... and harder still to want to admit its inevitable reality. But... no matter how weird experience may come to be - our inner-personal emotional experience and/or our mass-market cultural experience -

> *It is a miracle, but somehow, whatever happens all-ways contains the seeds of all that we need to make our next quantum leap into new levels of consciousness.... so... COME ON LEAP!*

PLAYING WITH TRUE GENIUS - There is another very important social and educational benefit that comes to us as a by-product of this high-tech yoga. Ultimately, and no matter how we may feel about video games in general, one truth is inescapable: it is hard to find any greater accumulation of applied innovative genius than that which is pooled to create commercial software that is available to virtually everyone today. Every powerful software package that is on the market is the end-product of thousands of hours of some the very best and clearest creative thinking that humankind can muster.

Of course, if we choose to consume 'killing games' then that is what we will learn. But if we chose to reach out a little further... there is *no limit* to the learning and the brilliant reflection that the computer can bring into even the most banal and otherwise limiting of our life environments.

Wherever we may encounter it, whenever we come face-to-face with the highest expressions of the *human-computer interface*, the mind power that shines out at us is often simply amazing!

Today, among so many of us who strive to get closer to the Earth and her simple wisdom, it is simply unfashionable to celebrate the riches of the mind. But *Mind* has its own medicine... and it is very magical and very power-full medicine, indeed! And nowhere is Mind flowering with more expansive creativity today than in the world of electronic intelligence and multi-dimensional communications technology.

Until very recently, this great mind-power was less obvious in the world of Nintendo-Sega than at the leading edge of more 'serious' programing for user-computers. Lately, things are changing even faster. The evolutionary curve is almost straight up! There are unimaginably amazing things to come... and the most amazing of all will come to those who are open to being... amazed!

So... let us look beyond the world of the video games of today... and take a peek at what lies just ahead:

THE WHOLE-EARTH SACRED CIRCLE

Every culture and every tribe has its own places of great ritual meaning. Highly charged places. Places of great Meaning. These are our *'sacred sites.'* These are the 'special places' where we naturally feel more centered, more peace-full, more receptive to our inner voices... more open to Spirit... and whatever medicine may come.

Today, some of us pick our sacred sites intellectually: picking them because they (are said to) fall on special energy grids (or ley lines); choosing them, perhaps, because they have certain plants growing there which are (said to be) important medicine plants; declaring that a particular site is important because it is located exactly half-way between two other places... (or whatever).

Once selected by this mental process - and no matter what criteria are used - we then use the power of Mind to *consecrate* the chosen place.

And, yes, we *can* choose to follow Mind's linear (straight line) path... and then hope that real Feeling and Meaning will come. Or... we can choose our sacred sites from feeling alone. For here, as everywhere,

Feeling, Intuition, Imagination, Guidance and Destiny
All become ONE whenever Mind can be put to rest!

Once a sacred site is consecrated by either Mind or Feeling (or both), we are free to celebrate its Meaning... and its Power. As we imbue the chosen place with our Trust and Hope and Celebration, it easily becomes the earth-plane repository for all that we value... and, if we are fortunate, the earth-channel for all that we need.

For those who can still the mind - for those who can trust a higher level of awareness to make such choice - sacred sites *become* sacred because of a confluence of many levels of experience: special sensory experience, spontaneous emotional feeling, subtle (intuitive) impressions, deep medicine vision, directly channeled guidance... as the site of meaningful events... and whatever else has Meaning.

There are places which are known as sacred sites to our own medicine family because we have felt Spirit there, once or many times; because we *'found place'* when we were not looking for any place at all; because we discovered that some place immediately felt special, 'loaded' with feeling and meaning... for every one; or perhaps because we always go there... but never had any feeling of 'why.' And these places naturally call us back. Each *Free-Ritual of Returning* brings more experience and increases meaning until the special place is steeped with deep medicine power, full of family feeling, rich with family history and so becomes woven into our ever-changing, free-ritual tradition.

The most powerful *Feeling of Place* often comes in the least likely situations: the place where we first found that we were in love... the place where we happened to be when we first heard tragic news... the place where we used to hide from the world when we were very small... or the earth-place of all our ancestors.

Now there is a new sacred site which has just opened up for us all. All who visit this place know that it is special: rich with Sign... full of Meaning... a place which can evoke the highest Spiritual Vision. And this new place of deep medicine is the *first* sacred site in the history of our planet that has the potential to be truly available to everyone, wherever we may live, anywhere on this planet... and in time, far beyond.

This is the sacred site of the *Net*: the Internet, the World Wide Web... and what is often called *'virtual community'* or, the *'Global Village.'* And this is *The Sacred Circle of the Electronic Medicine Wheel:*

VIRTUAL COMMUNITY - PLANETARY MEDICINE

Much of my life-work is with Circles: Ritual Circles - Shamanic Healing Circles - Community Council Circles - Family Circles... and Planetary Circles as well. Within the *Living Circle Process* as it is coming clear to me, there is a project which I am shepherding which is still in its embryonic stage: I am working to create a format for an emotionally viable (and mutually response-able) *Global Virtual Community** which is based upon my years of exploration and wonder with-in the one and only *Living Circle.*

The technology exists... and we are already communicating world-wide in various on-line 'conferences.' But the link-ups are still too difficult - artificially tied to keyboard channels, bearing real-time dollar costs... and dependent upon everyone's willingness to give long hours to the project(ion) at the same time that we all notice that 'spare time' is running out for our culture as a whole.

So it is still too early on in our technological evolution to be able to meet others in the great depth of our most open selves *and* to have the time to process-through *whatever* may arise - the good, the difficult, the magical, the painful - in *Open Global Circle Networks.*

Ok... so just now, we are limited by technology. It's always been like that. But at the cutting edge of human evolution (and consciousness), our *need* to be able to instantly communicate in-depth and on a global level is growing exponentially. And the *Ritual Medicine of Urgent Need* is all-ways good medicine, indeed!

Personally, I live in deep trust that electronic communications will meet that need *just* as it becomes real-time critical to the emotional and physical survival of our planet... and will open up an instantaneous - all-time - no-time - time-less link between whoever wishes to be 'on-line'... to share with others they may never actually meet... at the very deepest levels of human intimacy... and awareness... and medicine... and Spirit.

---

* Readers who are seriously interested in joining in this project are invited to contact the author via the publisher of this book.

Through this link we can begin to explore and evolve at last, worldviews and world futures that can account for and include *every* culture and every area, every localized condition and every local need. Whether we can ever raise our selfish human consciousness enough to actually *serve* the needs of all humanity remains, of course, to be seen. But before we had the *link* - the *network* - we could not even begin to do it at all! And today the Internet is growing exponentially every second and is already beginning to light up the Global Consciousness.

What we now call the Internet is, quite literally, a 'network of all networks.' And this specialized potential of the Internet to empower global consciousness is central to *'The Electronic Medicine Wheel.'*

We are entering a new possibility together: just now, humanity is poised on the very edge of a profound quantum leap of consciousness... into whole-planet communion.... into *one-ness* of Heart and Spirit. It will take time. After all, we have all lived with-in our illusion of separateness (of self, family, city, nation) for so many tens of thousands of years.

But look around! Taste the wind! Listen to the *Breath of the Earth* and you will feel it too: *Something is coming!* And just now, all Sign says:

"YES! WE CAN DO IT!... AND JUST IN TIME!"

"Is this Medicine?" you may well ask.

"How could it be anything else?" flashes the obvious answer.

But in the back of my head, that little voice which speaks to me of *Global Family Medicine Vision* says...

"Hey! Wait and see! JUST WAIT AND SEE!"

And so I do. And so we do. Awaiting what may be humankind's most profound Free-Ritual Initiation ever... all the Mother-Father Medicine Shamans of the Earth acting in every way we can to do whatever we can to guide the Process to the fulfillment of our highest Medicine Vision... for all the Children of the Earth... and for the Father Sky and the Mother Earth and their endless *Tantric Dance of Life.*

><><

CHAPTER 14

END IN' PEACE

We have walked a long journey together, you and I, your family and ours, from feeling the simple magic of a dewdrop on a leaf and sharing it with a newborn babe... to reveling in the world of Maya (the world of material illusion)... to plunging headlong into high technology... and there perhaps tasting the possibility of global planetary unity. And it is *all* 'Medicine.'

Medicine is everywhere. Medicine is in everything. The Path of the Shaman and the Medicine Wheel spans all time and space, all life and death, all that is known and all that will never be known. Wherever it takes us, we are committed to go. Wherever it leads, we feel privileged to follow.

There is no other Path... there is no other Way... that promises to wholly accept and so affirm *'the all'* of every one's experience. There is no other Process which is so finely tuned to learning from every one... and from every one's experience.

If you walk in Trust and Openness... you can walk in safety anywhere... and you will *'Walk in a Sacred Manner.'* You do not need a leader, a teacher or a *guru* to walk the Medicine Path. You need only two things: the *courage* to trust that Revelation and Guidance are all around you and all-ways flowing through you... and the *humility* to *LET GO* of all ego-control and simply *"LET IT BE."*

When we can learn to walk on this Mother Earth together, heart to heart, family within family, tribe within tribe, then we may finally begin to understand what it is to be Free - Earth-Free... Sky-Free... Heart-Free... Spirit-Free.

We hope that these tales of our Medicine Family's ongoing adventures of discovery have been inspiring in some way to you... that your own Medicine Family Vision may be expanded from this brush with ours. And we also hope that your own Medicine Family will find some of our experiences and processes to be useful.

However you feel this *Ritual of Word* and this *Ritual of Invitation*, we would welcome your feedback. Now you have heard our Story... and we would love to hear *your* family's Medicine Story as well!

Until then, our little circle will be 'making medicine' wherever we are... no doubt equally wonder-filled in a field of moonlit magic or in the dazzle of bright city lights.

And wherever you meet us I hope that you will know my children at once... by their open hearts... and their open spirits. And so we might all come to recognize each other by these signs.

Someday, perhaps, our families will meet as we each follow our paths in search of our same and separate Medicine Vision... perhaps one day coming to join our families together in ever expanding Medicine Circles, honoring the Dance of the Mother Earth and our Father Sun. For now we have walked together... our family and yours... and now we *know* for sure:

IN THE REALM OF MEDICINE... ANYTHING IS POSSIBLE!

><><

"O our Father, the Sky
O our Mother, the Earth
Behold a good Family
Walking in a Sacred Manner
In a good Land.

In a Sacred Manner shall we walk.
In a Sacred Manner shall we stand.
May the Tree again flower,
May the Good Road be shown.

In a Sacred Manner may we Walk Together...
As One Heart - As One Mind - As One Breath
And as One Family Circle...
From Now... in to Forever."

><>< **HO!** ><><

- AFTERWORD -

A LETTER FROM THE ELDEST DAUGHTER

Hello! This is Ami. Now I am seventeen... and I want to add something of my own experience of growing up with the 'Medicine Family Vision' -

Since these stories were written, I have been immersed in the trials and true loves of adolescence. Tasted the clear and murky sides of human existence. Bound my soul to a few very special people. Rebelled... returned. Discovered what it feels like to love, to be lost, to be left, to search. To steer my way through daily life - though at times clumsily, as though blindfolded - with a growing sense of autonomy. A deep sense of self.

I wonder how much I have changed, how much I am changing, how much I will change? Growing up feels so rapid and tumultuous sometimes... and yet I feel always the same in my soul.

At last my age is finally hospitable to my life's work. So now I am beginning... everything! It has been five years since my brief taste of professional performance (a feature film and stage and studio singing). I gave it all up because it terrified my fumbling, early teen identity... but also because I just wanted to be a kid.

But now I have re-emerged with a new born desire to work at what I know I am destined to become. It is not fame that I want, it is not fortune. It is the chance to express to the world the art that flows through me. To spread joy and hope - and most of all, *awareness*.

I am now living in an apartment with friends. I am currently acting 2-3 days per week in an Australian TV series. I have my own band which I am writing-composing and singing for. I am employed as a vocalist for techno acts and am developing some tracks of my own for an international release. These are very small beginnings of real work, I know, but it all requires great focus and discipline from me - even more because I am just starting my last year of high school and want to maintain excellent grades for college.

As all this energy swirls within and around me, I am continually thankful for the total preparation that I have been given by my family.

I feel that my highly focused relationship to my work and the constant feedback that I seem far more mature than my years is a direct result of the way I have been raised - i.e., *consciously*.

Because, above all else, I am aware of having been addressed as a *conscious being* - as a thinking, feeling, aware individual - from the moment of my conception onwards. And this has given me an invaluable depth of wisdom and understanding.

Now that I seem to have conquered the most confusing years of adolescence, I feel finally able to fully honor this Medicine Path that I have been given (and chosen for) with all the power that wells up within me.

From my 'medicine family' (and the Medicine Family Vision that guided us) I have gained instinctual relational intuition. The value of honesty. Surrender and strength in my growing sexuality. Reverence for the Divine. To address my life as a never-ending journey, a process of evolution, a realization of physical entity by a traveling soul. And in all I do, the ability to move through life with spiritual, mental, emotional Vision.

From the ways of my shaman father I have learned the power to integrate knowledge, surrender to magic, find my own ritual, ignite my assertive power, and how to use deep intuition as my guide.

Here is the Christmas card that I brought to my dad this year, after our longest separation ever:

Hello again Dear Father, Dear Friend...

I cannot believe I'm going to see you again. I can't believe a whole year of my life - our lives - has passed in absence. But now I am ready! And at last I'm bursting to connect with you. Show you who and what I have become - and oh, so *different. During this year away I have realized that no matter how far away we are or for ever how long... I feel it is my bound duty, whenever we meet, to give you a report... an account of everything. To get your guidance. Because now I can talk with you in absolute honesty, with absolute trust.*

You are my Oracle. A being who is my father, my soul's mentor, my protection, and the wisdom of my parental guidance. A channel for my growth.

I've come to revere the way in which you have nurtured my spirit. Given me depth - the room and willingness to attain power of heart, mind, body and soul. I'm having my first taste of where I'm going. And I feel prepared. Not totally ready, but very eager. For the first time in my life I feel really proud of my self.

SO THANK YOU, FATHER!

- ami, melbourne oz 12/96

- AND AFTER ALL -

A MESSAGE FROM THE MOTHER HEART

The stories you have just read evolved over many years. They are the stories of a father and a shaman who has found ways of teaching powerful spiritual concepts to children, while living close to the Earth.

For many years now, I have seen the benefits and greatness that Jai's deep sharing has given our children: fathering of a very powerful kind. His endless teaching, loving, celebrating and shepherding of our children was (and is) a powerful spiritual force in their lives, for which I am deeply thankful. And I know that I have grown immensely from it as well.

In this book I find a wonderful simplicity which flows through Jai's process. But as you take these stories into your heart and try to follow this Path you will also find great depth of feeling and new awareness.

I continually see the results of this in the open-heartedness and lasting wonder in my children's faces and in their capacity to understand, empathize, communicate and share with others, with a unique inner wisdom and joy.

And as you journeyed through this book and learned more of this gentle approach to Deep Fathering, you may well have wondered: "Where was the *Mother* of this family through all of this? Where was *she* while her children and their father were off exploring on the Medicine Path...?"

Well... when our children were very young, my yoga was very much 'being a Mother.' That was my life. Mothering was my inspiration: it was where I learned about surrender, Spirit, love, death, joy, suffering - about all of Life. However, 'medicine' as a spiritual path seemed foreign to me. It wasn't part of my (Australian) culture... and even though I shared many circles and learned and changed a lot through these medicine processes, I just did not embrace it as 'me.' Inner resistance. Lack of surrender. Limited vision... whatever.

Growing in more recent years through Bhakti Yoga - and through helping to edit this book - I have come to appreciate my family's natural path of Earth-centered spirituality more deeply. I lament, at times, my own resistance to fully embracing this process and know that had I been able to do so sooner, even greater family unity and growth would have flowered.

I wholly recommend this MEDICINE FAMILY VISION to any family as a way of sharing that is simultaneously a path of learning to love and explore Nature, a path of understanding and sharing each other's feelings and a way into deep bonding. It brings to families a process that is formative in expanding consciousness and, most of all, a journey toward our Inner Selves. And for children, it is a constant adventure and a source of real FUN!

- Leia Daemion, 1997

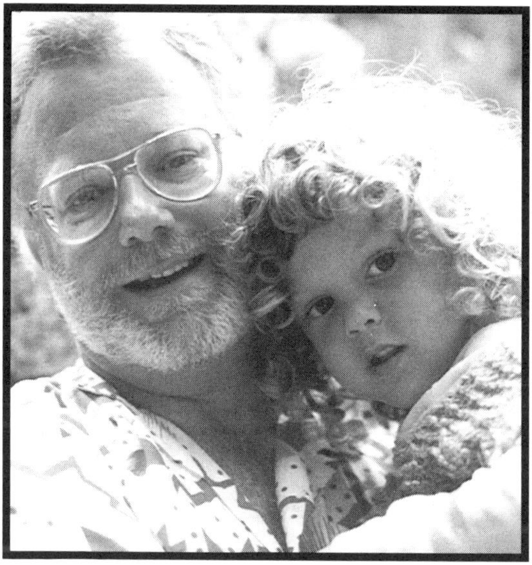

SOMETHING ABOUT THE AUTHOR...

So what is the 'medicine story' of this father who writes with such obvious bliss and joy at the privilege of guiding his child-gift, mini-shamans through their endless initiations and dis-coveries...?

Well, just as you have already seen. Just as he is. And just as he may yet become to be....

After a few early years of family life that carried me across many states and settings over my first six years, I was turned loose in the then-wild hills of California and there began a childhood of almost complete aloneness. Parents, yes. Siblings, yes... but still very much a self-nourishing, self-guiding and self-raising situation. And this can be an ecstatic state, even for a very young, would-be Indian warrior!

Free to follow my own desires and delights, I would walk for endless hours through the golden hills and dive into the mysteries of every valley stream. And all that space and natural wonder fed my naturally wild, out-rushing exploration... and softly nourished my deeper solitude. I had time and place to be intimate with Nature - and so the time (and the need) to find myself in those first Vision Quests.

And whenever the wilderness became disorienting or too dark... I would run to the shelter of our well-kept, well-fed (and emotionally sterilized) suburban, American scene, to stash the day's treasures and sit through an impersonal family dinner... and another night of waiting for the sun to rise again over a distant, beckoning mountain.

In these childhood wanderings (as in my yoga), I was always looking for 'secrets' - for what was somehow not 'supposed to be' revealed... always exploring as far as I could from the center of my cultural context... but never really understanding what led me on this strange, 'different drummer' path. It (and I) seemed different... and that just seemed to be how it was. Of course, I had peer-friends, and we roamed together, yes... but the Big Medicine, the power-full lessons, the true Initiations, always seemed to come when I was all alone in that vast magic-place. And come for me they certainly did!

And beyond all this... from those early years of secret shamanic initiation (usually secret even from me!) have emerged a few moments on this life-path that can be marked and labeled in the usual way:

JAI DAEMION spent the 'sixties studying psychology and philosophy, traveling in the U.S. and Europe and working as a professional musician. In 1969 he emigrated to London and there began his healing journey as a neo-Reichian Breath-Therapist.

Moving between London and the U.S. for several few years, by 1973 Jai was involved in leading workshops at growth centers (The Esalen Institute and others); had founded a new age development center ('Rainbows End') in Northern California; and was working to create New Age Festivals and spiritual lifestyle experiments... eventually becoming a prime mover of the Tribal Healing Festival Movement that flowered on the West Coast of the U.S. (and in other countries as well) from about 1973-1983.

In 1976 Jai was invited to India in response a gift of land intended for a Spiritual Center and then went on to Australia to share the 'California Healing Festival' energy with the vibrant alternative movement in Oz. There, love blossomed once again... and so his Deep-Fathering Journey began, with births from 1977-1987.

From 1982 onwards, Jai has been deeply involved in working with computers (at first to facilitate the writing process and later as an important tool for his work with electronic sound), eventually becoming involved with whole-planet 'virtual circle' networking via the A.P.C. nets in the early '90's. He also developed a unique human-computer 'experiential interface' and 'personal growth engine' - a project for some unimagined future.

In 1986, Jai returned to music with three releases of new age meditational keyboard music (1987-1990) - and soon afterward, began to record his unique 'Shamanic Chants' which had evolved through countless night-fire rituals and free-range howls at festivals all around the planet [see the new release by Ajna Media on CD/cassette: "SONGS FROM THE ANCIENT EARTH"]. During these years he also produced the book: THE HEALING POWER OF BREATH; wrote many magazine articles and monographs, including many on fine art photography; reveled in fathering and 'made circle' at gatherings along the East Coast of Australia and during occasional visits to the U.S. and Asia.

Since 1990 Jai's writing has been focused on three books that reveal his process of Living Circle Shamanism (THE POWERS OF THE LIVING CIRCLE, THE PROCESS OF THE LIVING CIRCLE and THE SONG OF THE LIVING CIRCLE); three books on male consciousness, culture and fathering (FATHER TIME, NEW MAN RISING and SPIRITUAL FATHERING); an exposition of his original philosophy of Wholistic Phenomenology (EMOTION AND CONSCIOUSNESS); a unique communications clearing process (RITUAL COMMUNICATIONS); and a magical exploration of DEEP-FATHERING THE FIRST MENSTRUATION.

To his every new project, then, Jai brings thirty years of innovative work with 'Tantric Breath Therapy' - Neo-Reichian Psychotherapy - 'The Emotional Continuum' - 'The Living Circle Process' - 'Free-Ritual Shamanism' - Ritual Healing Circles - group communications - community & educational networking processes - natural birthing - prenatal emotional development - conscious death and dying - 'Wholistic Integrative Therapy' - 'Co-Reflexive Massage Therapy' - the philosophy of Wholistic Phenomenology - shamanic chanting and toning - multi-dimensional electronic keyboard music - photographic fine art 'light-painting' - multi-media performance art - and global electronic networking.

[A little voice - maybe a frustrated would-be agent, maybe someone else's Mom - calls from far away in an incredulous tone: *"So? With all of this... what does he offer* you*? A little book on having 'happy time' with your kids...?"* To which he says, of course: *"'With all of this' ... what else is there to do...?"]*

Jai & his family have recently settled on the U.S. West Coast where Jai continues his writing-teaching and is now spending more time in his music studio, organizing publication of his many writings... while continuing to teach Free-Ritual Shamanism and creating unique *'FIRST CIRCLE INITIATIONS'* for individuals, families, groups and communities.

MUSIC & WORD AVAILABLE FROM AJNA MEDIA

- **THE MEDICINE FAMILY VISION** **$16.95**

  by Jai Daemion [Ajna Media, Eugene, OR. 1997. 400 pages]

- **THE HEALING POWER OF BREATH -** **$12.95**
  AN INTRODUCTION TO WHOLISTIC BREATH THERAPY

  by Jai Daemion [Prism Press, Dorset, UK. 1989. 235 pages]

** See reference on page 121 of this book **

NB: This book has been out of print since 1990. We have a limited number of fresh copies available. Please note: due to the type of paper used in the original printing, some yellowing of page edges may be present.

- **'SONGS FROM THE ANCIENT EARTH'** - by Jai Daemion
  Unique & Powerful 'Free-Sound Shamanic Chanting'

  CASSETTE: $10.95 - CD: $17.95

- **'WHAT ABOUT THE CHILDREN?'** - by Ami Daemion
  Primitive 'demo' recordings of 2 versions of Ami's eco-song.

  CASSETTE: $5.95

** See story on pages 360-368 of this book **

SEND ORDERS TO:

ajna media

PO Box 70133
Eugene, Oregon 97401
Phone/Fax (541) 937-1963
Please call or fax 11am-4pm PT
Email: ajna@sprintmail.com

- CREDIT CARD ORDERS - CALL TOLL-FREE: 1-888-255-2562 -
SEE ORDERING INFO & COUPON ON LAST PAGE OF THIS BOOK!

FIRST CIRCLE INITIATIONS

rites of passage - shamanic healing - vision - medicine path - breath
tantra - 'new-man-rising' - free-male consciousness - deep fathering
marriage - man-woman-child bonding - conscious conception
celebrations of birth - death - re-birth

LIVING CIRCLE RITUAL CELEBRATIONS

free-ritual shamanic healing circles
earth-spirit healing rituals
the father circle
communion councils

LECTURES & SEMINARS

culture and consciousness: the next frontier
deep-parenting the children of spirit
free-child development in an un-free world
living the archetypes of consciousness
integrating mind-body-emotion-spirit
self-integration beyond psychotherapy
wholistic-integrative healing

> < > <

FOR INDIVIDUALS, GROUPS, FAMILIES, COMMUNITIES

please contact

JAI DAEMION

c/o Ajna Media
PO Box 70133
Eugene Oregon 97401

YOU CAN ORDER DIRECT FROM AJNA MEDIA!

Please send the following books / CD's / cassettes:

THE MEDICINE FAMILY VISION (no.) ___x $16.95ea.=________

THE HEALING POWER OF BREATH ___x $12.95ea.=________

SONGS FROM THE ANCIENT EARTH CD ___x $15.95ea.=________

___CASSETTES x $10.95ea.=________

'WHAT ABOUT THE CHILDREN?' ___CASSETTES x $6ea.=________

TOTAL OF ALL ITEMS PURCHASED: $__________

PLEASE ADD SHIPPING & HANDLING (see below) $__________

TOTAL AMOUNT DUE: $__________

Indicate method of payment:

CHECK ☐ MONEY ORDER ☐ CREDIT CARD ☐

Name:______________________________________

Address:____________________________________

City: ______________________**State:**___ **Zip:**________

Phone (optional): Area Code ( ) ______________

VISA ☐ **MASTERCARD** ☐ **AMEX** ☐ **DISCOVER** ☐

CARD NO: __ __ __ __ __ __ __ __ __ __ __ __ __ __ __ __

NAME ON CARD:______________________**EXPIRY:**________

SIGNATURE:__________________________________

>< CREDIT CARD ORDERS- CALL TOLL-FREE! 1-888-255-2562 ><

☐ **Please add my name to the Ajna Media mailing list.**

SHIPPING OPTIONS

◊ DOMESTIC BOOK RATE - Please add $2.50 for first item ordered, plus $1 for each additional item. Allow 4-6 weeks for delivery.

◊ PRIORITY MAIL - For faster delivery, please add $4.00 for up to two items ordered, plus $2 for each additional item & specify "Priority Mail."

◊ PAYMENT - U.S./Canadian orders - Send check or money order in U.S. dollars payable to: **AJNA MEDIA**.

◊ INTERNATIONAL ORDERS - Send 'International Bank Money Order' payable in U.S. dollars to Ajna Media - Include air mail shipping & handling: US$13.00 per book, US$10 first cassette/CD, US$7 ea. add'l.

><>< IMPORTANT! SEE ADDRESS AND ORDER INFO 2 PAGES BACK! ><><